RESISTANCE TRAINING FOR HEALTH AND REHABILITATION

James E. Graves, PhD
Syracuse University

Barry A. Franklin, PhD
William Beaumont Hospital,
Wayne State University,
and the University of Michigan

Editors

Human Kinetics

Library of Congress Cataloging-in-Publication Data

Resistance training for health and rehabilitation / James E. Graves, Barry A. Franklin, editors.
   p. cm.
   Includes index.
   ISBN 0-7360-0178-6
     1. Weight training. 2. Exercise therapy. I. Graves, James E., 1954- II. Franklin, Barry A.
   RM725 .R395 2001
   615.8'2--dc21
                                             2001024450

ISBN: 0-7360-0178-6

Permission notices for material reprinted in this book from other sources can be found on pages x-xi.

Acquisitions Editor: Loarn D. Robertson, PhD; **Managing Editor:** Amy Stahl; **Assistant Editor:** Derek Campbell; **Copyeditor:** John Mulvihill; **Proofreader:** Jim Burns; **Indexer:** Betty Frizzéll; **Permission Manager:** Dalene Reeder; **Graphic Designer:** Robert Reuther; **Graphic Artist:** Kathleen Boudreau-Fuoss; **Photo Manager:** Clark Brooks; **Cover Designer:** Kristin Darling; **Photographers (interior):** Elizabeth DeBeliso, Peter Roberts; **Art Manager:** Craig Newsom; **Illustrator:** Dody Bullerman; **Printer:** Edwards Brothers

Printed in the United States of America   10   9   8   7   6   5   4   3   2   1

Human Kinetics
Web site: www.humankinetics.com

United States: Human Kinetics
P.O. Box 5076
Champaign, IL 61825-5076
800-747-4457
e-mail: humank@hkusa.com

Canada: Human Kinetics
475 Devonshire Road Unit 100
Windsor, ON N8Y 2L5
800-465-7301 (in Canada only)
e-mail: orders@hkcanada.com

Europe: Human Kinetics
Units C2/C3 Wira Business Park
West Park Ring Road
Leeds LS16 6TR, United Kingdom
+44 (0) 113 278 1708
e-mail: humank@hkeurope.com

Australia: Human Kinetics
57A Price Avenue
Lower Mitcham, South Australia 5062
08 8277 1555
e-mail: liahka@senet.com.au

New Zealand: Human Kinetics
P.O. Box 105-231, Auckland Central
09-523-3462
e-mail: hkp@ihug.co.nz

Dedicated to Michael L. Pollock, PhD (1936-1998),
preeminent scientist, clinician, researcher, teacher,
and friend. He chaired the writing group for the American
College of Sports Medicine's first Position Stand
on the quantity and quality of exercise in 1978,
and he coauthored its third revision two decades later!
These papers were vital in establishing aerobic
conditioning, resistance exercise, and flexibility training
as integral components of a healthy lifestyle.

Dr. Pollock was among the first to document the effects
of endurance exercise and weight training on aerobic
and musculoskeletal fitness. His tireless pursuit
of the optimal frequency, intensity, duration, and modes
of exercise training serve as the basis for contemporary
exercise prescription. Indeed, many of the concepts
and ideas in this text, Resistance Training for Health
and Rehabilitation, *were initially guided by his vision.*

Sir Isaac Newton said, "If I have seen further . . . it is
by standing upon the shoulders of giants."
Michael Pollock provided these "shoulders" to many
of his junior colleagues in exercise science and sports
medicine. We were among these colleagues.

Contents

Preface

This text originated from a symposium titled "Resistance Training for Health and Disease" organized by the late Dr. Michael Pollock (1936-1998). Presented at the 1995 Annual Meeting of the American College of Sports Medicine, the symposium reviewed exercise training guidelines for the elderly, acute responses to resistance training, safety issues, low back strengthening for the prevention and treatment of low back pain, the influence of resistance training on bone density, and the prescription of resistance training for health. The presenters at the symposium were internationally recognized experts in the field and, along with other preeminent authorities, provided valuable contributions to this text.

As one of the nation's most respected experts on the prescription of physical activity, Dr. Pollock was well aware of the emerging body of scientific evidence on the value of resistance training for health and rehabilitation. Indeed, recent statements on exercise by the American Heart Association, American Association of Cardiovascular and Pulmonary Rehabilitation, American College of Sports Medicine (ACSM), and the surgeon general promulgate resistance training as an integral component of preventive and exercise-based rehabilitative programs for a variety of disease states and orthopedic injuries.

The origin of resistance training can be traced to ancient Greek and Egyptian societies, and weightlifting as an athletic event was among the sports included in the first Modern Olympic Games in Athens (1896). Traditionally practiced by relatively few individuals interested in improving athletic performance or developing a bodybuilder's physique, resistance training is now considered an essential component of a comprehensive physical fitness program, with consistently increasing participation rates. It is required for the development and maintenance of muscular strength, muscular endurance, and muscle mass. Known health benefits of resistance training include: increased bone mineral density, lean body mass, insulin sensitivity, and basal metabolism; reduced insulin response to a glucose challenge; decreased resting diastolic blood pressure (especially among hypertensive individuals); and an improved serum lipid profile. There is also evidence that resistance training can prevent or attenuate musculoskeletal injury during physical activity. In recognition of the importance of resistance training to overall health and fitness, ACSM developed guidelines for the prescription of this complementary activity, which were added to its position stand on "The Recommended Quantity and Quality of Exercise for the Development and Maintenance of Health and Fitness in Healthy Adults" in 1990. These guidelines were further refined in ACSM's more recent position stand, published in 1998, to include recommendations for resistance training in the elderly.

Physical therapists and related orthopedic rehabilitation specialists have long recognized that improved functional capacity and morphological changes associated with resistance training have therapeutic value for the rehabilitation of orthopedic injuries. Only recently has resistance training been recognized as beneficial in the prevention and rehabilitation of chronic diseases and medical conditions, such as heart disease, diabetes, arthritis, and pulmonary disorders. This text is the first of its kind to address the emerging and expanding role of resistance training for health promotion, disease prevention, and rehabilitation. While there is a plethora of information available on resistance training for athletes and sedentary but otherwise healthy persons, until now there was no single source of information available on the prescription of resistance training for varied clinical populations. This is due to the fact that until recently, we have not understood the benefits of resistance training for clinical populations and information for the development of specific guidelines has been scarce. This text summarizes our current understanding of resistance training for health and rehabilitation and presents specific guidelines and considerations for the prescription of resistance training as part of our exercise armamentarium in a variety of clinical populations.

The text is designed for physicians, physical and occupational therapists, rehabilitation specialists, exercise professionals, and other health care providers who prescribe resistance training for individuals with and without chronic disease or multiple comorbidities. It is also designed for students of exercise science and exercise science faculty who are interested in clinical applications of exercise. It represents our current level of understanding of the acute and chronic physiological responses to resistance training and, for each of the diseases covered, presents a practical approach to the prescription of resistance training for the prevention and rehabilitation of that disease.

We believe that this virtual pharmacopoeia of resistance training guidelines will be a valuable addition to your practice or reference library, and we are excited that the benefits, rationale, safety, and prescription of this form of exercise are now available in a concise and practical format.

Acknowledgments

We wish to thank the authors who painstakingly worked to summarize, in a clear and concise manner, the latest research findings in each area, with specific reference to practical applications. It has been an honor and a privilege for us to collaborate with this prestigious group of scientists, clinicians, researchers, and teachers, who are authorities in their respective fields. Their contributions, both past and present, have largely structured the current practice of resistance training in the clinical setting.

Credits

Figure 2.1 Reprinted, by permission, from M.L. Pollock et al., 1995, "Exercise prescription for physical fitness," *Quest* 47 (3): 326.

Figure 9.1 Adapted, by permission, from Joseph et al., 1999, "Differential effect of resistance training on body composition and lipoprotein-lipid profile in older men and women," *Metabolism* 48: 1474-1480.

Figure 12.1 Adapted with permission from the American College of Cardiology (**Journal of the American College of Cardiology**), 1996, 28, 1471-1477.

Figures 12.2 and 12.5 Adapted, by permission, from K.J. Stewart et al., 1998, "Safety and efficacy of weight training soon after acute myocardial infarction," *Journal of Cardiopulmonary Rehabilitation* 18: 37-44.

Figure 12.3 Adapted with permission from American Journal of Cardiology, Vol. 65, K. Bertagnoli, P. Hanson, and A. Ward, Attenuation of exercise-induced ST depression during combined isometric and dynamic exercise in coronary artery disease, pp. 314-317, Copyright © 1990, with permission from Excerpta Medica Inc.

Figure 14.1 Adapted from Journal of Heart & Lung Transplantation, Vol. 12, Braith et al., Skeletal muscle strength in heart transplant recipients, pp. 1018-1023, Copyright © 1993, with permission from Elsevier Science.

Figures 14.2-14.4 Adapted, by permission, from Braith et al., 1998, "Resistance training prevents glucocorticoid-induced myopathy," *Medicine and Science in Sports and Exercise* 30 (4): 483-489.

Figure 14.5 Adapted, by permission, from Braith et al., 1996, "Resistance exercise training restores bone mineral density in heart transplant recipients," *Journal of the American College of Cardiology* 28: 1471-1477.

Table 2.2 Reprinted, by permission, from Starkey et al., 1996, "Effect of resistance training volume on strength and muscle thickness," *Medicine and Science in Sports and Exercise* 28 (10): 1311-1320.

Table 2.3 Reprinted, by permission, from DeMichele et al., 1997, "Effect of training frequency on the development of isometric torso rotation strength," *Archives of Physical Medicine and Rehabilitation* 27: 64-69.

I
PART

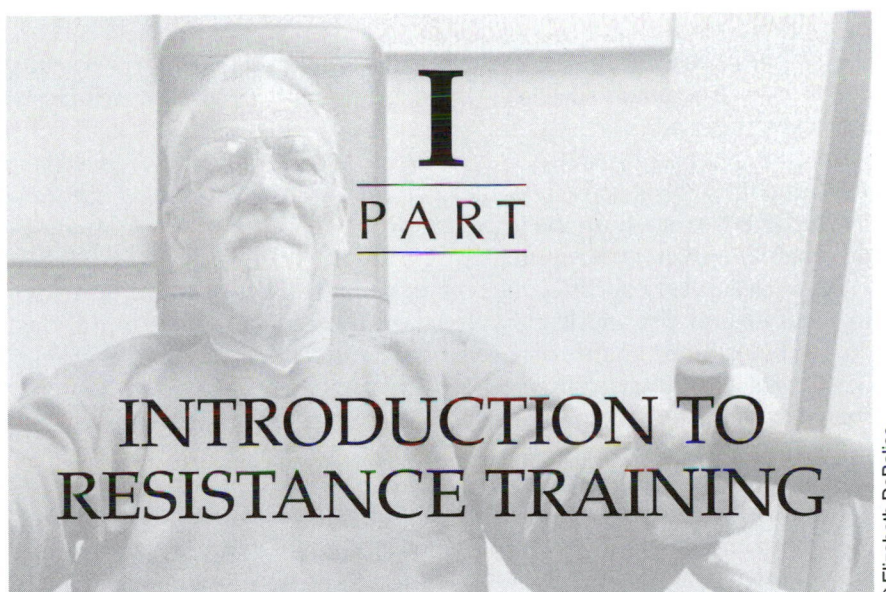

INTRODUCTION TO RESISTANCE TRAINING

Although exercise programs have traditionally emphasized dynamic lower-extremity exercise, research increasingly suggests that complementary resistance training, when appropriately prescribed and supervised, has favorable effects on muscular strength, cardiovascular endurance, hypertension, hyperlipidemia, and psychosocial well-being. These benefits are mediated by metabolic, cardiovascular, pulmonary, endocrine, and neuromuscular adaptations that are governed by the same set of parameters as endurance exercise (i.e., intensity, specificity, and volume of training).

Resistance exercise has value in the treatment of orthopedic injuries, low back pain, osteoporosis, overweight and obesity, sarcopenia (loss of skeletal muscle mass that may accompany aging), and diabetes mellitus. Moreover, resistance exercise may be helpful in reducing older persons' susceptibility to falls. Weight training has also been shown to attenuate the rate-pressure product when any given load is lifted. Thus, resistance training can improve myocardial efficiency by reducing cardiac demands during daily activities such as carrying groceries or lifting moderate-to-heavy objects. Indeed, many professional and government health associations, including the American College of Sports Medicine, American Heart Association, American Association of Cardiovascular and Pulmonary Rehabilitation, and the surgeon general's report on physical activity and health, now include resistance training as an integral component of a well-rounded physical conditioning program.

Heart rate and blood pressure responses are not elevated beyond clinically acceptable limits during resistance exercise. This fact attests to the safety of resistance exercise. Increased subendocardial perfusion, secondary to elevated diastolic blood pressure, may also contribute to the lower incidence of ischemic responses during isometric or isodynamic efforts. Furthermore, the myocardial oxygen supply/demand relationship appears to be favorably altered by superimposing static on dynamic effort so that the magnitude of ST-segment depression is lessened at any given rate-pressure product.

As with aerobic conditioning, cessation of resistance training results in a rapid and pronounced reversal of the physiologic adaptations. Nevertheless, the benefits of resistance training may be sustained for up to 12 weeks with a reduced training frequency, provided that the intensity of training is maintained. This suggests that individuals who are forced to reduce their resistance training volume have the opportunity to retain training benefits.

Because long-term exercise compliance remains a challenge in persons with and without chronic disease, resistance training can provide a means for maintaining interest and increasing diversity. Nevertheless, it should serve as a supplement to, rather than a replacement for, the aerobic exercise prescription.

CHAPTER 1

Introduction

James E. Graves, PhD
Syracuse University

Barry A. Franklin, PhD
William Beaumont Hospital, Wayne State University,
and the University of Michigan

Exercising to develop and maintain muscular strength (the ability to exert force), muscular endurance (the ability to exert force repeatedly), and muscle mass is commonly referred to as resistance training. Weightlifting with barbells, or specially designed weightlifting machines, is probably the most popular form of resistance training. Competitive athletes have long recognized that muscular strength and muscular endurance gained from resistance training have a positive influence on athletic performance. Today, resistance training is practiced by a wide variety of individuals with and without chronic disease, because it is also associated with favorable changes in cardiovascular function, metabolism, coronary risk factors, and psychosocial well-being (10).

The American College of Sports Medicine (ACSM), American Heart Association, American Association of Cardiovascular and Pulmonary Rehabilitation, and the U.S. surgeon general all include resistance training as an integral component of a well-rounded physical conditioning program (1, 4, 6, 11). In 1978, the ACSM published a position stand titled "The Recommended Quantity and Quality of Exercise for Developing and Maintaining Cardiorespiratory and Muscular Fitness in Healthy Adults" (2). *Fitness,* in this position stand, was defined as aerobic capacity (cardiorespiratory fitness) and healthy body composition. Although specific recommendations for developing muscular strength, muscular endurance, and muscle mass were not included in the paper, resistance training was not ignored. Based on the work of DeLorme in the mid-1940s (5), and later by Mayhew and Gross (8), Misner et al. (9), Wilmore (12), and Gettman et al. (7), the position stand stated that weight training "has significant value for increasing muscular strength and endurance, and lean body weight" (2, p. viii).

By the late 1980s there was enough information in the scientific literature to develop prescriptive guidelines for resistance training. In a revision of their 1978 position stand, the ACSM published "The Recommended Quantity and Quality of Exercise for Developing and Maintaining Cardiorespiratory and Muscular Fitness in Healthy Adults" (3). The revised position stand included the following statement on resistance training: "Strength training of a moderate intensity, sufficient to develop and maintain fat-free weight (FFW), should be an integral part of an adult fitness program. One set of 8-12 repetitions of eight to ten exercises that condition the major muscle groups at least $2 \text{ d} \cdot \text{wk}^{-1}$ is the recommended minimum." The revised position stand also described the following principles with respect to resistance training:

- Muscular strength and muscular endurance are developed by the overload principle. Overload refers to continually increasing the stress (resistance) placed on the muscles as they become capable of generating greater levels of force.
- The effect of resistance training is specific to the area of the body being trained (i.e., the principle of training specificity). Training the arms, for example, will have little or no effect on the muscles of the legs. This provides the rationale for the recommendation that 8-10 different exercises be used to condition the major muscle groups.
- Although resistance training can be performed in a variety of ways, dynamic resistance exercise at a slow to moderate speed, moving through a full range of motion, with normal breathing, is recommended.
- The expected improvement in muscular strength and muscular endurance from resistance training is dependent on the volume and intensity of the training as well as the participant's initial level of muscular fitness, which is inversely related to their potential for improvement.
- Multiple-set training regimens have little or no additional effect in the magnitude of improvement in muscular strength and endurance

when compared with single-set training regimens performed at the same intensity.

Another important concept discussed in the ACSM's 1990 position stand is the distinction between physical activity as it relates to health and as it relates to fitness (3). It is now recognized that the quantity and intensity of exercise needed to obtain health-related benefits may differ from what has been traditionally recommended for the development of physical fitness (athletic performance). Health-related benefits can occur at lower levels or intensities of exercise—amounts that may not necessarily improve cardiorespiratory fitness. Such programs, however, are usually associated with increased exercise duration, training frequency, or both.

The most recent ACSM position stand (1998), titled "The Recommended Quantity and Quality of Exercise for Developing and Maintaining Cardiorespiratory and Muscular Fitness, and Flexibility in Healthy Adults," promoted the concept that the health and fitness benefits of exercise are cumulative (minimum of 10 min bouts accumulated throughout the day), provided expanded prescriptive guidelines regarding resistance training, and advocated complementary flexibility exercises (static and/or dynamic techniques) to develop and maintain range of motion (4). It emphasized that, for the average adult beginning a resistance training regimen, single-set programs performed a minimum of 2 times a week are recommended over multiple-set programs because they are highly effective and less time consuming. Such regimens should include 8-10 different exercises at a load that permits 8-12 repetitions/set for healthy sedentary adults and 10-15 repetitions/set for older and more frail persons (approximately 50-60 years of age and above) or cardiac patients.

Although the physical performance benefits of resistance training have been recognized for many years, knowledge of its value for health and fitness, disease prevention, and rehabilitation is relatively new. Recognized adaptations to resistance training that promote health include the development and maintenance of muscle mass, increased bone mineral density, modest improvements in cardiorespiratory fitness, reductions in body fat, lowered blood pressure in hypertensive individuals, reduced glucose-stimulated plasma insulin concentrations, improved blood lipid-lipoprotein profiles, enhanced physical function, and a reduced risk of orthopedic injury. This text summarizes what is currently known about prescribing resistance training exercises for the development of health and prevention and rehabilitation of a variety of injuries, medical conditions, and chronic diseases. We believe this information will be a valuable complement to the guidelines established for prescribing resistance training programs.

The book is organized into four parts. The first part covers general principles and adaptations of resistance training that may be applied to all individuals. The authors of chapters in this section are preeminent applied scientists whose contributions to the current literature are widely recognized.

In chapter 2, Dr. Matt Feigenbaum gives a historical perspective of resistance training guidelines and discusses the application of these guidelines to specific populations. Included in this comprehensive overview is information from *Physical Activity and Health: A Report of the Surgeon General,* the most recent position stand published by the American College of Sports Medicine, the revised exercise standards of the American Heart Association, and the American Association for Cardiovascular and Pulmonary Rehabilitation's guidelines for the prescription of resistance training in populations with cardiovascular, pulmonary, or metabolic disease (1, 4, 6, 11). Guidelines for healthy adults, the elderly, and cardiac patients are also introduced in this chapter.

Next, Dr. Bill Brechue and colleagues have provided two detailed chapters that review the metabolic responses and adaptations to resistance exercise, highlighting the neuromuscular system. Each of these chapters represents a summary of our current understanding of the physiological adaptations to resistance training. Chapter 3, by James Brown and Dr. Brechue, reviews the acute and chronic cardiovascular, ventilatory, and endocrine responses to resistance training. The information contained in this chapter provides a solid foundation for understanding resistance training adaptations as they relate to specific established guidelines. In chapter 4, Matthew Beekley and Dr. Brechue describe how the nervous system interacts with skeletal muscle to produce movement. Sections in this chapter consider the production of force and movement, "adaptation strategies" to resistance exercise, and the neural and morphological adaptations that occur from resistance training.

In chapter 5, Dr. Neil McCartney discusses the safety of resistance training with respect to hemodynamic responses, abnormal signs/ symptoms (e.g., ischemic ST-segment depression, angina pectoris, and threatening arrhythmia), and their potential sequelae. He reviews dynamic and static resistance exercise, the acute circulatory responses to resistance exercise, the variable effects of load and repetitions, the influence of muscle mass, and the safety of resistance training based on the reported incidence of cardiovascular events. The key message conveyed is that appropriately prescribed resistance training is a safe form of exercise for the majority of the population, and is associated with minimal risk of cardiovascular complications, even in individuals with heart disease. Proscriptions and contraindications to traditional resistance training in clinical populations are presented.

The benefits of physical activity are maintained through continued participation. People often alter their frequency of participation for a variety of reasons. In chapter 6, Dr. James Graves addresses the volume of resistance training required to maintain muscular strength and endurance. This chapter points out that the benefits of resistance training can be maintained for short periods of time with a reduced training frequency; however, the complete cessation of training produces a rapid decline in physiological function. The chapter also addresses issues related to adherence to resistance training programs.

Chapter 7 presents detailed guidelines for prescribing resistance training to healthy adults. This chapter, authored by Dr. Feigenbaum, outlines the specific benefits associated with resistance training. Covered in this chapter are muscular strength and function, aerobic capacity, body composition, insulin resistance, serum lipid-lipoprotein profiles, fitness maintenance, safety considerations, and practical applications of the exercise prescription. This is an important chapter because it emphasizes that resistance training is one component of a well-rounded fitness program, which should also include exercises for developing and maintaining cardiorespiratory fitness and flexibility.

Part II of the text covers the benefits of resistance training for those people in special populations and those with medical conditions. Authors of chapters in this section are widely recognized experts on the prescription of physical activity in these special populations. In chapter 8, Dr. Lori Ploutz-Snyder discusses resistance training and women, especially issues that are unique to female participants. A section on basic physiological considerations examines cellular responses, protein synthesis, neuromuscular responses, and hormonal responses to resistance training. An additional section on applied physiological responses includes a discussion of muscular strength and hypertrophy, weight loss and body composition, functional tasks, menopause, secondary amenorrhea, and pregnancy. The chapter also covers the importance of resistance training for the prevention of osteoporosis and type 2 diabetes, the maintenance of functional capacity, healthy aging, and weight control.

With chapter 9, Dr. William Evans has authored a provocative examination of resistance exercise, aging, and weight control. He introduces the term *sarcopenia* to describe the age-related loss in skeletal muscle mass. The implications of sarcopenia relative to the age-associated decreases in basal metabolic rate, muscular strength, and activity levels are discussed with respect to the reduced energy requirements of the elderly. Increased body fat and abdominal obesity may be directly linked to the increased incidence of type 2 diabetes among the elderly. Dr. Evans' review discusses the extent to which regularly performed exercise affects the energy needs and adaptations by elderly people. Specific attention is given to muscle strength training in the elderly.

In chapter 10, Dr. Lorelee Stock, Ralph Requa, and Dr. James Garrick discuss the types of musculoskeletal injuries that are commonly associated with various forms of resistance training, risk factors associated with weight training injuries, and the types of musculoskeletal injuries that occur with weight training. Recommendations are given for specific types of resistance training, as well as considerations for preventing injuries.

In chapter 11, Dr. Maria Fiatarone Singh summarizes resistance training for health, disease prevention, and rehabilitation in elderly patients and frail individuals. Dr. Fiatarone Singh reviews the importance of exercise for the health of older persons and the anti-aging effects of resistance training. Many of the age-related declines in physiologic function and health status can be prevented or even reversed with appropriately prescribed resistance training. Dr. Fiatarone Singh discusses the physiological changes associated with the aging process and the potential benefits of resistance training in relation to these changes. These recognized benefits include increases in muscle strength, muscle mass, gait stability, flexibility, habitual physical activity, and gastrointestinal transit time; resistance to postural stress; improved balance, nutritional intake, functional status, and health-related quality of life; and decreased psychological dysfunction (e.g., depression).

Part III of the textbook discusses the application of resistance exercise to specific chronic visceral diseases. Contributors to these chapters, and the chapters in part IV, are well-known clinicians and basic and applied scientists who are recognized leaders in the application of resistance training for rehabilitation. In chapter 12, Dr. Kerry Stewart, Dr. Barry Franklin, and Dr. Ray Squires describe the role of resistance training in patients with coronary heart disease, specifically discussing its benefits, rationale, safety, and prescription. Additional sections discuss the advantages and limitations of types of resistance training equipment, summarize patient selection guidelines, and provide recommendations for the timing of participation post-event.

In chapter 13, Dr. Neil Gordon and Dr. Richard Leighton address the prescription of resistance training for hypertension and stroke patients. Following a brief pathophysiological, prevention, and therapeutic overview, the authors detail the benefits and cardiovascular risks of resistance training in this patient population and offer reasonable resistance training guidelines. Although there are currently no definitive guidelines for resistance training in stroke patients, Dr. Gordon recommends a prescriptive approach similar to that advocated for postmyocardial infarction patients.

In chapter 14, Dr. Randy Braith and Peter Magyari have produced an outstanding review of resistance training for solid organ transplant recipients. This chapter addresses the unique concerns of organ transplant recipients, including severe deconditioning prior to transplantation and the potential adverse effects of immunosuppressive pharmacological treatment, especially on lean body mass. The benefits of resistance training in addressing these concerns are reviewed, and specific guidelines for the safe and effective prescription of resistance exercise in organ transplant recipients are provided. Resistance training is advocated to reverse steroid-induced osteoporosis as well as to restore functional capacity.

Resistance training and chronic obstructive pulmonary disease (COPD) is presented by Dr. Michael Berry in chapter 15. Dr. Berry defines COPD and presents the epidemiology of the disease before addressing the functional impact of respiratory and peripheral skeletal muscle dysfunction on exercise tolerance. Ventilatory muscle training, upper-extremity resistance training, and whole-body resistance training are given considerable attention. Additional research is needed to make up for the relative lack of information defining the optimal resistance training prescription for patients with COPD. Dr. Berry identifies specific research questions that need clarification in this particular population.

Resistance exercise for patients with diabetes mellitus is summarized in chapter 16 by Dr. Otto Sánchez and Dr. Arthur Leon. Sections of this chapter include a discussion of the prevalence of diabetes mellitus, its classification and clinical presentation, as well as long-term complications of the disease. The authors describe exercise as an important tool in the management of diabetes mellitus, where the aims are to achieve glycemic control, reduce coexisting cardiovascular disease risk factors, and prevent or reduce the progression of chronic complications. Resistance exercise training for patients with diabetes mellitus is recognized as an important component of the overall exercise regimen. The authors discuss safety of resistance exercise in this patient population, list specific contraindications to this form of training, and provide general guidelines for prescribing resistance exercise for previously sedentary individuals with diabetes mellitus.

Part IV of the text addresses the use of resistance training for people with chronic physical disabilities. In chapter 17, Dr. James Rimmer has contributed an especially interesting description of resistance training for persons with physical disabilities, including those with special deficits or defects resulting from congenital deformities, injury, or chronic disease. Disability often leads to physical inactivity, which in turn is associated with a variety of secondary conditions that adversely impact health and result in further deterioration of the primary disabling condition. For example, a sedentary lifestyle may cause wheelchair users to experience secondary complications such as reduced aerobic fitness, muscle atrophy, osteoporosis, and impaired circulation to the lower extremities leading to eventual thrombus formation or decubitus ulcers. In addition, a diminished self-efficacy, greater dependence on others for daily living, and reduced ability for normal societal interactions can have a deleterious psychological impact. Prescribing resistance training for individuals with varied physical disabilities is extremely challenging, and this chapter covers much ground in addressing these issues. Primary sections include general resistance training guidelines for persons with physical disabilities and resistance training guidelines for specific disability groups. The latter include spinal cord injury, multiple sclerosis, post-polio syndrome, cerebral palsy, and stroke.

The favorable influence of resistance training on patients with arthritis and related musculoskeletal disorders is addressed in chapter 18 by Dr. Walter Ettinger. After a review of the different types of arthritis, Dr. Ettinger summarizes the limited evidence for resistance training as beneficial therapy for arthritis. Guidelines for exercise prescription are provided, with reference to special concerns for this escalating patient population.

In chapter 19, resistance training for low back pain and dysfunction is addressed by Dr. James Graves, Dr. John Mayer, Dr. Ted Dreisinger, and Dr. Vert Mooney. This chapter presents a historical perspective of the emergence of resistance training therapy for persons with low back pain, and the unique physiological responses associated with training the lumbar paraspinal muscles. Low back injuries occur when external forces of activity exceed the structural integrity of the lumbar spine. Properly prescribed resistance training can help to prevent as well as rehabilitate many low back disorders. Specific guidelines for the prescription of resistance exercise for low back pain patients include a relatively low frequency of exercise. The importance of lumbar health for the prevention of industrial injury and disability are also discussed.

The final chapter, by Jennifer Layne and Dr. Miriam Nelson, is on resistance training and osteoporosis. The significance of osteoporosis is addressed in several earlier chapters that cover physiological changes associated with aging. Layne and Nelson provide additional detail on the characteristics of this severely debilitating condition and bone response to resistance training. Specific recommendations for resistance training for patients with osteoporosis are given.

We believe that this virtual pharmacopoeia of resistance training indications, contraindications, and guidelines for health, disease prevention, and rehabilitation will be a valuable resource for primary care physicians, other members of the health care team (e.g., physical and occupational therapists), and exercise professionals who work with a wide range of individuals. To be noninjurious to the subject and effective for the purposes intended, resistance exercise must be prescribed specifically, after consideration of the subjects' goals and interests, age, physical characteristics, gender, previous exercise experience, unique deficits or defects, coexisting medical conditions, and functional status. This book has the special purpose of providing the reader with a single source of information for accomplishing this.

References

1. American Association of Cardiovascular and Pulmonary Rehabilitation. 1995. *Guidelines for cardiac rehabilitation programs*. Champaign, IL: Human Kinetics.
2. American College of Sports Medicine. 1978. The recommended quantity and quality of exercise for developing and maintaining cardiorespiratory and muscular fitness in healthy adults. *Medicine and Science in Sports* 10: vii-x.
3. American College of Sports Medicine. 1990. The recommended quantity and quality of exercise for developing and maintaining cardiorespiratory and muscular fitness in healthy adults. *Medicine and Science in Sports and Exercise* 22: 265-274.
4. American College of Sports Medicine. 1998. The recommended quantity and quality of exercise for developing and maintaining cardiorespiratory and muscular fitness, and flexibility in healthy adults. *Medicine and Science in Sports and Exercise* 30: 975-991.
5. DeLorme, T.L. 1945. Restoration of muscle power by heavy resistance exercise. *Journal of Bone and Joint Surgery* 27: 645-667.
6. Fletcher, G., G. Balady, V. Froelicher, L. Hartley, W. Haskell, and M. Pollock. 1995. Exercise Standards: A statement for healthcare professionals from the American Heart Association. *Circulation* 91: 580-615.
7. Gettman, L., J. Ayres, M. Pollock, and A. Jackson. 1978. The effect of circuit weight training on strength, cardiorespiratory function, and body composition of adult men. *Medicine and Science in Sports* 10: 171-176.
8. Mayhew, J., and P. Gross. 1974. Body composition changes in young women with high resistance weight training. *Research Quarterly* 45: 433-439.
9. Misner, J., R. Boileau, B. Massey, and J. Mayhew. 1974. Alterations in body composition of adult men during selected physical training programs. *Journal of the American Geriatrics Society* 22: 33-38.
10. Pollock, M., B. Franklin, G. Balady, et al. 2000. Resistance training in individuals with and without cardiovascular disease: Benefits, rationale, safety, and prescription. *Circulation* 101: 828-833.
11. U.S. Department of Health and Human Services. 1996. *Physical activity and health: A report of the surgeon general*. Atlanta, GA: U.S. Department of Health and Human Services, Centers of Disease Control and Prevention, National Center for Chronic Disease Prevention and Health Promotion.
12. Wilmore, J.G. 1974. Alterations in strength, body composition, and anthropometric measurements consequent to a 10-week weight training program. *Medicine and Science in Sports* 6: 133-138.

Rationale and Review of Current Guidelines

Matthew S. Feigenbaum, PhD
Furman University

Resistance training, also known as strength or weight training, has become popular during the past two decades and is now considered an integral component of a comprehensive fitness program for individuals interested in improving their health and fitness status as well as for those rehabilitating from an array of diseases and/or disabilities. Traditionally, resistance training programs have been designed to maximize adaptations contributing to muscle hypertrophy, strength, power, and athletic prowess (8, 32). Although these goals continue to govern competitive collegiate and professional athletic programs, research studies have also established that resistance training promotes health in adult fitness participants and patients in supervised rehabilitation settings (2, 5, 6, 66, 72). Given the increasing evidence that resistance training plays a significant role in many health factors, it is not surprising that both the exercise science and medical communities recommend that individuals of all ages and of both genders participate in comprehensive exercise programs. Within the past decade, the surgeon general and major health organizations—the American College of Sports Medicine (ACSM), the American Heart Association (AHA), and the American Association for Cardiovascular and Pulmonary Rehabilitation (AACVPR)—have developed resistance exercise guidelines appropriate for various segments of the population (see table 2.1) (2, 5, 6, 33, 72). This chapter addresses the rationale for, and reviews, current resistance training program guidelines as published by the major professional health organizations.

Historical Perspective: Resistance Training Guidelines

Resistance training programs were not recommended for enhancing athletic performance or rehabilitating from orthopedic injuries until the latter part of the 1940s, or for improving adult fitness until the 1970s. The evolution of formal guidelines can be traced to the post–World War II era, when army physician Captain Tom DeLorme incorporated heavy progressive resistance exercises in rehabilitation programs designed for orthopedically disabled veterans (22). After conducting a series of studies, Drs. DeLorme and Watkins recommended the use of heavy resistance and a low number of repetitions

TABLE 2.1   Standards, Guidelines, and Position Statements Regarding Resistance Training

	Sets; reps	Stations/devices	Frequency
HEALTHY SEDENTARY ADULTS			
1998 ACSM position stand (5)	1 set[a]; 8-12 reps	8-10 exercises[b]	2-3 d · wk^{-1}
1998 ACSM guidelines (6)[c]	1 set; 8-12 reps	8-10 exercises	2 d · wk^{-1} min.
1996 Surgeon general's report (72)	1-2 sets; 8-12 reps	8-10 exercises	2 d · wk^{-1}
ELDERLY PERSONS			
Pollock et al. (66)	1 set; 10-15 reps	8-10 exercises	2 d · wk^{-1} min.
CARDIAC PATIENTS			
1995 AHA Exercise Standards (33)	1 set; 10-15 reps	8-10 exercises	2-3 d · wk^{-1}
1995 AACVPR guidelines (2)	1 set; 12-15 reps	8-10 exercises	2-3 d · wk^{-1}

Note: ACSM = American College of Sports Medicine; AHA = American Heart Association; AACVPR = American Association of Cardiovascular and Pulmonary Rehabilitation; reps = repetitions; min. = minimum. [a] ACSM (5): multiple-set regimens may provide increased benefits. [b] Minimum one exercise per major muscle group: e.g., chest press, shoulder press, triceps extension, biceps curl, pull-down (upper back), lower back extension, abdominal crunch / curl-up, quadriceps extension, leg curls (hamstrings), calf raise. [c] ACSM (6): guidelines developed for healthy, sedentary, and low-risk diseased populations.

to develop muscular strength, and light resistance and a high number of repetitions to develop muscular endurance (23). As a result of the improved recovery from injuries and increases in muscle mass, strength, and function, resistance training gained formal recognition in the medical community. During the 1950s and 1960s, several researchers conducted short-term resistance training studies in which they manipulated and evaluated training volume variables (sets, repetitions, frequency of training, intensity, and rest periods), the results from which formed the basis for many of the early resistance exercise recommendations (10, 11, 12, 17, 54, 60, 75, 76).

Beginning in the 1940s and continuing through the 1970s, Dr. Tom Cureton and others (36) promoted the importance of a well-rounded program, including aerobic endurance exercise, calisthenics, and resistance training for adult fitness programs (20, 21). However, during the same time period, a growing body of epidemiological research indicated a strong link between activity patterns, sedentary lifestyles, and the incidence of cardiovascular disease (34, 48, 61). In his 1968 work, *Aerobics*, Ken Cooper stated: "The best exercises [for stimulating the cardiovascular system] are running, swimming, cycling, walking, stationary running, handball, basketball, and squash, and in just about that order. Isometrics, weight lifting, and calisthenics, though good as far as they go, don't even make the list, despite the fact that most exercise books are *based* on one of these three, especially calisthenics" (19, p. 15). With the development of master's track-and-field competition (first national meet in 1971), Frank Shorter winning the gold medal at the widely watched 1972 Olympic Games in Munich, and the numerous publications on running (e.g., *Runner's World*), health and fitness became synonymous with aerobic exercise, and the perceived need to incorporate resistance training into adult fitness programs declined.

In 1978, the ACSM issued its original position statement titled "The Recommended Quantity and Quality of Exercise for Developing and Maintaining Cardiorespiratory and Muscular Fitness in Healthy Adults" (3). Reflecting the trends and research available at the time, the focus of the statement was on establishing exercise guidelines for developing and maintaining cardiorespiratory fitness and body composition. The lack of research quantifying the amount of resistance training recommended for the average adult was the main reason for omitting resistance training guidelines in the 1978 ACSM statement, not because it was thought to be unimportant (M.L. Pollock, personal communication, May 1993). It was and remains the policy of the major professional organizations, including the ACSM, that position stands must be accompanied by research documentation. Unfortunately, the omission of resistance training guidelines from the 1978 ACSM statement was interpreted as meaning that this type of exercise was not important. In

1980, the American Alliance for Health, Physical Education, Recreation and Dance (AAHPERD) published its new *Health Related Fitness Test Manual* (1). The manual excluded upper-body strength test items, further implying their lack of importance.

In the mid- to late 1970s, professional and collegiate athletic programs and health clubs (e.g., YMCAs), recognizing the impact of resistance training on athletic performance, improved physique, and general fitness, added free weights and/or resistance exercise machines (e.g., Universal, Nautilus) to their facilities. In 1978, the National Strength and Conditioning Association (NSCA) was formed to bridge the gap between the scientific bases and practical applications of resistance training. Although the NSCA has predominantly focused on prescribing and designing strength and conditioning programs for improving athletic performance, the organization has been a strong advocate for incorporating resistance training into comprehensive fitness programs for all segments of the population. By the mid-1980s, the medical community began to recognize the potential health value of resistance training in relation to functional capacity and other health-related factors (e.g., bone mineral density, basal metabolism, weight control, and low back health) in patients with diseases/disabilities other than orthopedic. At this time, research into resistance training and its quantification for the average adult fitness participant intensified. In 1989, AAHPERD added upper-body strength training and testing as an integral component in its Physical Best program (57). In 1990, the ACSM formally recognized the importance of the comprehensive fitness program and added a resistance training component to the previously published 1978 position statement. In 1991, the AHA and AACVPR also incorporated resistance training into their exercise rehabilitation regimens, and now most major health organizations currently recommend resistance training as part of a comprehensive exercise program (see table 2.1). Thus, Dr. Tom Cureton's concept of recommending a comprehensive fitness program for all segments of the population had come full circle (see figure 2.1) (20, 21).

Scientific Basis for Resistance Exercise Prescription

Resistance training is well established as the most effective method available for improving muscular strength and endurance through the progressive overload principle (i.e., by increasing more than normal the resistance to movement or frequency and duration of activity) (22, 25, 32, 44, 67). Any magnitude of overload will result in strength development, but heavier resistance loads to maximal or near maximal effort will elicit a significantly greater training effect (32, 44, 52, 67). The intensity and volume of exercise can be manipulated by varying the weight load, the number of repetitions and sets com-

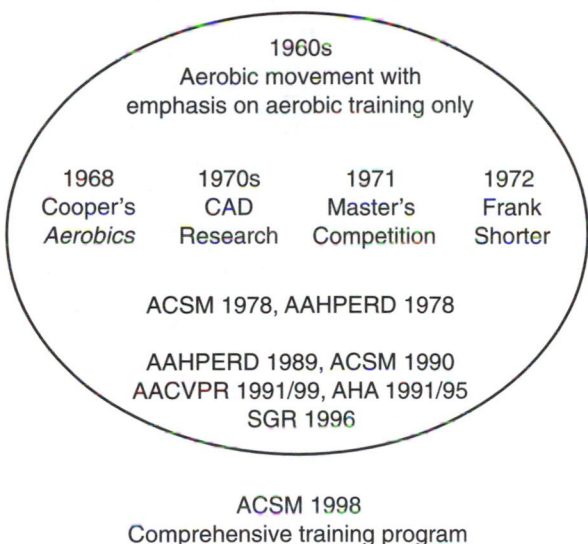

Well-rounded program
Tom Cureton: 1940-1965
Motor fitness: Endurance–strength–flexibility–
agility–balance–power

1960s
Aerobic movement with
emphasis on aerobic training only

1968	1970s	1971	1972
Cooper's	CAD	Master's	Frank
Aerobics	Research	Competition	Shorter

ACSM 1978, AAHPERD 1978

AAHPERD 1989, ACSM 1990
AACVPR 1991/99, AHA 1991/95
SGR 1996

ACSM 1998
Comprehensive training program
Aerobic–resistance–flexibility

Figure 2.1 By 1998, Cureton's recommendation for a comprehensive training program had come full circle.

Reprinted from Pollock et al. 1995.

pleted, and the rest interval between sets and exercises (32). When prescribing a resistance exercise program, the clinician, coach, or fitness instructor must decide what constitutes an optimal balance of these factors to maximize benefits, and must take into consideration the individual's health and fitness status, goals, access to an appropriate training environment, and understanding of the proper application of the basic underlying training principles and concepts. Programs prescribed for competitive athletes, which often include exercises designed specifically to improve the development of explosive power (e.g., Olympic lifts, plyometrics), are usually not appropriate for children, adult fitness enthusiasts, sedentary middle-aged adults, elderly persons, or patients with chronic disease(s), and vice versa. The major health organizations recognized the need for developing resistance exercise guidelines for specific segments of the population (see table 2.1). Although these guidelines constitute the basis for prescribing individualized exercise programs, the basic components common to all resistance training programs constitute the framework for resistance exercise prescription, regardless of the intended population.

Number of Repetitions

Muscular strength is best developed by using heavier weights (that require maximal or near maximal tension development) with few repetitions, and muscular endurance is best developed by using lighter weights with a greater number of repetitions (26, 32, 67). To some extent, both muscular strength and endurance are developed under each condition, but each loading scheme favors a more specific type of neuromuscular development (32, 67). Thus, 8-12 repetitions per set are recommended to elicit improvements in both muscular strength and endurance; however, a lower repetition range, with a heavier weight (e.g., 6-8 repetitions), may better optimize strength and power (32). Because orthopedic injury may occur in older and/or more frail participants when performing efforts to volitional fatigue using a high-intensity, low- to moderate-repetition maximum (RM) training regimen, the completion of 10-15 repetitions or RM is recommended (5, 66). The term RM refers to the maximal number of times a load can be lifted before fatigue using good form and technique. Caution is advised for training that emphasizes eccentric contractions during each repetition, compared with concentric or isometric contractions, as the potential for muscle soreness and injury is increased particularly in individuals beginning a resistance training program (7, 47).

Number of Sets

Although 3 or more sets of 6-12 repetitions per exercise (e.g., bench press, squat) performed 3 days per week as part of a periodized program is a traditional resistance exercise prescription for many athletic programs, the minimal and optimal number of sets required to elicit significant gains in health parameters is substantially less for adult fitness participants. There is a surprising lack of well-controlled long-term clinical trials reported in the peer-reviewed literature comparing single- versus multiple-set resistance training programs, particularly for the adult fitness model. The topic of single versus multiple sets and, in the broader scheme, what constitutes the optimal volume of resistance training, has generated much contention in the exercise science and medical communities (5, 32, 70). The existing ACSM recommendations regarding the number of sets to be performed (i.e., one set, although multiple-set regimens may provide greater benefits if time allows) are clearly directed at the adult fitness model, not collegiate or professional athletes, and reflect the empirical research conducted to determine the minimal and optimal levels of exercise needed to induce health- and fitness-related adaptations in the musculoskeletal systems (5, 6). Table 2.2 summarizes the results from resistance training studies that compare the volume of training using a variety of muscle groups.

To date, only one study, conducted by Berger, has found a multiple-set protocol to elicit greater strength gains than a single set (10); the majority of studies indicate there is not a significant difference in the first few months of an adult fitness program (40, 58, 65, 68, 69, 73, 74). The results

TABLE 2.2 Results From Studies Comparing Strength Gains Found Using Single or Multiple Sets of Resistance Exercise

Reference	Sex	Age	N	Exercise	d/wk	Duration	Sets × RM	% Increase
Berger (10)	M	C	177	Bench press	3	12 wks	1×6/10	22.4
							2×6/10	21.8 NS
							3×6/10	25.3[a]
Silvester (68)	M	C	48	Biceps curl	3	8 wks	1×10-12	24.6
							3×6	26.2 NS
Stowers (71)	M	C	28	Squat	2	7 wks	1×10	16.1
							3×10	21.1 NS
				Bench press			1×10	8.0
							3×10	10.6 NS
Westcott (73)	M/F	35	44	Nautilus circuit[b]	3	4 wks	1×10	11.2[b]
							2×10	10.8[b] NS
Westcott (74)	M/F	40	77	Dips/ chin-ups	3	10 wks	1×5/10/15	4.8[c]
							2×5/10/15	4.1[c] NS
							3×5/10/15	5.2[c] NS
Pollock (65)	M/F	26	78	Cervical extension	2	12 wks	1×8-12	40.9
							2×8-12	43.5 NS
Graves (39)	M/F	31	110	Lumbar extension	1	12 wks	1×8-12	19.0
							2×8-12	16.0 NS
Starkey (69)	M/F	35	49	Knee extension	3	14 wks	1×8-12	30.1
							3×8-12	26.8 NS
				Knee flexion	3	14 wks	1×8-12	18.7
							3×8-12	17.7 NS

Note: M = male; F = female; C = college undergraduates; NS = no significant difference vs. one set
[a] $p < 0.05$; 3 sets > 1 set
[b] Nautilus circuit—average strength increase of five exercises: leg extension, leg curl, torso pullover, arm extension, arm curl
[c] Data indicates the average increase in the *number* of dips and chin-ups combined
Reprinted from Starkey et al. 1996 (69).

of Berger's study, which formed the basis for prescribing multiple sets of 6-10 repetitions, indicated that 3 sets of 6-10 repetitions were superior to 1 or 2 sets with similar repetitions following 12 weeks of bench press exercise performed 3 days per week (10). When comparing Berger's analysis of covariance (ANCOVA) data, the groups started with a 1-RM (one-repetition maximum) bench press of 56.6 kg and finished with 69.3 kg (22.4% increase; 1-set group), 68.9 kg (21.8% increase; 2-set group), and 70.9 kg (25.3% increase; 3-set group). Although there was a statistically significant difference, the magnitude of difference between the groups training with 1 set versus 3 sets was small (2.9%). Furthermore, there are no studies existing in the literature, including the Berger study, that indicate that 2 sets are superior to 1 set for the first 3 to 4 months of a resistance training program.

With the exception of the Berger study (10), the literature supports the recommendation of single-set programs performed to fatigue and indicates that the quality (intensity) and not the quantity (volume) of resistance training may be the most important factor for developing muscular strength in sedentary persons during the first few months of a resistance training program (58, 68, 71). Despite the variety of muscle groups tested (pectorals, biceps, lumbar extensors, quadriceps, etc.), most studies in the literature have reached similar conclusions (see table 2.2). It should be noted that most of the studies were conducted over a period of 4-14 weeks, and studies of longer duration may show greater strength gains with multiple-set regimens. Although additional long-term clinical studies need to be conducted, the existing literature clearly indicates that for the first 3 to 4 months of resistance training, single-set programs are as effective as multiple-set programs for improving muscular strength in previously untrained persons.

In support of this recommendation, the amount of time required to complete a single-set program has also been shown to be substantially less than one-half the time required to complete multiple-set protocols. Messier and Dill reported that the time required to complete a 3-set free-weight training program averaged 50 min compared with only 20 min for 1 set (58). This time efficiency often translates into improved program compliance, as exercise programs that last longer than 1 hour are associated with higher dropout rates (41, 62). Considering the similarities in strength gains for single- and multiple-set programs, single-set programs are recommended for the adult fitness population because they are less time consuming, more cost efficient, and appear to produce similar health and fitness benefits (5, 29, 62).

Frequency of Training

The frequency of training for a muscle group is also an important component of the design of a resistance training program (16, 24, 32, 35,

39). The rest period must be sufficient to allow for muscular recuperation and development and to prevent overtraining. However, too much rest between training sessions can result in detraining. A 48 h rest period between concurrent training sessions is generally recommended, which corresponds with a 3 days per week frequency of training guideline for individual muscle groups (32). Although 3 days per week of resistance exercise is generally recommended for maximal strength gains, research studies indicate that isolated muscle groups are unique in their trainability and adaptability to resistance training (24, 39, 67). Table 2.3 summarizes the results from resistance training studies that compare frequency of training using a variety of muscle groups.

TABLE 2.3 Results From Studies Comparing Frequency of Training Using Resistance Exercise

Reference	N	Sex*	Exercise	Days/wk	Duration	Sets × RM	Increase %
Berger (13)	NA	NA	Bench press	2, 3	12 wk	1×10	NA[a]
Henderson (43)	117	M	Bench press	2, 3	6 wk	2×9 3×6	2×/wk = 12.8 lbs 3×/wk = 19.2 lbs[b]
Hunter (46)	14	M	Bench press	3	7 wk	3×10	M = 11.9% F = 19.5%
	11	F					
	10	M		4	7 wk	2×10	M = 16.7%[c]
	11	F					F = 33.3%[c]
Gillam (35)	15	M	Bench press	1	9 wk	18×1	1×/wk = 19.5%
	14			2			2×/wk = 24.2%
	15			3			3×/wk = 32.3%[d]
	13			4			4×/wk = 29.0%
	11			5			5×/wk = 40.7%[d]
Barham (9)	90	M	Full-knee bends	5, 3, 2	6 wk	3×5	NA[e]
Braith et al. (16)	28	M	Bilateral knee extension	2, 3	10 wk	1×7-10	2×/wk = 13.5% 3×/wk = 21.2%[f]
	33	F					
	31	M		2, 3	18 wk	1×7-10	2×/wk = 20.9% 3×/wk = 28.4%[f]
	25	F					
Graves et al. (39)	72	M	Lumbar extension	1×/2wk 1, 2, 3	12, 20 wk	1×8-12	1×/2wk = 26.6% 1×/wk = 38.9%[g] 2×/wk = 41.4%[g] 3×/wk = 37.2%[g]
	42	F					
Pollock et al. (65)	50	M	Cervical extension	1, 2	12 wk	1×8-12	1×/wk = 8.7% 2×/wk = 32.8%[h]
	28	F					

(continued)

21

TABLE 2.3 *(continued)*

Reference	N	Sex*	Exercise	Days/wk	Duration	Sets × RM	Increase %
Leggett et al.	54	M	Cervical	1×/2wk	12 wk	1×8-20	1×/2wk = 9.0%
(50)	26	F	rotation	1, 2, 3			1×/wk = 15.9%
							2×/wk = 24.3%[i]
							3×/wk = 38.4%[i]
Blanton	47	M	Torso	1, 2	12 wk	1×8-12	1×/wk = 17.4%[j]
(14)	34	F	rotation				2×/wk = 21.8%[j]
DeMichele	33	M	Torso	1, 2, 3	12 wk	1×11-15	1×/wk = 4.9%
et al. (24)	25	F	rotation				2×/wk = 16.3%[k]
							3×/wk = 11.9%[k]

NA = data not available; RM = repetition maximum
* Sex: M = male; F = female
[a] $p > 0.05$; 2 = 3×/wk
[b] $p < 0.05$; 3×/wk > 2×/wk
[c] $p < 0.01$; 4×/wk > 3×/wk
[d] $p < 0.05$; 5×/wk > 1-4 ×/wk, 3, 5×/wk > 1, 2×/wk
[e] $p < 0.05$; 5, 3×/wk > 2×/wk
[f] $p < 0.01$; 3×/wk > 2×/wk
[g] $p < 0.05$; 1, 2, 3×/wk > 1×/2wk
[h] $p < 0.05$; 2×/wk > 1×/wk
[i] $p < 0.05$; 2, 3×/wk > 1×/wk, 1×/2wk: 3×/wk > 2×/wk
[j] $p < 0.05$; 1 = 2×/wk
[k] $p < 0.01$; 2, 3×/wk > 1×/wk
Reprinted from DeMichele et al. 1997 (24).

Two studies evaluating the effects of frequency of training have shown that 4 or more training sessions per week produced optimal strength gains in several muscle groups (35, 46). Using the bench press exercise, Gillam indicated that training 5 days per week over a 9-week period was superior to training regimens of 1, 2, 3, or 4 days per week (35). Interestingly, training 3 or 4 days per week produced similar results that were significantly greater than those obtained by the groups training 1 or 2 days per week. Hunter and Henderson also found that increasing the frequency of bench press training to 4 and 3 days per week, respectively, produced greater strength gains than lesser-frequency protocols (43, 46). In contrast, Berger (12) found that bench pressing either 2 or 3 days per week produced similar strength gains over the course of 12 weeks. Similar findings have also been reported for studies evaluating strength gains in the lower limb muscles. Braith et al. found 3 days per week to be superior to 2 days per week in increasing quadriceps (knee extension) strength, and an earlier study by Barham showed that performing the squat exercise 3 days per week was as effective as 5 days per week, and that both training frequencies were superior to performing the squat exercise 2 days per week (9, 16).

While the chest, arms, and legs may require a training frequency of 3 days per week or more to develop optimal strength gains, additional studies suggest that the muscles supporting the spine (e.g., lumbar extensors) and smaller muscles of the torso may respond as well with fewer training sessions per week (39, 63). For example, Graves et al. found no significant differences in dynamic and isometric strength generated by isolated lumbar extensor muscles among groups training 1, 2, or 3 days per week for 20 weeks (39). When assessing cervical rotation strength, Leggett et al. found that training frequencies of 2 and 3 days per week were superior to 1 day per week or 1 day every 2 weeks over a 12-week training period (50). Pollock et al. indicated that training 2 days per week is superior to 1 day per week for increasing cervical extension strength, but because training 3 days per week was not evaluated, no inferences can be made in this regard (65). As for the muscles involved in torso rotation, DeMichele et al. concluded that the 2 days per week training frequency obtained better adherence and equal strength gains compared to 3 days per week; both of these groups elicited greater improvements than the group training 1 day per week (24).

Based on the findings of these studies, we can say that there is no single optimal frequency of resistance training for all muscle groups. Whether the differences in the strength gains occurring in isolated muscle groups are due to variations in neuromuscular integration, muscle morphology, or other mechanisms warrants further investigation. Although clinicians and other health professionals must consider the specific needs and goals of individual participants (e.g., time needed to recover from a training session), particularly for those who are frail or who have orthopedic limitations, the conservative frequency-of-training guideline of a minimum of 2 days per week seems appropriate (see table 2.2). Participants who have time and want to achieve more benefits may choose to weight train 3 days per week. In addition, in prescribing traditional resistance exercise programs (8-10 exercises for the major muscle groups—e.g., chest, back, shoulders, arms, abdomen, legs, hips), the minimum of 2 days per week training frequency allows more time for recuperation, is less time consuming, and thus may enhance adherence. Programs of 2 days per week also appear to produce 80-90% of the strength benefits of programs of higher frequency in the untrained person for the first few months.

Modality of Exercise

Muscular strength and endurance can be developed by means of static (isometric) or dynamic (isotonic or isokinetic) exercises. Although each type of training has its advantages and limitations, for healthy adults, dynamic resistance exercises are recommended, as they best mimic activities associated with daily living. Resistance training for the average participant should be rhythmical and performed at a moderate-to-slow controlled speed, through a pain-free range of motion, and with a normal breathing pattern during the lifting movements. Heavy resistance exercise can cause a dramatic acute increase in both systolic and diastolic blood pressure, especially during a Valsalva maneuver (51, 53).

The expected improvement in strength from resistance training is difficult to assess because increases in strength are affected by the participant's initial level of strength and potential for improvement (32, 42, 44, 59). For example, Mueller and Rohmert found increases in strength ranging from 2% to 9% per week depending on initial strength levels (59). In comparison, studies involving elderly participants (30, 31) and young to middle-aged persons using lumbar extension exercise (63) have shown greater than 100% improvement in strength after 8-12 weeks of training. Although the literature reflects a wide range of improvement in muscular strength with resistance training programs, the average improvement for sedentary young and middle-aged men and women for up to six months of training is 25-30%. In a review of 13 studies representing various forms of isotonic training, Fleck and Kraemer reported an average improvement in bench press strength of 23.3% when subjects were tested on the equipment with which they were trained and 16.5% when tested on special isotonic or isokinetic ergometers. These investigators also reported an average increase in leg strength of 26.6% when subjects were tested with the equipment that they trained on and 21.2% when tested with special isotonic or isokinetic ergometers (32). Improvements in strength resulting from isometric training have been of the same magnitude as found with isotonic training (16, 32, 37, 38).

Current Resistance Training Guidelines for Healthy Adults

The guidelines/statements shown in table 2.1 reflect the scientific-based research conducted to determine minimal and optimal levels of exercise needed to induce health- and fitness-related adaptations in the musculoskeletal systems. The addition of resistance training as a component of the comprehensive fitness program was an important inclusion by ACSM, and subsequent statements and guidelines published by the ACSM, AHA, AACVPR, and the surgeon general recommend resistance training for both healthy and diseased populations (2, 4, 5, 6, 33, 72). At first glance, the ACSM recommendation for resistance training for healthy adults may appear minimal, but these minimal standards were based on the following premises: "First, the time it takes to complete a comprehensive, well-rounded program is important. Programs lasting more than 60 min per session are associated with higher dropout rates (62). Second, although greater frequencies of training (16, 32, 35) and additional sets or combinations of sets and repetitions may elicit larger strength gains (10, 22, 32, 44, 76), the magnitude of difference is usually small" (4). Taking these assumptions into consideration, the minimal standard appears acceptable for most healthy adults beginning a resistance training program.

The guidelines recommended by the various health organizations are very similar in their application of exercise prescription variables. For safety and in consideration of time allotments, most resistance training programs should incorporate variable-resistance machines and traditional calisthenics and flexibility exercises. Intensity should start low and progress slowly, allowing time for adaptation. If a 1-RM test is administered for the purposes of assessing muscular strength at the beginning of a resistance training program, then 30-40% of the 1-RM for the upper body and 50-60% of 1-RM for the hips and legs should be used as the starting weight for the first exercise training session. When the participant can comfortably lift the weight 12 repetitions using good form and perceives it to be light to somewhat hard (12-13 on the Borg RPE scale), 5% can be added to the next training session (15). Although completing one set of 8-12 repetitions at a comfortably hard level (RPE = 12-13) is the initial goal, the participant should strive to progress to a higher intensity (RPE = 15-16, hard). Since the level of fatigue (intensity) is an important factor for attaining a maximal benefit, exercising to a maximal effort gives the best results (RPE = 19-20; cannot complete another repetition using good form) (6, 32). At this level of training, progression to a higher weight should occur every 1-2 weeks. If a subject cannot lift the weight a minimum of 8 times, then the weight should be reduced 5% for the next training session. Although the current minimal standard recommended by the ACSM (5) seems appropriate, most of the research used to formulate the resistance training guidelines was based on data from healthy adults under 50 years of age.

Current Resistance Training Guidelines for the Elderly

As described previously, resistance training is well established as an essential training modality for proper musculoskeletal development and maintenance and improves physical functional capacity and quality of life, especially in the elderly and more frail low-fit individuals (31). The ACSM exercise prescription guidelines for young adults and middle-aged adults are also appropriate for the elderly (see table 2.1), with slight but distinct differences in exercise prescription application (5, 6, 49, 55,

66). Due to the natural course of physiological degradation (e.g., loss of bone mineral density), elderly adults may be more fragile and thus more susceptible to fatigue, orthopedic injuries, and cardiovascular and pulmonary complications, and these factors need to be taken into consideration when prescribing physical activity programs (6, 18, 27, 33, 45, 64, 66). In addition, elderly adults are generally more sedentary, and lowering the intensity of the activity and progressing more slowly than in programs prescribed for younger adults may be more beneficial over the long term. The mode of exercise is also an important consideration when designing resistance exercise programs for the elderly. From a safety standpoint, variable-resistance machines with selectorized weight stacks are generally recommended for several reasons (66):

1. The initial weight can be applied at a low level and increased in small increments (1 kg or less).
2. The equipment is usually designed to stabilize the hips and protect the lower back, thus reducing the risk of injury.
3. Many machines are designed to avoid handgripping, which reduces the risk of exercise-induced hypertension.
4. The machines are usually designed to allow the resistance to be applied evenly through the participants' full range of motion (ROM).
5. Many types of equipment can be double pinned to allow the subject to exercise through their pain-free ROM.
6. Many resistance machines do not require the participant to balance or control the weight, as do dumbbells and barbells, which may reduce the likelihood of injury.

In addition to being safer, variable-resistance machines generally require less time to use when compared to free-weight exercises. Allowing participants to complete their exercise sessions in a minimal amount of time often translates into improved program compliance. Given the inherent risk of orthopedic injury in the elderly population, exercise sessions should begin at a lower intensity level (10-15 repetitions) and progress more slowly (every 2-4 weeks) than programs designed for younger adults (every 1-2 weeks), allowing time for adaptation. Since the fastest growing segment of the U.S. population is the elderly, further research is needed to determine the health and fitness benefits of resistance training as well as exercise guidelines for the elderly.

Current Resistance Training Guidelines for the Cardiac Patient

Like healthy adults, cardiac patients require a minimum level of muscular exertion to accomplish activities associated with daily living, but they often lack the physical strength, muscular endurance, and/or confidence to perform these tasks. Comprehensive rehabilitation programs for cardiac patients, however, have traditionally emphasized dynamic aerobic exercise for maintaining and improving cardiovascular fitness as well as for the known health benefits. The AHA, ACSM, and AACVPR described the importance of muscular fitness in preparing the cardiac patient to return to work and to participate in household and leisure activities (2, 6, 33). Many of these vocational and recreational activities place demands on the body that more closely resemble resistance exercise than aerobic exercise. Therefore, it seems prudent to incorporate resistance training into the patient's exercise program, especially since recent research indicates that complementary resistance training has many favorable health and fitness benefits.

Updated resistance training guidelines for cardiac patients developed by the AHA and AACVPR have been published (see table 2.1) and are similar to the guidelines established for healthy adults (2, 5, 6, 33). The primary differences involve reduced exercise intensity, slower progression of the training volume variables, and increased patient monitoring and program supervision. Guidelines for cardiac patients include the use of a lighter weight performed with 10-15 or 12-15 repetitions (2, 33). Although resistance training has been shown to be a safe procedure in regard to precipitating a cardiovascular event (28, 56), recommendations vary greatly as to the level of fatigue (moderate to maximum) required in such programs (2, 6, 33). Thus, it appears that low-risk patients who have a metabolic equivalent (MET) capacity greater than 7 can be cleared for heavy resistance training (10/12-15 repetitions to fatigue), while other more high-risk patients should keep their fatigue to a moderate level (RPE $\leq$ 15). An additional point to consider when prescribing exercise programs for cardiac patients, and other patient populations, is that pharmacotherapy (e.g., beta blockers) may alter the normal hemodynamic responses to exercise. In recognition of this, the RPE scale developed by Borg is gaining increasing acceptance as an effective method for monitoring the cardiac patient's level of exertion during resistance exercise testing and training (15, 33).

Summary of Current Resistance Training Guidelines

The surgeon general's report on physical activity and health, the updated versions of the ACSM position stand on exercise training, the *Guidelines for Exercise Testing and Prescription* developed by ACSM, the revised "Exercise Standards" of AHA, and the AACVPR *Guidelines for Cardiac Rehabilitation Programs* serve as the foundation for most recommendations regarding physical activity program design (see table 2.1) (2, 5, 6, 33, 72). These guidelines/statements reflect the scientific-based research conducted to determine minimal and optimal levels of exercise needed to induce health- and fitness-related adaptations in the cardio-vascular-respiratory and musculoskeletal systems. Although these recommendations may appear minimal, clinicians should emphasize that resistance training needs to be incorporated into a comprehensive fitness program (including aerobic training and flexibility exercises). The comprehensive fitness program should be designed so that it can be performed 2-3 days per week, with each session not lasting more than 60 min. Although research indicates that greater frequencies of training and/or larger training volumes may elicit larger strength gains, the magnitude of difference within the first few months is usually small and is often associated with an increased incidence of injuries and/or a decrease in program adherence (5). Taking these assumptions into consideration, the minimal guidelines are acceptable for the healthy sedentary person or chronic disease patient beginning a resistance training program or for those who do not desire to attain the highest level of strength. For safety and in consideration of time allotments, most resistance training programs should incorporate 8-10 exercises that condition the major muscle groups a minimum of 2 days per week. Intensity should progress slowly, allowing time for adaptation. To develop or maintain range of motion, special calisthenic and flexibility exercises should be included. The goal is to be able to complete 1 set of 8-12 repetitions to volitional fatigue (8-12 RM) for healthy persons under 50 years of age. The AHA and AACVPR guidelines for cardiac patients and that of Pollock et al. for persons over 50 years of age recommend a lower-intensity program, which may reduce the risk of orthopedic injury (2, 33, 66). For the more fragile populations, 1 set of 10-15 repetitions is recommended. Depending on patient status, this lower-intensity program would be performed to a level perceived as moderate/comfortably hard or to volitional fatigue. It is interesting to note that both the ACSM and AACVPR have reduced the recommendation for number of sets from 2 or 3 to 1 (minimal standard) in their latest statements (2, 6). Further research is needed to determine the ideal number of repetitions for fragile populations as well as for persons participating in rehabilitation programs.

When prescribed appropriately, resistance training is effective for developing fitness, health, and for the prevention and rehabilitation of orthopedic injuries. Although recent studies indicate that resistance training may reduce the risks for several debilitating diseases (e.g., cancer, heart disease, diabetes, low back pain, osteoporosis), further research is clearly warranted in this area. There is enough existing evidence to conclude that resistance training, particularly when incorporated into a comprehensive fitness program, can offer substantial health benefits for persons of all ages. These benefits, including improvements in functional capacity, translate into an improved quality of life.

References

1. American Alliance for Health, Physical Education, Recreation and Dance. 1980. *AAHPERD health related fitness test manual*, 9-22. Washington, DC: American Alliance for Health, Physical Education, Recreation, and Dance.
2. American Association of Cardiovascular and Pulmonary Rehabilitation. 1995. *Guidelines for cardiac rehabilitation programs*. 2d ed., 27-56. Champaign, IL: Human Kinetics.
3. American College of Sports Medicine. 1978. The recommended quantity and quality of exercise for developing and maintaining cardiorespiratory and muscular fitness in healthy adults. *Medicine and Science in Sports and Exercise* 10: vii-x.
4. American College of Sports Medicine. 1990. The recommended quantity and quality of exercise for developing and maintaining cardiorespiratory and muscular fitness in healthy adults. *Medicine and Science in Sports and Exercise* 22: 265-274.
5. American College of Sports Medicine. 1998. The recommended quantity and quality of exercise for developing and maintaining cardiorespiratory and muscular fitness, and flexibility in healthy adults. *Medicine and Science in Sports and Exercise* 30: 975-991.
6. American College of Sports Medicine. 1998. *ACSM's resource manual for guidelines for exercise testing prescription*. 3d ed., 448-455. Baltimore: Williams & Wilkins.
7. Armstrong, R.B. 1984. Mechanisms of exercise-induced delayed onset muscular soreness: A brief review. *Medicine and Science in Sports and Exercise* 16: 529-538.
8. Atha, J. 1981. Strengthening muscle. *Exercise and Sport Sciences Reviews* 9: 1-73.
9. Barham, J.N. 1960. A comparison of the effectiveness of isometric and isotonic exercise when performed at different frequencies per week. Unpublished doctoral dissertation, Louisiana State University, Baton Rouge.
10. Berger, R.A. 1962. Effect of varied weight training programs on strength. *Research Quarterly* 33: 168-181.
11. Berger, R.A. 1962. Optimum repetitions for the development of strength. *Research Quarterly* 33: 334-338.
12. Berger, R.A. 1965. Comparison of the effect of various weight training loads on strength. *Research Quarterly* 36: 141-146.
13. Berger, R.A. 1965. Application of research findings in progressive resistance exercise to physical therapy. *Journal of the Association of Physical and Mental Rehabilitation* 19: 200-203.
14. Blanton, J.H. 1990. Quantitative strength assessment and trainability of the torso rotation musculature. Unpublished master's thesis, University of Florida, Gainesville.
15. Borg, G.A.V. 1982. Psychophysical bases of perceived exertion. *Medicine and Science in Sports and Exercise* 14: 377-381.
16. Braith, R.W., J.E. Graves, M. Pollock, S.H. Leggett, D.M. Carpenter, and A.B. Colvin. 1989. Comparison of two versus three days per week of variable resistance training during 10 and 18 week programs. *International Journal of Sports Medicine* 10: 450-454.
17. Capen, E.K. 1950. The effect of systemic weight training on power, strength and endurance. *Research Quarterly* 21: 83-89.
18. Carpenter, D., and B. Nelson. 1999. Low back strengthening for health, rehabilitation, and injury prevention. *Medicine and Science in Sports and Exercise* 31: 18-24.
19. Cooper, K.H. 1968. *Aerobics*. New York: Evans.
20. Cureton, T. 1945. Physical fitness: A no. 1 health problem. *Hygeia* 23: 186-187, 224.
21. Cureton, T. 1969. *The physiological effects of exercise programs upon adults*, 3-18. Springfield, IL: Charles C Thomas.
22. DeLorme, T. 1945. Restoration of muscle power by heavy resistance exercise. *Journal of Bone and Joint Surgery* 27: 645-667.

23. DeLorme, T., and A. Watkins. 1948. Technics of progressive resistance exercise. *Archives of Physical Medicine* 29: 263-273.

24. DeMichele, P.D., M.L. Pollock, J.E. Graves, D.N. Foster, D. Carpenter, L. Garzarella, W. Brechue, and M. Fulton. 1997. Effect of training frequency on the development of iso-metric torso rotation strength. *Archives of Physical Medicine and Rehabilitation* 28: 64-69.

25. Dishman, R.K. 1994. Prescribing exercise intensity for healthy adults using perceived exertion. *Medicine and Science in Sports and Exercise* 26: 1087-1094.

26. Edstrom, L., and L. Grimby. 1986. Effect of exercise on the motor unit. *Muscle and Nerve* 9: 104-126.

27. Evans, W.J. 1999. Effect of exercise on body composition and functional capacity of the elderly. *Medicine and Science in Sports and Exercise* 31: 12-17.

28. Faigenbaum, A.D., G.S. Skrinar, W.F. Cesare, W.J. Kraemer, and H.E. Thomas. 1990. Physiologic and symptomatic responses of cardiac patient to resistance exercise. *Archives of Physical Medicine and Rehabilitation* 71: 395-398.

29. Feigenbaum, M.S., and M.L. Pollock. 1999. Prescription of resistance training for health and disease. *Medicine and Science in Sports and Exercise* 31 (1): 38-45.

30. Fiatarone, M.A., E.C. Marks, D. Ryan, C.N. Meredith, L.A. Lipsitz, and W.J. Evans. 1990. High intensity strength training in nonagenarians. *Journal of the American Medical Association* 2630: 3029-3034.

31. Fiatarone, M.A., E.F. O'Neill, N.D. Ryan, M. Clements, G.R. Solares, M.E. Roberts, S.B. Kehayias, J.J. Lipsitz, and W.J. Evans. 1994. Exercise training and nutritional supplementation for physical frailty in very elderly people. *New England Journal of Medicine* 330: 1769-1775.

32. Fleck, S.J., and W.J. Kraemer. 1997. *Designing resistance training programs.* 2d ed., 1-115. Champaign, IL: Human Kinetics.

33. Fletcher, G.F., G. Balady, V.F. Froelicher, H. Hartley, W.L. Haskell, and M.L. Pollock. 1995. Exercise Standards: A statement for healthcare professionals from the American Heart Association. *Circulation* 91: 580-615.

34. Fox, S.M., and J.S. Skinner. 1964. Physical activity and cardiovascular health. *American Journal of Cardiology* 14: 731-746.

35. Gillam, G.M. 1981. Effects of frequency of weight training on muscle strength enhancement. *Journal of Sports Medicine* 21: 432-436.

36. Golding, L.A., C.R. Myers, and W.E. Sinning. 1973. *Y's way to fitness: The complete guide to fitness testing and instruction,* 67-96. Champaign, IL: Human Kinetics.

37. Graves, J.E., M.L. Pollock, S.H. Leggett, R.W. Braith, D.M. Carpenter, and L.E. Bishop. 1988. Effect of reduced training frequency on muscular strength. *International Journal of Sports Medicine* 9: 316-319.

38. Graves, J.E., M.L. Pollock, A.E. Jones, A.B. Colvin, and S.H. Leggett. 1989. Specificity of limited range of motion variable resistance training. *Medicine and Science in Sports and Exercise* 21: 84-89.

39. Graves, J.E., M.L. Pollock, D.N. Foster, S.H. Leggett, D.M. Carpenter, R. Vuoso, and A. Jones. 1990. Effect of training frequency and specificity on isometric lumbar extension strength. *Spine* 15: 504-509.

40. Graves, J.E., B.L. Holmes, S.H. Leggett, D.M. Carpenter, and M.L. Pollock. 1991. Single versus multiple set dynamic and isometric lumbar extension strength training. In *Proceedings (book III): World Confederation for Physical Therapy 11th International Congress,* 1340-1342. London.

41. Haas, C.J., L. Garzarella, D. Dehoyas, and M.L. Pollock. 2000. Single versus multiple sets and long-term recreational weightlifters. *Medicine and Science in Sports and Exercise* 32 (1): 235-242.

42. Hakkinen, K. 1985. Factors influencing trainability of muscular strength during short term and prolonged training. *National Strength and Conditioning Association Journal* 7: 32-34.

43. Henderson, J.M. 1970. The effect of weight load and repetitions, frequency of exercise, and knowledge of theoretical principles of weight training on changes in muscular strength. Unpublished doctoral dissertation, North Texas State University.

44. Hettinger, R. 1961. *Physiology of strength*, 18-40. Springfield, IL: Charles C Thomas.

45. Holloszy, J.O. 1995. Sarcopenia: Muscle atrophy in old age. *Journal of Gerontology* 50A: 1-161.

46. Hunter, G.R. 1985. Changes in body composition, body build, and performance associated with different weight training frequencies in males and females. *National Strength and Conditioning Association Journal* 7: 26-28.

47. Jones, D.A., D.A. Newman, M. Round, and S.E.L. Tolfree. 1986. Experimental human muscle damage: Morphological changes in relation to other indices of damage. *Journal of Physiology (London)* 375: 435-438.

48. Kannel, W.B. 1970. Physical exercise and lethal atherosclerotic disease. *New England Journal of Medicine* 282: 1153-1154.

49. Lampman, R.M. 1987. Evaluating and prescribing exercise for elderly patients. *Geriatrics* 42: 63-73.

50. Leggett, S.H., J.E. Graves, M.L. Pollock, M. Shank, D.M. Carpenter, B. Holmes, and M. Fulton. 1991. Quantitative assessment and training of isometric cervical extension strength. *American Journal of Sports Medicine* 19: 653-659.

51. Lewis, S.F., W.F. Taylor, R.M. Graham, W.A. Pettinger, J.E. Shutte, and C.G. Blomqvist. 1983. Cardiovascular responses to exercise as functions of absolute and relative work load. *Journal of Applied Physiology* 54: 1314-1323.

52. MacDougall, J.D., G.R. Ward, D.G. Sale, and J.R. Sutton. 1977. Biochemical adaptation of human skeletal muscle to heavy resistance training and immobilization. *Journal of Applied Physiology* 43: 700-703.

53. MacDougall, J.D., D. Tuxen, D.G. Sale, J.R. Moroz, and J.R. Sutton. 1985. Arterial blood pressure response to heavy resistance training. *Journal of Applied Physiology* 58: 785-790.

54. MacQueen, I.J. 1954. Recent advances in the technique of progressive resistance exercise. *British Medical Journal* 11: 1193-1198.

55. McCartney, N., A.L. Hicks, J. Martin, and C.E. Webber. 1995. Long-term resistance training in elderly: Effects of dynamic strength, exercise capacity, muscle, and bone. *Journal of Gerontology* 50A: B97-B104.

56. McCartney, N. 1999. Acute responses to resistance training and safety. *Medicine and Science in Sports and Exercise* 31: 31-37.

57. McSwegan, P., C. Pemberton, C. Petray, and S. Going. 1989. *Physical best: The AAHPERD guide to physical fitness education and assessment*, 20-24. Reston, VA: American Alliance for Health, Physical Education, Recreation and Dance.

58. Messier, S.P., and M.E. Dill. 1985. Alterations in strength and maximal oxygen uptake consequent to Nautilus circuit weight training. *Research Quarterly for Exercise and Sport* 56: 345-351.

59. Mueller, E.A., and W. Rohmert. 1963. Die Geschwindigkeit der Muskelkraft zunahme Bein isometrischen Training. *Internationale Zeitschrift für Angewandte Physiologie* 19: 403-419.

60. O'Shea, P. 1966. Effects of selected weight-training programs on the development of strength and muscle hypertrophy. *Research Quarterly* 37: 95-102.

61. Paffenbarger, R.S., and W.E. Hale. 1975. Work activity and coronary heart mortality. *New England Journal of Medicine* 292: 545-550.

62. Pollock, M. 1988. Prescribing exercise for fitness and adherence. In *Exercise Adherence: Its Impact on Public Health*, edited by R. Dishman, 259-282. Champaign, IL: Human Kinetics.

63. Pollock, M.L., S.H. Leggett, J.E. Graves, A. Jones, M. Fulton, and J. Ciruili. 1989. Effect of resistance training on lumbar extension strength. *American Journal of Sports Medicine* 17: 624-629.

64. Pollock, M.L., J.F. Carroll, J.E. Graves, S.H. Leggett, R.W. Braith, M. Limacher, and J.M. Hagberg. 1991. Physical fitness and performance: Injuries and adherence to walk/jog and resistance training programs in the elderly. *Medicine and Science in Sports and Exercise* 23: 1194-1200.

65. Pollock, M.L., J.E. Graves, M.M. Bamman, S.H. Leggett, D.M. Carpenter, C. Carr, J. Cirulli, J. Matkozich, and M. Fulton. 1993. Frequency and volume of resistance training: Effect of cervical extension strength. *Archives of Physical Medicine and Rehabilitation* 74: 1080-1086.

66. Pollock, M.L., J.E. Graves, D.L. Swart, and D.T. Lowenthal. 1994. Exercise training and prescription for the elderly. *Southern Medical Journal* 87: S88-S95.

67. Sale, D.G. 1987. Influence of exercise and training on motor unit activation. In *Exercise and Sport Sciences Reviews,* edited by D.B. Pandolf, 95-152. New York: Macmillan.

68. Silvester, L.J., C. Stiggins, C. McGown, and G.R. Bryce. 1984. The effect of variable resistance and free weight training programs on strength and vertical jump. *National Strength and Conditioning Association* 5: 30-33.

69. Starkey, D.B., M.L. Pollock, Y. Ishida, M.A. Welsch, W.F. Brechue, J.E. Graves, and M.S. Feigenbaum. 1996. Effect of resistance training volume on strength and muscle thickness. *Medicine and Science in Sports and Exercise* 28: 1311-1320.

70. Stone, M.H., S.S. Plisk, M.E. Stone, B.K. Schilling, H.S. O'Bryant, and K.C. Pierce. 1998. Athletic performance development: Volume load—1 set vs. multiple sets, training velocity and training variation. *National Strength and Conditioning Association Journal* 20: 22-31.

71. Stowers, T., J. McMillan, D. Scala, V. Davis, D. Wilson, and M. Stone. 1983. The short-term effects of three different strength-power training methods. *National Strength and Conditioning Association Journal* 5: 24-27.

72. U.S. Department of Health and Human Services. 1996. *Physical activity and health: A report of the surgeon general,* 22-29. Atlanta, GA: U.S. Department of Health and Human Services, Centers for Disease Control and Prevention, National Center for Chronic Disease Prevention and Health Promotion.

73. Westcott, W. 1986. 4 key factors in building a strength program. *Scholastic Coach* 55: 104-105, 123.

74. Westcott, W.L., K. Greenberger, and D. Milinus. 1989. Strength-training research: Sets and repetitions. *Scholastic Coach* 58: 98, 100.

75. Withers, R.T. 1970. Effect of varied weight-training loads on the strength of university freshman. *Research Quarterly* 41: 110-114.

76. Zinovieff, A.N. 1951. Heavy-resistance exercise: The Oxford techniques. *British Journal of Physical Medicine* 14: 129-132.

3
CHAPTER

Metabolic, Cardiovascular, Pulmonary, and Endocrine Responses and Adaptation to Resistance Exercise

James B. Brown, MS
William F. Brechue, PhD
Indiana University

Energy homeostasis in a cell or the whole body is based on the relationship that energy supply equals energy demand. Muscle contraction(s) impose an increased energy demand that requires an up-regulation of energy metabolism to provide ATP (adenosine triphosphate) and restore energy homeostasis at the new energy demand. Metabolic up-regulation requires an increased delivery of nutrients and oxygen to the working muscle cell and removal of carbon dioxide and waste from it. Responses by the cardiovascular, pulmonary, and endocrine systems provide the needed substrate and waste removal, allowing the cell to meet the metabolic demand. The purpose of this chapter is to examine the acute and adaptive responses of the systems constituting the metabolic response to resistance exercise. This chapter is divided into four sections: metabolic, cardiovascular, pulmonary, and endocrine response to resistance exercise. Within each section, the response of that system to acute resistance exercise is covered, followed by the adaptive response to resistance exercise, divided into changes in variables at rest and in response to an acute bout of resistance exercise.

Metabolism

During a muscle contraction, the energy (ATP) demand is based on the energy requirement for the various components of the contraction: cross-bridge kinetics (myosin ATPase), calcium handling (Ca^{2+} ATPase), and membrane repolarization (Na^+—K^+ ATPase). ATP demand is directly related to the number of cross-bridge interactions, be it force generation (isometric contractions) or work performance (force generation with changes in muscle length). Thus, the metabolic response is dictated by the overall energetic demands of force production and work.

Metabolic Response to Resistance Exercise

A muscle contraction is inherently nonoxidative (anaerobic); energy for a single contraction is supplied by cellular ATP "stores" and creatine phosphate (CrP). Recovery from a single contraction is aerobic; oxygen uptake ($\dot{V}O_2$) increases in proportion to the ATP and CrP used during the contraction. Single maximum voluntary isometric contractions, 1-RM (one-repetition maximum) contractions, or single submaximal contractions represent a relatively low energy demand that is dependent on the intensity of the contraction and the particular exercise being performed (amount of muscle mass incorporated in the exercise). The contraction is fueled by ATP present at the initiation of contraction and by CrP. There is some breakdown of glycogen and glucose utilization, as ATP production from glycolysis is known to begin from the onset of contraction (14, 50, 91) and is likely involved in meeting single contraction energy demand. Muscle lactate has been shown to accumulate without appearance in the blood unless the contraction lasts longer than approximately 5 s (14, 91). Post-contraction $\dot{V}O_2$ is theoretically proportional to the ATP and CrP used during the contraction. The magnitude of the recovery $\dot{V}O_2$ ranges from a peak of two to four times the pre-exercise level, with a duration of 5-10 min depending on the intensity of the contraction and the amount of muscle mass involved (unpublished observations). The purpose and dynamics of recovery $\dot{V}O_2$ are discussed in the following paragraphs.

Energy Demand

With multiple muscle contractions, the metabolic strategy remains the same: recovery must follow each contraction. The problem here is providing recovery ATP so that the next contraction can be performed. That is, recovery must take place during the contractions. It is this signal that drives the metabolic rate to increase ATP production during the contractions. If the supply of ATP is unable to meet demand, the ability to produce force is reduced (fatigue) or additional motor units must be recruited to meet the expected force/work. The latter is of diminishing return if ATP production cannot be incremented. Thus, the recovery process during the bout is the metabolic response to exercise: the elevation of glycolytic and oxidative metabolism during the bout.

The typical set of resistance exercise would incorporate 2-12 repetitions and would be completed in less than 2 min. $\dot{V}O_2$ mechanisms are slow, as oxidative phosphorylation takes time to become fully active, thus, there is a gradual incrementing of $\dot{V}O_2$ as work continues over time. $\dot{V}O_2$ increases to twice rest values during the completion of a single set of resistance exercise (bench press, squat, curl, and press; 68). If the contractions (exercise) cease before full activation of oxidative metabolism, then $\dot{V}O_2$ will rise during the postexercise period (see "Metabolic Recovery," p. 36). On cessation of the single set, $\dot{V}O_2$ continues to rise to levels that are four to five times rest values after the completion of a brief isometric contraction or an 8-repetition set of exercise (68). Thus, ATP production must proceed during the contractions independent of oxygen and oxidative phosphorylation, and the majority of ATP supplied during the contractions must come from CrP and glycolysis (glycogen to lactic acid). Creatine phosphate declines during this phase to provide ATP, but would soon be depleted if ATP were not provided by glycolysis (recovery during contractions) (14, 50, 91). Evidence of glycolytic involvement is seen from small but significant increases in blood lactate concentration (~2 mmol) after a single set (50, 91) and decreased glycogen (108) without a change in blood glucose concentration (34). The energy demand for a single set of resistance exercise is related to the load (intensity), number of repetitions, and the amount of muscle mass incorporated in the exercise (13, 47, 56, 92).

With multiple sets of resistance exercise, the energetic strategy now includes recovery per contraction and recovery per set. In multiple-set programs, $\dot{V}O_2$ increases and remains elevated throughout the workout. The average sustained levels of $\dot{V}O_2$ range from 35 to 55% of treadmill maximal $\dot{V}O_2$ (16, 44, 92, 101), with the highest levels seen between sets (94). The magnitude of the $\dot{V}O_2$ response is determined by the load (intensity), number of sets and reps, and the amount of rest between sets (12, 13, 47, 92). There is a "sawtooth" pattern to the $\dot{V}O_2$ response to resistance exercise; longer rest periods between sets (>3 min) will result in greater oscillations in $\dot{V}O_2$ (112) and more recovery during the rest period, while shorter rest periods (15-60 s) will have a $\dot{V}O_2$ response that looks more like continuous work (102, 109). These patterns may explain the effect, or lack thereof, of resistance exercise on $\dot{V}O_2$max (discussed in "Metabolic Adaptations to Resistance Exercise," p. 37). The energy supply during each set is still provided primarily by oxygen-independent metabolism as blood lactate levels continue to rise (108). Multiple-set work bouts elicit blood lactate concentrations between 5 and 30 mmol, which, like $\dot{V}O_2$, are ultimately determined by amount of work performed (load, number of sets and repetitions) and the duration of the rest period (34, 52, 71, 92, 108). Longer rest periods (2-5 min) are associated with lower blood lactate levels as more lactate is oxidized between sets (52). The progressive increment in lactate is associated with a progressive decline in muscle glycogen and increases in blood glucose (71, 108, 114).

Mobilization of free fatty acids during multiple sets of resistance reflects the increasing energy demands and aerobic nature of the exercise and recovery from exercise (71). This reflects the increased drive for oxidative metabolism during the work in an attempt to recover after each individual set of exercise. Low volumes of resistance exercise or multiple sets with longer rest periods fail to show this fat mobilization response (34, 114).

Metabolic Recovery

Recovery after a contraction or multiple contractions is proportional to the energy requirement to do the work and how much was provided through aerobic metabolism during the work. This metabolic recovery is typically equivalent to the amount of depletion of ATP and CrP and utilized oxygen stores (e.g., myoglobin), plus a little extra to support the energy demands of recovery (elevated postexercise heart rate and breathing frequency, etc.). When resistance exercise ceases, there is a steep decrease in energy demand; however, $\dot{V}O_2$ decreases exponentially to pre-exercise levels. This appears to be the case for single-bout resistance exercise, where $\dot{V}O_2$ increases in the first minute postexercise, but declines to near rest values by 4 min (68). Multiple-set resistance exercise results in a significant elevation in postexercise uptake compared to rest values, which may remain elevated for up to 24 h (32, 82). Further, when performing resistance and endurance-type exercises (50% $\dot{V}O_2$max for 1 h) with the same total caloric expenditure, the postexercise oxygen consumption following exercise is similarly elevated above rest for at least 14 h (32). However, resistance exercise results in a significantly higher uptake at ~1 h postexercise. It is clear that the postexercise $\dot{V}O_2$ is significantly greater in magnitude and duration than predicted for metabolic recovery.

Aside from metabolic recovery, there are several factors that are known to drive mitochondrial respiration, and are likely mediators of the uncoupling of postexercise $\dot{V}O_2$ from metabolic recovery, and of the development of the significant excess postexercise oxygen consumption (EPOC) associated with resistance exercise.

The factors involved in setting EPOC have been reviewed (26). Temperature (heat from work or futile substrate cycling), catecholamines, and cortisol are indirect mediators of EPOC. Each is known to increase within a bout of resistance exercise. Administration of beta-blockers after a bout of resistance exercise significantly attenuates the magnitude and duration of EPOC, accelerating the return to pre-exercise levels (82). The high levels of fat metabolism following resistance exercise (34, 71) may also play a role in EPOC by somehow uncoupling oxidative phosphorylation (as reviewed by 26). Oxidation of lactate during recovery appears to serve as a substrate (carbon) source rather than playing any role in driving metabolic rate (26).

The magnitude of EPOC following endurance-type exercise appears to be related to the duration and intensity of the exercise performed (e.g., 3, 33). This apparently holds true for resistance exercise as well. The greater the intensity and duration of activity, the greater the perturbation of facultative stimulators of metabolic rate during and following the resistance exercise.

In summary, the energy demand for a single contraction is dependent on the intensity of the contraction and the muscle mass involved (e.g., dead lift versus bench press). The total energy demand for a single set of resistance exercise is dependent on the load (intensity), the number of repetitions performed, and the amount of muscle mass used. In multiple-set workouts, the energy demand will be determined by the single-set characteristics, as well as the number and combination of sets and the duration of the rest interval. The magnitude and duration of EPOC is related to the intensity and duration of the exercise, similar to that seen with endurance-type exercise.

Metabolic Adaptations to Resistance Exercise

Quite simply, the metabolic responses to an acute bout of resistance exercise are increased in resistance-trained individuals, as they are capable of performing more work and creating greater energetic demands (59). Thus, greater exercise $\dot{V}O_2$, depletion of CrP, lactate levels (muscle and blood), and EPOC are observed.

Changes in $\dot{V}O_2$max following resistance training are related to the intensity of the training and the duration of the rest period between sets. When the rest intervals are short (<30 s), as in circuit weight training protocols, post-training increases in $\dot{V}O_2$max average about 10% (as reviewed by 28, 49). The magnitude of change is small compared to that observed with endurance-type exercise training, but significant when considering that the energetic demands of resistance exercise (~50% of treadmill $\dot{V}O_2$max) are below the threshold for inducing changes in $\dot{V}O_2$max. Bodybuilders have a higher $\dot{V}O_2$max than untrained individuals, and typically train with high volume (high number of sets with 8-12 repetition range) and relatively short rest intervals. $\dot{V}O_2$max does not change in response to heavy resistance exercise training that promotes large strength gains—for example, powerlifting or Olympic-style weightlifting—and involves relatively longer rest periods.

The effects of resistance exercise on aerobic capacity are reflected in the morphologic and biochemical changes in skeletal muscle (46, 64, 93, 107, 110-113). In general, various muscle fiber characteristics are altered by resistance exercise training, but the findings are not consistent. This is undoubtedly related to the wide variation in training strategies and training experience of the individuals studied. In general, heavy resistance exercise training reduces the relative oxidative capacity of skeletal muscle. Mitochondrial density is reduced (64), and oxidative enzyme activity (citrate synthase, succinate dehydrogenase, 3-hydroxyacyl-CoA-dehydrogenase) are unaltered or reduced in powerlifters and Olympic-style weightlifters compared to untrained individuals (46, 112). Additionally, muscle hypertrophy in powerlifters or Olympic-style weightlifters leads to a reduction in capillary density, despite unaltered capillary per fiber ratios (107). These changes support the lack of response in $\dot{V}O_2$max in powerlifters or Olympic-style weightlifters. In addition, heavy resistance exercise does not appear to alter phosphofructokinase or lactate dehydrogenase activity. Bodybuilder-style weightlifters have slightly higher citrate synthase activity in slow-twitch muscle (110) than untrained individuals and similar capillary density (107). Despite the extreme muscle enlargement, bodybuilders maintain capillary density by inducement of new capillary growth (93). These changes appear to support the noted elevation in $\dot{V}O_2$max compared to untrained individuals.

Creatine phosphate (62, 63) and glycogen (62, 108) concentrations appear to increase in resting muscle, indicating a greater energy storage, although this response is not consistent (109). Resting blood glucose is unaltered (34), but blood free-fatty acid levels appear to be increased (52, 91).

The Cardiovascular System

The cardiovascular system responds to increased metabolic demand during exercise by increasing blood flow. This function supports metabolism by delivering oxygen and nutrients to the working muscle cell and removing carbon dioxide and waste.

Cardiovascular Response to Resistance Exercise

Blood flow through the cardiovascular system can be represented by a simplification of Poiseuille's law (100):

$$F \text{ (flow)} = \Delta P \text{ (driving pressure)}/R \text{ (resistance to flow)}$$

For blood flow to occur, a driving pressure (ΔP) sufficient to overcome systemic resistance to flow (R) must be attained. In the closed cardiovascular system where blood flow to and from the heart must be equal, flow may be represented by cardiac output (Q) and driving pressure by mean arterial pressure (MAP). MAP is a function of systolic and diastolic pressure, and thus changes in MAP may be inferred from changes in systolic and diastolic pressure. Although Poiseuille's law describes flow in a cylindrical tube, it may be generalized to estimate vascular resistance to flow (R) in the intact cardiovascular system. This resistance to flow is referred to as total peripheral resistance (TPR). Thus, the equation may be rewritten as

$$\text{Cardiac output (Q)} = \text{MAP}/\text{TPR}$$

and rearranged as:

$$\text{MAP} = Q \times \text{TPR}$$

This arrangement of the equation illustrates the direct proportional relationship of MAP to both Q and systemic resistance to flow, TPR. Thus, although a pressure gradient is required for flow to occur, changes in MAP during exercise are more a response to changes in the cardiovascular system, mediated by alterations in Q or TPR.

Cardiac Output

Cardiac output increases during resistance exercise (5, 76, 106). Cardiac output is determined by the product of heart rate and stroke volume. Heart rate is determined intrinsically by an autorhythmic rate of firing of pacemaker cells in the heart (~80 b/min). Resting heart rate is typically less than 80 b/min due to extrinsic parasympathetic influence, termed vagal tone. Heart rate increases significantly with resistance exercise (e.g., 44, 68, 102). Typical values range between 70 and 80% of treadmill maximum heart rate. Increases in heart rate with activity are primarily achieved by modulation of extrinsic influences on the heart. At the onset of exercise, vagal release (decreased acetylcholine stimulation) decreases K^+ conductance and increases pacemaker cell membrane potential slope, allowing the predominance of intrinsic pacing mechanisms. Sympathetic stimulation by norepinephrine, neural and hormonal, activates B_1 receptors in the heart and increases both chronotropic and inotropic properties of the myocardial contraction. Thus, with continuation of exercise, a combination of vagal release and sympathetic stimulation contributes to increases in heart rate. Additionally, centrally mediated modifications from group III and IV afferent neurons originating from contracting muscle impose a pressor reflex that contributes to increasing heart rate (70). Discharge from these fibers is apparently mediated by products of energy metabolism and mechanoreceptors (87).

The heart rate response to resistance exercise is exaggerated compared to endurance-type exercise (16, 44, 65, 68, 102). Heart rate per $\dot{V}O_2$ is significantly greater in resistance exercise. The exaggerated response is attributed to several mechanisms:

1. As will be discussed in the next section, stroke volume does not increase during resistance exercise; thus, increments in cardiac output can be achieved only through increases in heart rate.
2. The catecholamine response is greater in resistance exercise.
3. Use of the Valsalva maneuver will impact heart rate (see "Valsalva Maneuver and the Cardiovascular Response to Resistance Exercise," p. 45).
4. Gripping the bar results in sustained isometric contractions, which add to the pressor reflex drive.

Stroke volume is the volume of blood pumped by the heart in one contraction and equals end-diastolic volume (EDV) minus end-systolic volume (ESV). Stroke volume is influenced by several factors, including preload, afterload, and inotropic state of the myocardium (contractility).

Preload is the volume load placed on the heart as indicated by ventricular EDV, and is dependent on venous return and the factors that influence venous return. The observed phenomenon of increasing volume in this closed system making more blood available to the heart at any given workload (demand) indicates that blood volume is a primary effector of preload. In the nondiseased heart, increasing preload increases stroke volume through the Frank-Starling mechanism: increased ventricular force through ventricular wall stretching and optimized actin-myosin cross-bridge interaction. Increased sympathetic outflow at the onset of exercise leads to reduced venous compliance and shifts blood toward the heart. This acute response is effectively an increased blood volume that increases venous return and stroke volume. This principle is also demonstrated by the low resting heart rates and increased stroke volume of endurance-trained athletes whose blood volume increases as a result of their training.

Most indices of ventricular function are dependent on resistance exercise duty cycle. During sustained isometric contractions, the relaxation phase of the exercise duty cycle is eliminated and ventricular function is affected accordingly. Increases in TPR through vascular compression (see "Total Peripheral Resistance," p. 42) and reductions in diastolic ventricular filling resulting from decreased diastolic ventricular inflow reduce venous return (5, 76, 106). Additionally, echocardiographic studies have demonstrated a reduced posterior ventricular wall thickness and increased left-ventricular ESV (5). Thus, reductions in EDV and increases in ESV result in an exercise stroke volume that is below pre-contraction levels. In one case, initial decreases in stroke volume and ejection fraction were shown to gradually recover to pre-contraction levels late in the exercise bout (106). Improved venous return and preload, and the Frank-Starling mechanism appear responsible. Despite the recovery observed in the latter study, stroke volume is either reduced *or* maintained at pre-contraction level; thus, increases in cardiac output associated with resistance exercise can be achieved only by drastic increases in heart rate (5, 11, 65, 106).

During multiple-repetition resistance exercise, the duty cycle imparts a phasic nature to ventricular performance. Due to the intermittent nature of contractions and muscle pump action during dynamic exercise, venous return and EDV are maintained better than in equivalent isometric efforts. Thus, stroke volume is better maintained throughout exercise. Determinants of stroke volume (EDV, ESV) demonstrate a phase-dependent response to dynamic exercise. Stroke volume shows little or no reduction, compared to pre-exercise levels, during 95% maximum voluntary leg extension efforts to failure (60). This is due primarily to the recovery of EDV and ESV values to near pre-exercise levels at the lockout point and during the eccentric phase of a lift. Despite this, increments in heart rate remain the primary mechanism for increasing cardiac output during resistance exercise (65, 88). Table 3.1 summarizes indices of cardiac performance during isometric and dynamic resistance exercise.

Several other factors are known to affect venous return and myocardial preload. Intrathoracic pressure fluctuations as a result of ventilatory cycle affect venous return by improving the gradient for blood flow back to the heart. On inspiration, intrathoracic pressures decrease below atmospheric pressure such that there is a greater AP toward the heart. During dynamic exercise, vascular compression and relaxation cycles of working skeletal muscle serve as a pump to direct blood toward the heart. Posture plays an important role in determining preload. Exercising in a supine compared to an upright position leads to dramatic increases in venous return due in large part to reduced gravitational effects on blood volume.

Afterload is resistance to blood flow out of the ventricle, and it increases with increases in aortic pressure. This has the effect of limiting stroke volume by decreasing ventricular emptying time and ejection velocity. Afterload is increased during resistance exercise as blood pressure rises. The heart attempts to compensate for increased afterload during resistance exercise by increasing myocardial contractility. Catecholamines are positive inotropic effectors; increased sympathetic outflow and hormonal release associated with resistance exercise increase contractility in an effort to increase stroke volume (34, 57, 71).

However, it is of little quantitative value, because venous return is somewhat limited.

Total Peripheral Resistance

The vascular system can be viewed as a single tube whose diameter is indicative of the periphery's relative state of resistance to flow, TPR. TPR is determined intrinsically by the relative vasomotor tone, which is the summation of vasodilation and vasoconstriction on the entire vascular system. Extrinsically, TPR can be altered by vascular compression.

Local changes in vasomotor tone are responsible for distributing blood flow. At rest, only about 20% of cardiac output is directed toward skeletal muscle (97). During exercise as much as 80% of cardiac output may be directed toward active skeletal muscle. With the onset of exercise, increased sympathetic drive participates in a redistribution of blood flow through both an adrenergic-mediated, general vasoconstriction and increased venous tone. The latter shifts blood to the "arterial side," effectively increasing EDV and stroke volume. In active tissue, auto-regulatory mechanisms and local vasoactive metabolites serve to dilate the vasculature, increasing local blood flow. This process allows the cardiovascular system to match blood flow to metabolic demand locally.

Muscular contraction results in a mechanical compression of vascula-ture. If these compressive forces are great enough, they may overwhelm local vasodilation and impede or even occlude blood flow. Impedance

TABLE 3.1 Comparison of Left-Ventricular Performance in Sustained Isometric vs. Repetitive Shortening Exercise

Index	Isometric contraction	Dynamic exercise		
		Concentric	Lockout	Eccentric
Stroke volume	Initial decrease with some recovery	Little or no decrease	Return to pre-exercise values	Little or no decrease
Eject fraction	Initial decrease with some recovery	Increased	Increased	Increased
MAP	Increased	Increased	Increased	Increased
EDV	Increased	Decreased	Increased	Decreased
ESV	Increased	Decreased	Some increase	Decreased
SBP/ESV	No change	Increased	Increased	Increased

Increased, decreased, and no change are relative to pre-exercise values. MAP = mean arterial pressure; EDV = end-diastolic volume; ESV = end-systolic volume; SBP = systolic blood pressure to blood flow, and therefore effects on TPR and blood pressure, is achieved when a muscle contracts at an intensity as low as 15% of maximum voluntary contraction (MVC), while complete occlusion is possible at 30% of MVC (99). The effect of muscular force generation on TPR is further illustrated in the effects of muscle architecture on vascular compression (99). The greater force-generating capacity of a pennate muscle results in greater intramuscular fluid pressures and compression than observed in fusiform muscle.

Isometric contraction is constant force over time with no relaxation phase; therefore, it applies a constant compressive force to the vasculature. The magnitude of the effect is dependent on the intensity of contraction. During typical resistance exercise (shortening and lengthening contractions), muscular force is altered throughout the range of motion, as is vascular compression. Muscular force is typically greater during the shortening phase, and thus TPR and blood pressure would be higher during the shortening phase. During low-load (low-force) contractions or exercise there is little compression, and TPR is a function of vasomotor tone exclusively. During high-load (high-force) contractions or exercise, compression has maximal effects, overwhelming vasodilation and occluding blood flow during the shortening phase. TPR and blood pressure are dramatically increased. In addition, contraction-relaxation cycles of muscular effort (whether individual contractions are isometric or work performing) generate a contraction duty cycle that dictates the overall compressive force effect on blood flow, TPR, and blood pressure. The longer the contraction phase (longer the compression is present) relative to the relaxation phase, the greater the impact on TPR, blood flow, and blood pressure (8, 86). Employing a longer relaxation phase, relative to the contraction phase, minimizes the overall effect of vascular compression on TPR, total blood flow, and blood pressure (8). However, length of relaxation phase, in most cases, is dictated by the activity and is not easily altered. Thus, TPR, during resistance exercise, is a function of the relative vasomotor tone and the muscle compressive forces and the contraction duty cycle.

The extent of vasodilation during resistance exercise is evidenced by a postexercise blood pressure that is lower than pre-exercise (65). This is explained by local vasodilation that is no longer countered by mechanical compression (65). The net result is a postexercise decline in MAP due to a reduction in TPR in conjunction with decreasing cardiac output. Further, TPR has been shown to be lower than pre-exercise values at the lockout point of a bilateral leg extension (95% MVC) where vascular compression is at its lowest (60). Consequently, systolic blood pressure decreases despite unchanged cardiac output. Thus generalized vasoconstrictor and local vasodilator mechanisms operate similarly in endurance-type exercise and resistance exercise. With endurance-type exercise, TPR is typically reduced (11). However, increases in TPR with resistance exercise are entirely related to vascular compression overriding local vasodilation. Perhaps the single greatest determinant of the blood pressure response to resistance exercise is increased TPR due to vascular compression (11, 60, 65, 66).

Blood Pressure

Both systolic and diastolic blood pressure, and thus MAP, increase abruptly at initiation of an isometric contraction in an intensity-dependent (% MVC) fashion (1, 11, 43, 61, 65, 90, 97). With maintenance of the isometric contraction (>5 s), blood pressure remains elevated. This likely reflects increased cardiac output due to increasing energetic demands and maintenance of muscular compression and increased TPR during the contraction. As the isometric contraction is sustained, systolic and diastolic pressures begin to drift upward (66). With the development of muscular fatigue (reduction in force-generating capacity), "effort" is increased to maintain steady-level isometric force. This increase in relative effort to maintain force output leads to the blood pressure drift (66). The time to onset of this drift is dependent on the amount of relative force (% MVC) generated and the induction of fatigue.

During a single concentric muscle contraction, systolic and diastolic pressure rise and peak rapidly with onset of effort and subsequently decline through the range of motion, returning to pre-contraction levels at or near the end of the contraction (60, 90). In a single muscle contraction with both resisted concentric and eccentric phases (such as observed during traditional weightlifting exercise), arterial systolic and diastolic pressures are modulated in a phase-dependent manner. Pressures rise with concentric effort and decline through the range of motion to the lockout position. Pressures subsequently rise with onset of the eccentric phase and continue to rise until transition from concentric to eccentric movement. In the transition from eccentric phase to concentric phase, pressures again peak abruptly concomitant with the onset of the next concentric phase (60, 65, 90). These pressure peaks are associated with the highest compressive forces in the muscle.

Single bouts (multiple repetitions) of resistance exercise also result in gradual upward drift in arterial pressures such that pressures are significantly higher at the end of the bout compared to the pressures at initiation of the first contraction (65). Depending on the relative effort of the movement, pressure can be extremely high: systolic pressures as high as 480 mmHg and diastolic pressures as high as 350 mmHg during exercise to failure at 95% MVC; mean pressure changes represent a fourfold increase above resting values (65). The dramatic increase in pressure with repetitive contractions, as in the sustained isometric contraction, is likely a function of increased cardiac output in response to increasing energy demands, increased TPR due to compression and the "fatigue-effort" mechanism, and increased drive of the pressor reflex (65).

Thus, the magnitude of the blood pressure response at initiation of a brief isometric contraction, a single concentric contraction, or a single contraction with a concentric and eccentric phase is similar if the contractions involve a comparable muscle mass and force generation (11, 61, 66, 90, 97). Further, it is generally accepted that different types of contraction (concentric vs. eccentric or isometric) produce differing amounts of force. However, most researchers have demonstrated that the relative force production, rather than absolute force production, determines the blood pressure response to resistance exercise (66). In fact, most research has been able to demonstrate a strong linear relationship between the blood pressure response and the relative effort (% MVC). Therefore, the actual extent of the increase in blood pressure appears to be dependent on the relative effort (% MVC) involved and, to a lesser extent, the muscle mass involved.

In summary, during resistance exercise, cardiac output is determined by changes in heart rate, while TPR is determined by vascular compression overriding local vasodilation. The level and impact of vascular compression is related to the intensity of the contraction(s) and the contraction duty cycle. MAP (both systolic and diastolic pressure) increases due to increased cardiac output and TPR.

Pressor Reflex and the Cardiovascular Response to Resistance Exercise. Another mediator of cardiovascular and ventilatory responses to resistance exercise is the pressor reflex. This reflex is responsible for increases in heart rate and blood pressure during muscle contraction. Mediation of the reflex includes a central component originating in the supraspinal areas of the brain as well as a peripheral reflex component originating from mechanoreceptors and metaboreceptors in contracting muscle (70). The central component is generally thought to be related to central activation and motor unit recruitment and perceived effort (94). The afferent arm of the reflex arc is believed to include group III and IV thin fibers. Mechanical and metabolic stimuli from active muscle, such as lactic acid and cyclooxygenase products of arachidonic acid (prostaglandins and thromboxanes), have been shown to induce discharge from these afferents (87). Additional evidence for this peripheral control mechanism comes from studies in diseased populations where increases in vascular resistance alone can result in pressor reflex-mediated increases in heart rate, cardiac output, and blood pressure. This has been demonstrated in heart transplant patients without central input to the heart (42) and in patients with impaired myocardial function (21).

Valsalva Maneuver and the Cardiovascular Response to Resistance Exercise. The Valsalva maneuver involves forceful expiration against a closed glottis and is a normal involuntary action invoked during coughing, vomiting, defecation, or strenuous work. The influences of this maneuver on blood pressure consist of four phases (84). Increases in intrathoracic and intra-abdominal pressures with the onset of physical exertion lead to increases in systolic and diastolic blood pressures (phase I). Venous return is reduced due to increases in right atrial pressure (phase II), which decreases stroke volume. Increased heart rate and peripheral vasoconstriction mediated by the baroreflex follow to maintain blood pressure. With termination of effort (phase III), blood pressure decreases concomitantly with decreases in intrathoracic pressure. Right atrial pressure decreases and venous return increases, causing an "overshoot" of ventricular filling and stroke volume as phase IV begins. The maintenance of peripheral vasoconstriction and an augmented stroke volume result in increased cardiac output and arterial blood pressure. Baroreflex mediated vagal outflow leads to bradycardia to minimize the overshoot.

During heavy resistance exercise (efforts in excess of ~80% MVC), it is common for an individual to perform a Valsalva maneuver. Essentially, phase I is extended and the hypotensive phase II is shortened or eliminated during resistance exercise. As effort moves through the range of motion, the glottis is opened and intrathoracic pressures drop quickly to pre-exercise levels. However, if the glottis is not opened, then venous return and stroke volume will be affected (phase II). The phase I changes in intrathoracic and intra-abdominal pressures with onset of contraction have the biggest effect on the cardiovascular response to resistance exercise. Intrathoracic pressure changes with the Valsalva maneuver are superimposed on the pressure alterations produced by the exercise itself. This results in higher peak systolic and diastolic blood pressures than when there is no Valsalva.

It has been suggested that the extreme blood pressures exhibited during the combination of severe effort and a Valsalva maneuver lead to risk of cardiovascular injury (79). However, there are several suggested benefits to the Valsalva maneuver. Increases in intrathoracic and intra-abdominal pressures may serve to stabilize the torso during lifting. Additionally, some researchers suggest that use of a Valsalva maneuver during heavy resistance exercise may reduce the risk of cerebrovascular damage by equilibration of transmural pressures across cerebral blood vessels (65). Increased diastolic pressure would act to improve perfusion of the myocardium (coronary vessels; 60). Lastly, the greater cardiac output and arterial pressure (perfusion pressure) during phase IV may aid in movement of blood out of the thoracic cavity by overcoming the impedance to flow imposed by mechanical compression (9). Experimental manipulation of perfusion pressure (above levels seen during unperturbed muscle contractions) improves blood flow distribution within working muscle and improves metabolism-perfusion matching (9, 10). Thus, the increased pressure associated with the Valsalva maneuver, as compared to without it, may have a similar effect during resistance exercise.

Plasma Volume Shifts During Resistance Exercise. Endurance-type exercise results in significant decreases in plasma volume (98). The magnitude of these fluid shifts has been shown to be directly proportional to increases in MAP and relative exercise intensity (% VO_2max; 19, 73). Additionally, these plasma volume decreases and associated hormonal responses have been shown to elicit a subsequent 24 h postexercise plasma volume expansion (31). Plasma volume decreases (~13%) when subjects perform a series of resistance exercises at 70-80% 1-RM (16, 17, 53, 54). The volume of plasma lost during resistance exercise increases with intensity of resistance exercise (% 1-RM; 17). As in endurance-type exercise, the decrease in plasma volume is highly correlated with the increase in MAP associated with the resistance exercise. The magnitude of plasma volume shifts and the apparent mechanisms appear comparable to those seen with endurance-type exercise.

Most investigations into the plasma volume shifts associated with resistance exercise have demonstrated a return of plasma volume to preexercise levels within 30 min to 3 h (16, 17, 53, 54). However, plasma volume expansion (20%) was seen when plasma volume was evaluated 24 h after resistance exercise (83). The mechanism behind the volume expansion is likely the same as that seen in endurance-type exercise, but specific data are not available.

Cardiovascular Adaptation to Resistance Exercise

Increases in muscle mass and body size associated with resistance exercise result in a larger demand for cardiac output in order to supply an increased resting metabolic rate. As will be discussed later, these increases in body size are paralleled by proportional increases in resting stroke volume. This larger stroke volume enables the heart to meet demand for cardiac output without increasing heart rate. Indeed, cross-sectional studies of highly trained weightlifters have demonstrated mean resting heart rates ranging from 60 to 75 b/min and electrocardiogram rhythms (R-R intervals) that are not significantly different from those of sedentary individuals (5, 15, 23, 48, 85, 114). Longitudinal studies utilizing less highly trained individuals have demonstrated a trend toward lower (~4-13%) resting heart rates after resistance exercise training (104, 105). Two scenarios may account for this observation. Resistance training in previously untrained individuals may induce an early adaptation similar to that from endurance training. Endurance training results in an increased stroke volume secondary to blood volume expansion. Without a concomitant increase in resting metabolic rate and demand for cardiac output, resting heart rate is lowered (5). However, bradycardia may possibly reflect increased parasympathetic and decreased sympathetic influences on the heart (24). Cross-sectional studies of functional cardiovascular indexes show that absolute resting stroke volume is greater in elite weightlifting athletes compared to control individuals or recreational weightlifters (73). Differences between these groups lie in the elite weightlifters' significantly larger diastolic left-ventricular internal dimension in conjunction with a normal ejection fraction. However, when stroke volume is expressed relative to lean body mass or body surface area, the two groups are similar (24). Thus, it appears that resistance exercise training has minimal if any effect on stroke volume other than increases attributable to increases in body size. This adaptation allows an increase in resting cardiac output to meet increased metabolic demand without increasing heart rate and the rate-pressure product or work of the heart.

Resistance-trained individuals can perform higher-intensity isometric force or work bouts than untrained individuals, which increase energy demand. Consequently, exercise cardiac output must be higher (5). The heart rate response to an acute resistance exercise may be attenuated in resistance-trained individuals compared to untrained individuals. As discussed previously, untrained or endurance-trained individuals experience a reduction of venous return (decreased EDV) and stroke volume (increased ESV) during isometric exercise (5). As a consequence, the change in cardiac output is due entirely to increases in heart rate. However, resistance-trained individuals can defend stroke volume during resistance exercise better than untrained individuals because of increased myocardial contractility resulting in decreased ESVs (5). Accordingly, the higher levels of cardiac output necessary to meet the greater energy demand, secondary to greater forces or more external work, are achieved at lower heart rates.

Blood Pressure

Recently, resistance exercise has been prescribed not only for healthy individuals but for elderly and cardiac patients (2, 7, 29). Previous studies have established that endurance exercise is effective in reducing resting blood pressures in hypertensive individuals (18, 93). However, the effectiveness of resistance exercise for reducing resting blood pressures is still in doubt. When previously untrained males were trained for 16 weeks in a high-intensity resistance exercise program, resting diastolic blood pressure decreased 5 mmHg in the trained group, while the nontraining control group showed no change (47). Eight weeks of unilateral isometric handgrip exercise (4 sets at 30% MVC, 3 times per week) reduced systolic and diastolic blood pressures by 13 and 15 mmHg, respectively, in mildly hypertensive individuals (118). In contrast, resistance exercise training has been shown to have little effect on resting blood pressure in normotensive or mildly hypertensive individuals (4, 6, 28, 30, 96, 115, 116). In a comparison of resistance training modalities in previously untrained elderly individuals, 6 months of training led to decreased blood pressure only in endurance-trained individuals.

While present data appear controversial, a recent meta-analysis suggests that resistance exercise training may ultimately have a beneficial effect on blood pressure, showing 3-4% reductions in resting systolic and diastolic pressure (51). Although the magnitude appears small, it could represent significant reduction in cardiovascular morbidity for individuals suffering from essential hypertension (51). More importantly, however, the inclusive nature of this study firmly establishes that resistance exercise training does not result in increases in resting systolic or diastolic blood pressures.

Although resistance training does not increase resting blood pressure, the blood pressure response during an acute bout of resistance exercise is increased (10.8% and 8.8% for systolic and diastolic pressure, respectively) in resistance-trained individuals compared to untrained individuals. This is primarily due to increased central activation and higher muscular force (89). Increased motor unit activation contributes to a greater central pressor reflex component (75). Additionally, increased strength of respiratory musculature results in increased intrathoracic pressures attained with the Valsalva maneuver. The projection of these two changes onto the cardiovascular system contributes to the overall increase in blood pressure response.

Conversely, the peripheral portion of the pressor response seems to be reduced with resistance exercise training. Without the interference of a Valsalva maneuver, arterial pressures are lower in resistance-trained individuals compared to untrained individuals who lift similar relative loads (23). Thus, resistance exercise training appears to shift the regulation of the pressor reflex from peripheral to central mechanisms. Therefore, with resistance exercise training, greater blood pressures will be seen during exercise as a consequence of greater training loads and increased centrally driven pressor reflex.

Left-Ventricular Morphology

Changes in left-ventricular morphology are a consequence of athletic training and are specific to training mode. Endurance-type exercise training is associated with increases in left-ventricular internal dimensions with a minimum of wall thickening (5, 20). These changes are attributed to increased volume load (preload) on the heart. Although resistance training can alter diastolic function through ventricular remodeling and cardiac hypertrophy, diastolic function is enhanced rather than reduced as in a pathologic case (15, 80). Cross-sectional studies investigating adaptive ventricular morphology in resistance-trained athletes indicate that it follows a different course than with endurance-type exercise. Typically, resistance exercise duty cycling involves an isometric component that induces severe afterload stress on the heart. Accordingly, increases in diastolic posterior wall thickness and diastolic interventricular septal wall thickness occur as a consequence of resistance exercise training (22, 24, 27, 81). However, ventricular wall thickening occurs without significant changes in diastolic left-ventricular dimension, which are generally associated with the volume overloading effect of endurance training. A meta-analysis suggests that absolute and relative values of left-ventricular dimension (systolic or diastolic) are not affected by resistance training (24). In conjunction with increasing thickness in the diastolic posterior wall and interventricular septal wall, resistance exercise training results in absolute increases in left-ventricular mass (22, 24, 27, 81). However, when expressed as a function of lean body mass or body surface area, the differences between training modes are reduced. Indeed, meta-analysis of left-ventricular mass and the thickness of the diastolic posterior wall and diastolic interventricular septal wall indicates that changes in these parameters induced by resistance training are appropriate for the observed increases in body size (24).

The Pulmonary System

There has been little direct work on the ventilatory response to resistance exercise. Ventilation increases during exercise to participate in increased oxygen delivery and carbon dioxide removal. The acute response of ventilation to exercise has been well reviewed (67, 117).

Ventilatory Response to Resistance Exercise

In general, the ventilatory response to exercise occurs in three phases. Ventilation increases rapidly during the initial phase (first 20 s) due to increased central drive (stimuli originating in the cerebral cortex) and afferent nerve traffic from the working muscle. This includes "anticipatory" central drive. During the second, or slow phase, ventilation rises exponentially. Responsiveness of medullary neurons to stimuli is augmented, allowing a greater response to stimuli. Afferent signals from peripheral chemoreceptors are also integrated to ensure maintenance of pulmonary gas exchange parameters. The central drive and peripheral afferent stimulus components of phase I are maintained during phase II. The *final* phase of the response is the steady-state response where central and peripheral sensory feedback modulates ventilation to maintain alveolar gas pressures. The total ventilatory response requires about 3-5 min to reach steady level.

To consider the respiratory response to resistance exercise, it is necessary to consider the duration and intensity of the exercise bout. The duration of a typical set of resistance exercise (2-12 repetitions) is approximately 5-120 s. Therefore, the drive to breathe comes primarily from the first two phases of ventilatory control. In conjunction with cortical stimuli, initial afferent stimulus for increased ventilation comes from the pressor reflex: mechanoreceptor traffic along group III and IV afferent nerve fibers originating in muscle (25). As the exercise bout continues, and the metabolic demand is incremented, additional input from metaboreceptors, located in the active muscle, drives ventilation (25). This level of afferent drive is dependent on and directly proportional to the relative force (% MVC) generated by the muscle (74).

A ventilatory response can be seen with a contraction intensity as low as 15% of MVC (25). Increasing the effort to 30% MVC leads to a proportional increase in ventilation. At only 30% MVC, the ventilatory response is severe enough to elicit a hyperventilation as indicated by reductions in end-tidal partial pressure of carbon dioxide. That is, the drive to breathe is greater than the metabolic demand of the muscle. Resistance exercise performed at 70-80% of 1-RM elicits a moderate ventilatory response (50-60 L/min; 68, 102).

As with endurance-type exercise, initial increases in ventilation in response to resistance exercise are achieved through increases in tidal volume without much change in breathing frequency (25, 68). The predominance of tidal volume and limited change in breathing frequency may have as much to do with enforced duty cycle of lifting weights as the physiological regulation. Given the mechanics of breathing during performance of a lift (exhalation with effort and inhalation with recovery to starting position), it is not surprising that changes in the frequency of breathing would be limited and entrained to the lifting duty cycle. Additionally, breath holding is performed to aid stabilization of the torso during lifting. If the breath hold and lifting effort is intense enough (~80% MVC) to induce a Valsalva maneuver, breathing is necessarily interrupted until the release of the glottis. On release of the glottis, breathing is restored and ventilation increases rapidly, in part due to the ventilatory drive supplied by the Valsalva mechanism.

Ventilatory Adaptation to Resistance Exercise

The ventilatory response to resistance exercise following resistance exercise training has not been investigated, to our knowledge. However, there would likely be no ventilatory adaptations to resistance exercise, as there is none with endurance-type exercise. Changes in resting ventilation following resistance training would likely result from a greater resting metabolic rate secondary to increased muscle mass rather than any change in regulation. Likewise, changes in ventilation during a bout of resistance exercise would likely be due to changes in energy demand of performing greater work post-training.

The pressor reflex has been shown to be blunted after resistance exercise training (23). This may reduce the drive to breathe during a particular bout of exercise and perhaps lessen the hyperventilation seen during resistance efforts (25).

The Endocrine System

The nervous and endocrine systems are the main communication networks in the body responsible for integrating responses to changing environments. They work in concert to formulate this response; many nervous system functions are mediated by hormones. Resistance exercise represents two unique stresses on the body: an acute metabolic stress and a developmental stress based on the structural adaptations that accompany resistance exercise. Thus, integration and regulation of energy metabolism and development of skeletal muscle form the basis of the response of the neuroendocrine system to resistance exercise.

Endocrine Response to Resistance Exercise

In general, the magnitude of the neuroendocrine response to resistance exercise will be based on the amount of work performed as it interacts with load (intensity), muscle mass involved, number of sets and repetitions, and rest period between sets (40, 45, 55-57, 95). However, there are some exceptions (38, 39), which will be noted.

Adrenal hormones respond to stress. Resistance exercise results in elevated levels of serum cortisol, norepinephrine, epinephrine, and dopamine in both males and females (34, 39, 40, 45, 55, 57, 71, 73, 86). Increases in cortisol during resistance exercise appear to reflect the metabolic stress of the exercise. Cortisol and catecholamines are responsible for mobilization of free fatty acids and are glucogenic, supporting glucose metabolism by stimulating gluconeogenesis (amino acids to glucose). Norepinephrine and epinephrine play a role in vascular control and vasomotor tone. Epinephrine stimulates glycogen breakdown and glycolytic flux. Catecholamines also play a role in muscle function through greater central nervous system activation; and although they alter excitation-contraction coupling and increase the rate of force development in skeletal muscle, they do not appear to have direct affects on force production (unpublished observation in isolated skeletal muscle with intact circulation).

Plasma levels of insulin decrease during resistance exercise (34, 71). This response is not unlike that seen during prolonged endurance-type activity and may be related to changes in cell sensitivity to insulin (58). Further, muscle contraction alone has been shown to stimulate GLUT-4 transport of glucose independent of insulin (77).

Several androgenic hormones are known to increase in plasma as a result of resistance exercise. In males, serum levels of both total testosterone and free testosterone increase dramatically with resistance exercise and remain elevated more than 30 min postexercise (30, 36, 39, 45, 57, 58, 95). Little or no testosterone response is elicited in females (34, 45, 56, 57, 72). Serum growth hormone levels increase in both males (36, 56, 57) and females (55) performing heavy resistance exercise, though the magnitude of response is greater in men (55). In addition, the growth hormone response to resistance exercise in males and females appears to be dependent on the exercise protocol utilized (55, 56). Hypertrophy-inducing protocols that typically have a higher energy demand result in significantly higher levels of hGH (human growth hormone) than strength protocols. This may reflect the role of hGH in both tissue development and energy metabolism. The acute effects of hGH include stimulation of glucose uptake and inhibition of lipid metabolism, whereas prolonged elevation of hGH has opposite effects (78).

Many of the growth effects of hGH are mediated through insulin-like growth factors, which have been shown to increase with resistance exercise (55-57). The origin of these changes, while apparently secondary to hGH, are suspicious, as hGH stimulation and release of insulin-like growth factors requires more than 8 h, and these changes were seen within 2 h (55-57).

Endocrine Adaptation to Resistance Exercise

There have been few studies and there are little data regarding adaptations of the endocrine system to resistance exercise. The effects of resistance exercise training on resting hormone levels have been investigated in individuals with ability levels ranging from elite-level competitive lifters to previously untrained recreational lifters. At rest, hGH, catecholamines, insulin, insulin-like growth factors, and cortisol have been shown to be unaltered by resistance training (35, 37, 38, 41, 69). One study shows reduced cortisol levels after resistance exercise training (69). Given the nature by which hormone levels are regulated through feedback mechanisms, by other hormones, release and transport factors, inhibition/potentiation, diurnal variation, changing receptor sensitivity, and so on, it is not surprising that studies show no changes in blood hormone profiles, at rest, after resistance training. However, there is some evidence to suggest that cortisol, when elevated, may be a marker of overtraining (103). Chronic elevations in cortisol would be indicative of pathological stress and reflect a catabolic balance in the body.

Testosterone appears to be the one difference to the trend described above. Early studies showed that testosterone levels did not change with resistance training (35, 37, 38). Transient elevations in serum testosterone were noted only during periods of high-intensity training and seen only in the highest-level athletes. However, several reports show increases in resting testosterone levels after resistance training. Increased resting levels of testosterone and decreased levels of cortisol have been observed in non-elite and previously untrained lifters in response to resistance exercise (36, 41, 56, 101). Further, elevated testosterone levels have been reported following a two-year training period in trained athletes (37). These changes were coincident with increases in lutenizing hormone (LH) and follicle-stimulating hormone (FSH), which are higher brain center stimulators of testosterone production. Thus, with limited data, it appears that training experience and duration of training play a major role in determining the testosterone response to training.

In conclusion, the metabolic, cardiovascular, pulmonary, and endocrine responses to an acute bout of resistance exercise are inherently similar to those observed with endurance-type exercise. Differences in the magnitude and the pattern of responses represent differences in external loading, vascular compression, and contraction duty cycle. Adaptations to resistance exercise are governed by the same set of parameters as in endurance-type exercise: intensity, specificity, and duration/volume of training. However, the adaptations to resistance exercise are quite different from those to endurance-type training given the differences in external loading, vascular compression, and contraction duty cycle used in the training.

References

1. Alexander, T., D.B. Friedman, B.D. Levine, J.A. Pawelczyk, and J.H. Mitchell. 1994. Cardiovascular responses during static exercise. *Circulation* 89: 1643-1647.
2. American Association for Cardiovascular and Pulmonary Rehabilitation. 1995. *Guidelines for cardiac rehabilitation programs*. 2d ed. Champaign, IL: Human Kinetics.
3. Bahr, R., I. Inges, O. Vaage, O. Sejersted, and E.A. Newsholme. 1987. Effect of duration on excess postexercise O_2 consumption. *Journal of Applied Physiology* 62: 485-490.
4. Ballor, D.L., and E.T. Poehlman. 1992. Resting metabolic rate and coronary-artery-disease risk factors in aerobically and resistance-trained women. *American Journal of Clinical Nutrition* 56 (6): 968-974.
5. Ben-Ari, E., R. Gentile, H. Feigenbaum, D. Hess, E.Z. Fisman, A. Pines, Y. Drory, and M. Motro. 1993. Left ventricular dynamics during strenuous isometric exercise in marathon runners, weight lifters and healthy sedentary men: Comparative echocardiographic study. *Cardiology* 82: 75-80.
6. Blumenthal, J.A., W.C. Siegel, and M. Applebaum. 1991. Failure of exercise to reduce blood pressure in patients with mild hypertension. Results of a randomized controlled trial. *Journal of the American Medical Association* 262: 2395-2401.
7. Brechue, W.F., and M.L. Pollock. 1996. Exercise training for coronary artery disease in the elderly. *Clinics in Geriatric Medicine* 12 (1): 207-229.
8. Brechue, W.F., J.K Barclay, D.M. O'Drobinak, and W.N. Stainsby. 1991. Differences between $\dot{V}O_2$maxima of twitch and tetanic contractions are related to blood flow. *Journal of Applied Physiology* 71: 131-135.

9. Brechue, W.F., B.T. Ameredes, G.M. Andrew, and W.N. Stainsby. 1993. Blood flow elevation increases $\dot{V}O_2$ maximum during repetitive tetanic contractions of dog muscle in situ. *Journal of Applied Physiology* 74: 1499-1503.

10. Brechue, W.F., B.T. Ameredes, J.K. Barclay, and W.N. Stainsby. 1995. Blood flow and pressure relationships which determine $\dot{V}O_2$max. *Medicine and Science in Sports and Exercise* 27: 37-42.

11. Brechuza, G.R., M.C. Lenser, P.G. Hanson, and F.J. Nagle. 1982. Comparison of hemodynamic responses to static and dynamic exercise. *Journal of Applied Physiology* 53 (6): 1589-1593.

12. Brown, S.P., J.M. Clemons, Q. He, and S. Liu. 1994. Prediction of the oxygen cost of the deadlift exercise. *Journal of Sport Science* 12: 371-375.

13. Byrd, R., P. Hopkins-Price, J.D. Boatright, and K.A. Kinley. 1988. Prediction of the caloric cost of the bench press. *Journal of Applied Sports Science Research* 2: 7-8.

14. Christensen, E.H., R. Hedman, and B. Saltin. 1960. Intermittent and continuous running. *Acta Physiologica Scandinavica* 50: 269-286.

15. Colan, S.D., S.P. Sanders, D. McPherson, and K.M. Borrow. 1985. Left ventricular diastolic function in elite athletes with physiologic cardiac hypertrophy. *Journal of the American College of Cardiology* 6: 545-549.

16. Collins, M.A., K.J. Cureton, D.W. Hill, and C.A. Ray. 1989. Relation of plasma volume change to intensity of weight lifting. *Medicine and Science in Sports and Exercise* 21 (2): 178-185.

17. Collins, M.A., D.W. Hill, K.J. Cureton, and J.J. DeMello. 1986. Plasma volume change during heavy-resistance weight lifting. *European Journal of Applied Physiology* 55: 44-48.

18. Cononie, C.C., J.E. Graves, M.L. Pollock, M.I. Phillips, C. Sumners, and J.M. Hagberg. 1991. Effect of exercise training on blood pressure in 70-79-yr-old men and women. *Medicine and Science in Sports and Exercise* 23 (4): 505-511.

19. Convertino, V.A., L.C. Keil, E.M. Bernauer, and J.E. Greenleaf. 1981. Plasma volume, osmolality, vasopressin and renin activity during graded exercise in man. *Journal of Applied Physiology* 50 (1): 123-128.

20. Fagard, R., A. Aubert, J. Stassen, E.E. Vanden, L. Vanhees, and A. Amery. 1984. Cardiac structure and function in cyclists and runners. Comparative endocardiographic study. *British Heart Journal* 52: 124-129.

21. Fisher, M.L., D.O. Nutter, W. Jacobs, and R.C. Schlant. 1973. Haemodynamic responses to isometric exercise (handgrip) in patients with heart disease. *British Heart Journal* 35 (4): 422-432.

22. Fisman, E.Z., P. Embon, A. Pines, A. Tenenbaum, Y. Drory, I. Shapira, and M. Motro. 1997. Comparison of left ventricular function using isometric exercise Doppler echocardiography in competitive runners and weightlifters versus sedentary individuals. *American Journal of Cardiology* 79: 355-359.

23. Fleck, S.J., and L.S. Dean. 1987. Resistance-training and experience and the pressor response during resistance exercise. *Journal of Applied Physiology* 63 (1): 116-120.

24. Fleck, S.J. 1988. Cardiovascular adaptations to resistance training. *Medicine and Science in Sports and Exercise* 20 (suppl. 5): S146-S151.

25. Fontana, G.A., T. Pantaleo, F. Bongianni, F. Cresci, R. Manconi, and P. Pueccio. 1993. Respiratory and cardiovascular response to static handgrip exercise in humans. *Journal of Applied Physiology* 75 (6): 2789-2796.

26. Gaesser, G.A., and G.A. Brooks. 1984. Metabolic bases of excess post-exercise oxygen consumption: A review. *Medicine and Science in Sports and Exercise* 16: 29-43.

27. George, K.P., A.M. Batterham, and B. Jones. 1988. Echocardiographic evidence of concentric left ventricular enlargement in female weight lifters. *European Journal of Applied Physiology* 79: 88-92.

28. Gettman, L.R., and M.L. Pollock. 1981. Circuit weight training: A critical review of its physiological benefits. *Physician and Sportsmedicine* 9: 44-60.

29. Ghilarducci, L.E., R.G. Holly, and E.A. Amterdam. 1989. Effects of high resistance training in coronary artery disease. *American Journal of Cardiology* 64 (14): 866-870.
30. Gilders, R.M., E.S. Malicky, J.E. Falkel, R.S. Staron, and G.A. Dudley. 1991. Effect of resistance training on blood pressure in normotensive women. *Clinical Physiology* 11 (4): 307-314.
31. Gillen, C.M., R. Lee, G.W. Mack, C.M. Tomaselli, T. Nishiyasu, and E.R. Nadel. 1991. Plasma volume expansion in humans after a single intense exercise protocol. *Journal of Applied Physiology* 71 (5): 1914-1920.
32. Gillette, C.A, R.C. Bullough, and C.L. Melby. 1994. Postexercise energy expenditure in response to acute aerobic and resistive exercise. *International Journal of Sports Nutrition* 4: 347-360.
33. Gore, C.J. and R.T. Withers. 1990. Effect of exercise intensity and duration on postexercise metabolism. *Journal of Applied Physiology* 68: 2362-2368.
34. Guezennic, L., F. Leger, M. Shoste, M. Aymound, and P. Pesquies. 1986. Hormone and metabolite response to weightlifting training sessions. *International Journal of Sports Medicine* 7: 100-105.
35. Hakkinen, K., A. Pakarinen, M. Alen, H. Kauhanen, and P.V. Komi. 1987. Relationships between training volume, physical performance capacity, and serum hormone concentrations during prolonged training in elite weight lifters. *International Journal of Sports Medicine* 8: 61-65.
36. Hakkinen, K., A. Pakarinen, M. Alen, and P.V. Komi. 1985. Serum hormones during prolonged training of neuromuscular performance. *European Journal of Applied Physiology* 53: 287-293.
37. Hakkinen, K., A. Pakarinen, M. Alen, H. Kauhanen, and P.V. Komi. 1988. Neuromuscular and hormonal adaptations in athletes to strength training in two years. *Journal of Applied Physiology* 65 (6): 2406-2412.
38. Hakkinen, K., L. Keskinen, M. Alen, P.V. Komi, and H. Kauhanen. 1989. Serum hormone concentrations during prolonged training in elite endurance-trained and strength-trained athletes. *European Journal of Applied Physiology* 59: 233-238.
39. Hakkinen, K., and A. Pakarinen. 1991. Serum hormones in male strength athletes during intensive short term strength training. *European Journal of Applied Physiology* 63: 194-199.
40. Hakkinen, K., and A. Pakarinen. 1993. Acute hormonal responses to two different fatiguing heavy-resistance protocols in male athletes. *Journal of Applied Physiology* 74 (2): 882-887.
41. Hakkinen, K., and A. Pakarinen. 1995. Acute hormonal responses to heavy resistance exercise in men and women at different ages. *International Journal of Sports Medicine* 16 (8): 507-513.
42. Haskell, W.L., W.M. Savin, J.S. Schroeder, E.A. Alderman, N.B. Ingles Jr., G.T. Daughters II, and E.B. Stinson. 1981. Cardiovascular responses to handgrip isometric exercise in patients following cardiac transplantation. *Circulation Research* 48 (6, pt. 2): 1156-1161.
43. Haslam, D.R.S., N. McCartney, R.S. McKelvie, and J.D. MacDougall. 1988. Direct measurements of arterial blood pressure during formal weightlifting in cardiac patients. *Journal of Cardiopulmonary Rehabilitation* 8: 213-225.
44. Hempel, L.S., and C.L. Wells. 1985. Cardiorespiratory cost of the Nautilus express circuit. *Physician and Sportsmedicine* 13: 82-97.
45. Hickson, R.C., K. Hidaka, C. Foster, M.T. Falduto, and R.T. Chatterton Jr. 1994. Successive time courses of strength development and steroid hormone responses to heavy-resistance training. *Journal of Applied Physiology* 76: 663-670.
46. Houston, M.E., E.A. Froese, StP. Valeriote, H.J. Green, and D.A. Ranney. 1983. Muscle performance, morphology, and metabolic capacity during strength training and detraining. A one leg model. *European Journal of Applied Physiology* 51: 25-35.
47. Hunter, G., L. Blackman, and L. Dunnam. 1988. Bench press metabolic rate as a function of exercise intensity. *Journal of Applied Sports Science Research* 2: 1-6.

48. Hurley, B.F., D.R. Seals, A.A. Ehsani, L.-J. Cartier, G.P. Dalsky, J.M. Hagberg, and J.O. Holloszy. 1984. Effects of high-intensity strength training on cardiovascular function. *Medicine and Science in Sports and Exercise* 16: 483-488.

49. Hurley, B.F., J.M. Hagberg, A.P. Goldberg, D.R. Seals, A.A. Eshani, R.E. Brennan, and J.O. Holloszy. 1988. Resistive training can reduce coronary risk factors without altering $\dot{V}O_2$max or percent body fat. *Medicine and Science in Sports and Exercise* 20 (2): 150-154.

50. Jacobs, I., P.A. Tesch, O. BarOr, J. Karlsson, and R. Dotan. 1983. Lactate in human skeletal muscles after 10s and 30s of supramaximal exercise. *Journal of Applied Physiology* 55: 365-368.

51. Kelley, G. 1997. Dynamic resistance exercise and resting blood pressure in adults: A meta-analysis. *Journal of Applied Physiology* 82 (5): 1559-1565.

52. Keul, J., G. Haralambie, M. Bruder, and H.J. Gottstein. 1978. The effect of weightlifting exercise on heart rate and metabolism in experienced weightlifters. *Medicine and Science in Sports and Exercise* 10: 13-15.

53. Knowlton, R.G., R.K. Hetzler, L.A. Kaminsky, and J.J. Morrison. 1987. Plasma volume changes and cardiovascular responses associated with weight lifting. *Medicine and Science in Sports and Exercise* 19 (5): 464-468.

54. Kraemer, R.R., J.L. Kilgore, and G.R. Kraemer. 1993. Plasma volume changes in response to resistive exercise. *Journal of Sports Medicine and Physical Fitness* 33: 246-251.

55. Kraemer, W.J., S.J. Fleck, J.E. Dziados, E.A. Harman, L.J. Marchitelli, S.E. Gordon, R. Mello, P.N. Frykman, L.P. Koziris, and N.T. Triplett. 1993. Changes in hormonal concentrations after different heavy-resistance exercise protocols in women. *Journal of Applied Physiology* 75 (2): 594-604.

56. Kraemer, W.J., J.F. Patton, S.E. Gordon, E.A. Harman, M.R. Deschenes, K. Reynolds, R.U. Newton, N.T. Triplett, and J.E. Dziados. 1995. Compatibility of high-intensity strength and endurance training on hormonal and skeletal muscle adaptations. *Journal of Applied Physiology* 78 (3): 976-989.

57. Kraemer, W.J., J.S. Volek, J.A. Bush, M. Putukian, and W.J. Sebastianelli. 1998. Hormonal responses to consecutive days of heavy resistance exercise with or without nutritional supplementation. *Journal of Applied Physiology* 85 (4): 1544-1555.

58. Krotkiewshi, M., and J. Gorski. 1986. Effect of muscular exercise on plasma C-peptide and insulin in obese non-diabetics and diabetics, Type II. *Clinics in Physiology* 6: 499-506.

59. Laritcheva, K.A., N.I. Yalovaya, V.I. Shubin, and K. Smimov. 1978. Study of energy expenditure and protein needs of top weight lifters. In *Nutrition, physical fitness, and health*, edited by J. Parizkva and V.A. Rogozkin. International Series on Sports Sciences, vol. 7, 144-163. Baltimore: University Park Press.

60. Lentini, A.C., R.S. McKelvie, N. McCartney, C.W. Tomlinson, and J.D. MacDougall. 1993. Left ventricular response in healthy young men during heavy-intensity weightlifting exercise. *Journal of Applied Physiology* 75 (6): 2703-2710.

61. Lewis, S.F., P.G. Snell, W.F. Taylor, M. Hamra, R.M. Graham, W.A. Pettinger, and C.G. Blomqvist. 1985. Role of muscle mass and mode of contraction in circulatory response to exercise. *Journal of Applied Physiology* 58 (1): 146-151.

62. MacDougall, J.D., J.R. Ward, D.G. Sale, and J.R. Sutton. 1977. Biochemical adaptation of human skeletal muscle to heavy resistance training and immobilization. *Journal of Applied Physiology* 43: 700-703.

63. MacDougall, J.D., D.G. Sale, G.C.B. Elder, J.R. Sutton, and H. Howald. 1979. Mitochondrial volume and density in human skeletal muscle following heavy resistance exercise training. *Medicine and Science in Sports and Exercise* 11: 164-166.

64. MacDougall, J.D., D.G. Sale, G.C.B. Elder, and J.R. Sutton. 1982. Muscle ultrastructural characteristics of elite powerlifters and bodybuilders. *European Journal of Applied Physiology* 48: 117-126.

65. MacDougall, J.D., D. Tuxen, D.G. Sale, J.R. Moroz, and J.R. Sutton. 1985. Arterial blood pressure response to heavy resistance exercise. *Journal of Applied Physiology* 58 (3): 785-790.

66. MacDougall, J.D., R.S. McKelvie, D.E. Moroz, D.G. Sale, N. McCartney, and F. Buick. 1992. Factors affecting blood pressure during heavy weight lifting and static contractions. *Journal of Applied Physiology* 73 (4): 1590-1597.

67. Mateika J.H., and J. Duffin. 1995. A review of the control of breathing during exercise. *European Journal of Applied Physiology* 71: 1-27.

68. McAardle, W.D., and G.F. Foglia. 1969. Energy cost and cardiorespiratory stress of isometric and weight training exercises. *Journal of Sports Medicine* 9: 23-29.

69. McCall, G.E., W.C. Byrnes, S.J. Fleck, A. Dickinson, and W.J. Kraemer. 1999. Acute and chronic hormonal responses to resistance training designed to promote muscle hypertrophy. *Canadian Journal of Applied Physiology* 24 (1): 96-107.

70. McCloskey, D.I., and J.H. Mitchell. 1972. Reflex cardiovascular and respiratory responses originating in exercising muscle. *Journal of Physiology* 224:173-186.

71. McMillan, J.L., M.H. Stone, J. Sartin, R. Keith, D. Marple, C. Brown, and R.D. Lewis. 1993. 20-hour physiological responses to a single weight-training session. *Journal of Strength and Conditioning Research* 7: 9-21.

72. McMurray, R.G., T.K. Eubank, and A.C. Hackney. 1995. Nocturnal hormonal responses to resistance exercise. *European Journal of Applied Physiology* 72: 121-126.

73. Miles, D.S., M.N. Sawka, R.M. Glaser, and J.S. Petrofsky. 1983. Plasma volume shifts during progressive arm and leg exercise. *Journal of Applied Physiology* 54 (2): 491-495.

74. Mitchell, J.H., F.C. Payne, B. Saltin, and B. Schibye. 1980. The role of muscle mass in the cardiovascular response to static contractions. *Journal of Physiology* 309: 45-54.

75. Mitchell, J.H., M.P. Kayfinan, and G.A. Iwamoto. 1983. The exercise pressor reflex: Its cardiovascular effects, afferent mechanisms, and central pathways. *Annual Reviews of Physiology* 45: 229-242.

76. Mizushige, K., H. Matsuo, S. Nozaki, O.L. Kwan, and A.N. DeMaria. 1996. Differential responses in left ventricular diastolic filling dynamics with isometric handgrip versus isotonic treadmill exertion. *American Heart Journal* 131: 131-137.

77. Mueckler, M. 1990. Family of glucose transported genes: Implication for glucose homeostasis and diabetes. *Diabetes* 39: 6-11.

78. Munck, A., P.M. Guyre, and N.J. Holbrook. 1984. Physiological functions of glucocorticoids in stress and their relation to pharmacological actions. *Endocrine Reviews* 5: 25-44.

79. Narloch, J.A., and M.E. Brandstater. 1995. Influence of breathing technique on arterial blood pressure during heavy weight lifting. *Archives of Physical Medicine and Rehabilitation* 76: 457-462.

80. Pearson, A.C., M. Schiff, E. Mrosek, A.J. Labovitz, and G. Williams. 1986. Left ventricular diastolic function in weight lifters. *American Journal of Cardiology* 58: 1254-1259.

81. Pelliccia, A., A. Spataro, G. Caselli, and B.J. Maron. 1993. Absence of left ventricular wall thickening in athletes engaged in intense power training. *American Journal of Cardiology* 72 (1): 1048-1054.

82. Phillips, M.D., J.S. Skinner, W.F. Brechue, and R. Pourmand. 1998. Acute effect of high-intensity resistance training on resting metabolic rate. *Medicine and Science in Sports and Exercise* 30 (suppl. 5): S57.

83. Ploutz-Snyder, L.L., V.A. Convertino, and G.A. Dudley. 1995. Resistance exercise induced fluid shifts: Change in active muscle size and plasma volume. *American Journal of Physiology* 269 (38): R536-543.

84. Port, C., V. Bamrah, F. Tristani, and J. Smith. 1984. The Valsalva maneuver: Mechanisms and clinical implications. *Heart and Lung* 13: 507-518.

85. Ricci, G., D. Lajoie, R. Petitclerc, F. Pemonnet, R.J. Ferguson, M. Fournier, and A.W. Taylor. 1982. Left ventricular size following endurance, sprint and strength training. *Medicine and Science in Sports and Exercise* 14 (5): 344-347.

86. Robergs, R.A., M.V. Icenogle, T.L. Hudson, and E.R. Greene. 1997. Temporal inhomogeneity in brachial artery blood flow during forearm exercise. *Medicine and Science in Sports and Exercise* 29 (8): 1021-1037.

87. Rotto, D.M., and M.P. Kaufman. 1988. Effect of metabolic products of muscular contraction on discharge of group III and IV afferents. *Journal of Applied Physiology* 64 (4): 2306-2313.

88. Sagiv, M., P. Hanson, E. Goldhammer, D. Ben-Sira, and J. Rudoy. 1988. Left ventricular and hemodynamic responses during upright isometric exercise in normal young and elderly men. *Gerontology* 34: 165-170.

89. Sale, D.G., D.E. Moroz, R.A. McKelvie, J.D. MacDougall, and N. McCartney. 1994. Effect of training on the blood pressure response to weight lifting. *Canadian Journal of Applied Physiology* 19 (1): 60-74.

90. Sale, D.G., D.E. Moroz, R. McKelvie, J.D. MacDougall, and N. McCartney. 1993. Comparison of blood pressure response to isokinetic and weight-lifting exercise. *European Journal of Applied Physiology* 67: 115-120.

91. Saltin, B., and B. Essen. 1971. Muscle glycogen, lactate, ATP, and CP in intermittent exercise. In *Muscle metabolism during exercise*, edited by B. Pernow and B. Saltin, 419-424. New York: Plenum Press.

92. Scala, D., J. McMillan, D. Blessing, R. Rozenek, and M. Stone. 1987. Metabolic cost of a preparatory phase of training in weightlifting: A practical observation. *Journal of Applied Sports Science Research* 1: 48-52.

93. Schantz, P. 1982. Capillary supply in hypertrophied human skeletal muscle. *Acta Physiologica Scandinavica* 114: 635-637.

94. Schibye, B., J. H. Mitchell, F.C. Payne, and B. Saltin. 1981. Blood pressure and heart rate response to static exercise in relation to electromyographic activity and force. *Acta Physiologica Scandinavica* 113 (1): 61-66.

95. Schwab, R., G.O. Johnson, T.J. Housh, J.E. Kinder, and J.P. Weir. 1993. Acute effects of different intensities of weight lifting on serum testosterone. *Medicine and Science in Sports and Exercise* 25 (12): 1381-1385.

96. Schwartz, R.S., and V.A. Hirth. 1995. The effects of endurance and resistance training on blood pressure. *International Journal of Obesity* 19 (suppl. 4): S52-S57.

97. Seals, D.R., R.A. Washburn, P.G. Hanson, P.L. Painter, and F.J. Nagle. 1983. Increased cardiovascular response to static contraction of larger muscle groups. *Journal of Applied Physiology* 54 (2): 434-437.

98. Senay, L.C., Jr., and J.M. Pivarnik. 1985. Fluid shifts during exercise. *Exercise and Sport Sciences Reviews* 13: 335-387.

99. Serjersted, O.M., A.R. Hargens, K.R. Kardel, P. Blom, O. Jensen, and L. Hermansen. 1984. Intramuscular fluid pressure during isometric contraction of human skeletal muscle. *Journal of Applied Physiology* 56 (2): 287-295.

100. Smith, J.J., and S.P. Kampine. 1990. *Circulatory physiology: The essentials*. 3d ed. Baltimore: Williams & Wilkins.

101. Staron, R.S., D.L. Karapondo, W.J. Kraemer, A.C. Fry, S.E. Gordon, S.E. Falkel, F.C. Hagerman, and R. S. Hikida. 1994. Skeletal muscle adaptations during early phase of resistance training in men and women. *Journal of Applied Physiology* 76 (3): 1247-1255.

102. Stone, M.H., T. Ward, D.P Smith, and M. Rush. 1978. Olympic weightlifting: Metabolic consequences of a workout. In *Science in weightlifting*, edited by J. Terauds, 54-67. Del Mar, CA: Academic.

103. Stone, M.H., R. Keith, J.T. Kearny, S.J. Fleck, G.D. Wilson, and N.T. Triplett. 1991. Overtraining: A review of the signs and symptoms of overtraining. *Journal of Applied Sports Science Research* 5: 35-50.

104. Stone, M.H., J.K. Nelson, S. Nader, and S. Carter. 1983. Short-term weight training in young men. *Athletic Training* 18: 69-71.

105. Stone, M.H., G.H. Wilson, D. Blessing, and R. Rozenek. 1983. Cardiovascular responses to short-term Olympic style weight-training in young men. *Canadian Journal of Applied Sports Science* 8: 134-139.

106. Sullivan, J., P. Hanson, P.S. Rajko, and J.D. Folts. 1992. Continuous measurement of left ventricular performance during and after maximal isometric deadlift exercise. *Circulation* 85: 1404-1413.

107. Tesch, P.A., A. Thorsson, and P. Kaiser. 1984. Muscle capillary supply and fiber type characteristics in weight and power lifters. *Journal of Applied Physiology* 56: 35-38.

108. Tesch, P.A., E.B. Colliander, and P. Kaiser. 1986. Muscle metabolism during intense, heavy resistance exercise. *European Journal of Applied Physiology* 45: 363-366.

109. Tesch, P.A. 1987. Acute and long-term metabolic changes consequent to heavy resistance exercise. *Medicine and Science in Sports and Exercise* 26: 67-89.

110. Tesch, P.A., A. Thorsson, and B. Essen-Gustavsson. 1989. Enzyme activities of FT and ST muscle fibers in heavy-resistance trained athletes. *Journal of Applied Physiology* 67: 83-87.

111. Tesch, P.A., A. Thorsson, and E.B. Colliander. 1990. Effects of eccentric and concentric resistance training on skeletal muscle substrates, enzyme activities, and capillary supply. *Acta Physiologica Scandinavica* 140: 575-580.

112. Tesch, P.A., P. Buchanan, and G.A. Dudley. 1990. An approach to counteracting long-term microgravity-induced muscle atrophy. *Physiologist* 33 (suppl.): 77-79.

113. Thorstensson, A., B. Hulten, W. von Dobeln, and J. Karlsson. 1976. Effect of strength training on enzyme activities and fibre characteristics in human skeletal muscle. *Acta Physiologica Scandinavica* 96: 392-398.

114. Van Helder, W.P., M.W. Radomski, and R.C. Goode. 1984. Growth hormone responses during intermittent weightlifting exercise in men. *European Journal of Applied Physiology* 53: 31-34.

115. Van Hoof, R., F. Macor, P. Linjen, J. Stassem, L. Thijs, L. Vanhees, and R. Fagard. 1996. Effect of strength training on blood pressure measured in various conditions in sedentary men. *International Journal of Sports Medicine* 17 (6): 415-422.

116. Verrill, D., E. Shoup, G. McElveen, K. Witt, and D. Bergey. 1992. Resistive exercise training in cardiac patients. *Sports Medicine* 13 (3): 171-193.

117. Wasserman, K., B.J. Whipp, and R. Casaburi. 1986. Ventilatory control during exercise. In *Handbook of physiology, the respiratory system*, vol. 2, edited by A.P. Fishman, N.S. Chemiack, and J.G. Widdicombe, 595-620. Bethesda, MD: American Physiological Society.

118. Wiley, R.L., C.L. Dunn, R.H. Cox, N.A. Hueppchen, and M.S. Scott. 1992. Isometric exercise training lowers resting blood pressure. *Medicine and Science in Sports and Exercise* 24 (7): 749-754.

4

Resistance Training and the Neuromuscular System

Matthew D. Beekley, MS
William F. Brechue, PhD
Indiana University

The purpose of this chapter is to review the basic strategies by which the neuromuscular system controls skeletal muscle activity and adapts to overload (resistance exercise). Initially, we discuss the principles by which the neuromuscular system produces force and performs work. Then we review the adaptive strategies employed by the neuromuscular system to respond to resistance exercise. When applicable, animal studies are included that highlight possible adaptive responses of the human neuromuscular system to resistance training.

Function of Skeletal Muscle: Force Production and Movement Production

The purpose of skeletal muscle is to produce force. If the force produced is greater than the load (or resistance) on the muscle, the muscle will shorten, producing work (the product of force and displacement, or $F \cdot d$). If the work (W) is measured over a particular time period, it is expressed as power: $P = W/t$. Power is also determined by the product of the generated force and the velocity of shortening ($F \cdot d/t$). In this section, we discuss the factors that regulate force generation and velocity of shortening in the neuromuscular system.

Determinants of Force Production

Force generation is ultimately determined by the number of cross bridges formed within the skeletal muscle cell and the duration of activation of these cross bridges. There are a number of neural and structural factors within the neuromuscular system that modulate cross-bridge number and activation.

Force-Length Relationship

Because the number of cross bridges determines force, the overlap of the myofilaments (actin and myosin) is important. There is an ideal sarcomere length (~2.2 μ) at which the myofilaments overlap to produce the most cross bridges, and hence the most force (28). This is commonly designated optimal length (L_O). Isometric force increases linearly with length to L_O. At muscle lengths beyond L_O, force production decreases due to fewer cross bridges formed, as there is less myofilament overlap.

In humans, skeletal muscles are attached to bone(s), and they cross one or more joints where they function to produce force and/or movement. The force rotates about the joint(s). The rotational force produced is referred to as torque and is equal to the product of the force and the perpendicular distance from the line of force to the axis of rotation. Torque can be measured in humans during isometric contractions at various angles of the joint, producing a torque-by-angle relationship. This torque-by-angle relationship is often referred to as a torque curve. Changing the joint angle changes myofilament overlap and torque production. The angle at which the greatest torque is produced represents the optimal angle. Note that this optimal angle represents the optimal muscle length within the particular lever system and not necessarily the L_O of the muscle(s). Further, expression of the optimal angle in vivo typically involves several synergistic muscles (e.g., knee extensors), each with an individual L_O, that produce a "composite" L_O of the system (51). In other words, in vivo torque production depends not only on L_O, but also on the biomechanical arrangement of the bony lever system on which skeletal muscles act.

The shape of the in vivo human torque by joint-angle relationship is approximately the same as an isolated muscle but also depends on the range of motion of the system. Some muscle groups have only an ascending limb (lumbar extensors [29] and cervical extensors [85]) while others have both ascending and descending limbs (e.g., knee extensors, knee flexors, arm flexors [60]). The isometric torque by angle (force-length) relationship does not predict force-generating consequences of muscle that shorten.

Force-Frequency Relationship

Skeletal muscle force generation is incremented by recruiting additional motor units; small motor units are recruited first. To produce more force, larger motor units are recruited (Henneman's size principle; 39). Motor units have a threshold frequency of stimulation for recruitment: small motor units have a lower threshold, while larger motor units have a greater threshold. Thus, additional motor units can be recruited by increasing the frequency of stimulation.

Frequency of stimulation also affects force generation by altering cross-bridge activation. Force generation of a given motor unit increases linearly with increasing frequency of stimulation up to a maximum stimulation frequency (termed *fusion frequency*). Further increases in stimulation frequency do not result in additional force, and may actually decrease force (neuromuscular block). The summation of force is the result of prolonged saturating concentrations of intracellular calcium. Increased frequency of stimulation continually depolarizes the sarcoplasmic reticulum, such that calcium is not re-sequestered, resulting in continual activation of cross bridges. Therefore, frequency of stimulation modulates force generation through an interaction between motor unit recruitment (cross-bridge number) and a right shift in the force-frequency curve (cross-bridge activation).

Contractions of isolated muscles at stimulus frequencies less than fusion frequency result in "choppy" force production, termed *unfused tetanic contractions*. In humans, most voluntary contractions are unfused tetanic contractions (14). However, the actual contraction and movement of muscle are smooth. This is accomplished through asynchronous motor unit recruitment. Typically only a fraction of the total number of motor units available are recruited at once. Motor units are recruited and derecruited throughout a task, resulting in a smooth, controlled contraction or movement. As motor unit recruitment becomes more synchronous, as in very high force contractions, the movements become less refined.

There appears to be an interaction between the force-length and force-frequency relationships in muscle (5, 38, 46, 87, 100). As frequency of stimulation (in isolated muscle) or calcium concentration (in single fibers) is increased during isometric contractions, L_O (and hence peak force production) shifts to shorter sarcomere lengths (87, 100). How this is related to force production in vivo is not understood. Computer modeling suggests that the steepness (i.e., stiffness) of the force-length curve is increased at higher frequencies of stimulation (38). Given that intact skeletal muscle does not generally operate at L_o, but tends to operate on the ascending or descending limbs of the force-length curve, a change in stimulation frequency could substantially increase the predicted in vivo force.

Muscle architecture refers to the arrangement of muscle fibers relative to the axis of force generation. This arrangement is important in determining a muscle's force and shortening velocity capabilities, as it directly affects "fiber packing" density and cross-bridge number (73, 83). The impact of muscle architecture on force-generating capacity is described by the physiologic cross-sectional area (PCSA). The equation for PCSA is given below:

$$\text{PCSA (cm}^2) = \frac{\text{Muscle mass (g)} \times \cosine\ \theta}{\rho\ (g/cm^3) \times \text{Fiber length (cm)}}$$

where ρ = muscle density (commonly taken as 1.06 g/cm^3) and θ = muscle pennation angle. Pennate muscles have fibers oriented at angles to the force-generating axis; the angle of pennation typically varies between 0 and 40°. Muscles with fibers that run parallel to the muscle force-generating axis are termed parallel or fusiform. PCSA is usually considered proportional to maximal tetanic tension of the muscle. This is not true in the strict sense, because myofibrillar density and extracellular volume can vary, especially in aging and disease states (26). Muscle pennation angle plays a role in force production, because a force generated at an angle to the tendon will always be less than that same force at no angle; pennation angle results in less force transmitted along the axis of force production. A pennation angle of 30° results in ~15% reduction in force. However, the loss of force can be overcome by packing more fibers into a given space. Therefore, greater force can actually be generated by pennate muscle because of more cross bridges. The so-called space-saver entity of pennate muscle is to allow large force-generating capacity without a prohibitively large muscle mass.

Neuromuscular Reflexes

Force generation by a skeletal muscle can be modulated extrinsically by several reflexes and related phenomenon.

Renshaw cells are located in the spinal cord in close association with motor neurons. These inhibitory cells transmit inhibitory signals to nearby motor neurons. Stimulation of a motor neuron tends to inhibit surrounding motor neurons, referred to as *recurrent inhibition*. Likely, this allows the motor system to sharpen, or focus its signals and suppress unwanted signal "spillover." Thus, when using several muscles around a joint, the Renshaw cell may prevent all the intended muscles from contracting maximally, limiting force production.

Muscle spindles are connective tissue capsules implanted between muscle fibers, with afferent (via Ia and II nerve fibers) and efferent (via gamma nerve fibers) innervation, and specialized intrafusal fibers. Muscle spindles (intrafusal fibers) monitor muscle fiber length and rate of change of fiber length. Changes in length result in a concentric contraction of the muscle to limit length changes. Spindle reflexes limit force production in a muscle by evoking a contraction in the antagonist muscle, which is being lengthened during movement.

Golgi tendon organs are receptors embedded in tendons and respond to tension rather than length. When loaded, these organs exhibit inhibitory effects on agonist muscles and facilitatory effects on antagonist muscles. This prevents a muscular contraction from generating too much force that could possibly result in injury to the muscle, tendon, or bone.

Crossed-extensor reflexes refer to a phenomenon that is part of the withdrawal reflex. In response to painful stimuli, a limb will withdraw reflexively (typically by activation of a flexor muscle). The crossed-extensor reflex extends the opposite limb concurrently to support the body during withdrawal of the limb receiving noxious stimuli.

In some movements in untrained subjects, it is more difficult to achieve full motor unit activation in bilateral (both limbs acting together) than in unilateral contractions. The force produced in bilateral contractions is less than the sum of the forces produced by unilateral contractions (21, 95). This is termed *bilateral deficit*. The crossed-extensor reflex has been suggested as the mechanism for the bilateral deficit in skeletal muscle force production (65). The reduced force during the bilateral contraction is associated with a reduced motor unit recruitment in the prime movers (45, 109). Although the specific mechanism remains unknown, the deficit appears to be of neural origin. Although the bilateral deficit does not appear in all bilateral movements (21, 95), it does appear in both isometric and rapid ballistic contractions (109).

Co-Contractions

Simultaneous activation and contraction of antagonist muscles occurs in response to agonist muscle stimulation (22, 97). These co-contractions appear to have several purposes, including joint stabilization (6), precision of movement, and as a braking mechanism during rapid, ballistic movements (68, 74). These can be considered protective mechanisms as well (107). Antagonist activation and contraction is known to limit force production in agonists through reductions in motor unit recruitment (107) and motor unit firing rates (31). The mechanism is especially active in novel tasks or movements (82).

Each of these reflexes serves a protective role in vivo. Extreme expressions of force or strength as experienced in resistance exercise and athletics are potentially "dangerous" to the structural integrity of the neuromuscular system. In essence, each of these reflexes acts to limit force generation. Thus, these reflexes are often considered counterproductive when maximal force is desired, such as in athletic competition.

Determinants of Movement Production—Work and Power

When the force generated by a skeletal muscle is greater than the load on the muscle, the muscle shortens. The velocity at which muscle shortens is determined by the rate of cross-bridge turnover. This in turn is determined by myosin ATPase activity, the load on the muscle, and the muscle architecture. Myosin ATPase is responsible for the hydrolysis of ATP during a cross-bridge cycle. The greater the enzyme activity, the faster energy can be harvested for cross-bridge cycling. In skeletal muscle, maximal velocity of shortening is closely related to the level of myosin ATPase activity. This has been shown to be true in isolated muscle (18), and human muscle in vivo (112).

The greater the load on a muscle, the greater the force required before shortening can occur. Hill showed the relationship between force and velocity in isolated animal muscle to be hyperbolic, with higher forces (higher loads) associated with slower velocity of shortening (43). The velocity-force relationship is bound at its extremes by maximal force production without muscle shortening (isometric force) and maximal velocity of shortening without a load (no appreciable force generation) on the muscle. Subsequent research has focused on the nature of the relationship (shape of the curve) and has shown that while the relationship is defensible in both isolated and intact in vivo muscle, the mathematical expression of the relationship is debatable (19).

In vivo torque-velocity relationships in humans do not necessarily follow a hyperbolic pattern. For instance, the knee extensors, knee flexors, plantar flexors, and dorsiflexors all exhibit a plateau or even a depression in tension at slow contractile speeds (86, 112). It has been suggested that this is due to neural inhibition associated with Golgi receptor firing at high force production.

When a muscle shortens, it produces work or power as a function of the force generated and the velocity of shortening. Expressed graphically against force, the power curve is an inverted U with its peak typically ~30% of maximal isometric force. Given the shape of the velocity-force curve, it appears that the optimal conditions for producing power occur when the load on the muscle results in a force production and a velocity of shortening that are about 30% of the respective maximal values (67).

Muscle Architecture
The effect of muscle architecture on velocity of shortening is related to muscle fiber length (or the number of sarcomeres in series). Fiber length

is rarely identical to whole muscle length and can vary in humans by a large amount (<20 mm to >450 mm). Typically, muscle fascicle (bundles of fibers) length measured in vivo is equivalent to muscle fiber length, although the two are not necessarily synonymous (62, 106). Maximal velocity of shortening is proportional to fiber length at a given ATPase activity (89, 115). It has been suggested that muscle architecture is the critical variable for determining maximal velocity of shortening (9, 89, 92). The more sarcomeres in series, the faster the shortening, and the less shortening each sarcomere has to do for a given length change. Fiber length varies with pennation angle: the larger the pennation angle, the shorter the fiber lengths. Pennation angle also affects velocity. Velocity is reduced as a function of the cosine of the pennation angle. Sprinters have greater fascicle lengths and smaller pennation angles in the vastus lateralis and gastrocnemius compared to long-distance runners (1). Further, among sprinters, greater fascicle lengths and smaller pennation angles in vastus lateralis and gastrocnemius muscles are associated with better sprint performance (62). Both are suggestive of greater velocity of shortening.

While muscle fiber length clearly determines maximal velocity of shortening, sarcomeric length (myofilament overlap) plays no role. The number of cross bridges is unrelated to velocity of shortening; speed of shortening is dependent on the maximal cross-bridge cycling rate (17).

Response to Resistance Training: The "Adaptation Strategy"

Invoking adaptations in the neuromuscular system follows three overlapping principles: overload, novelty, and specificity.

Overload

To provide an adaptive response, the neuromuscular system must be exposed to loads beyond those typically encountered in normal activity; this is the basic premise behind the overload principle. The stimuli needed to provoke an adaptive response to resistance training can be provided in several ways: increased intensity, increased duration, or some combination of each. Increased intensity can be provided by increasing the load, changing the order of the exercises done, decreasing the rest time, or some combination of these. Increased duration can be provided by completing additional sets or repetitions, decreasing speed of movement during the resistance exercise, or some combination of the two. Note that once the muscle adapts to the overload, more intense or additional overloads (progression of loading) must be provided to provoke a new adaptation response.

Novelty

The neuromuscular system will adapt to "new" stimuli. Normally, we consider this principle important after an individual trains for an extended period of time. Early on in resistance training, simply adding more weight can be used as a load progression; later on, "wave" sets, pyramid sets, or use of new equipment can represent a novel stimuli independent of overload. New exercises or "new twists" to old exercises (e.g., altered grip) can also provide new stimuli.

Periodization also plays a role in novelty. Periodization refers to the organization of training into distinct time periods. Typically, the aim of each cycle (time period) is to allow the athlete to peak at a critical time (e.g., competition). Variation or novelty is included in the cycle, and can involve alterations in load, exercises used, intensity, volume, and so on. The goals of both periodization and novelty include preventing staleness and overtraining in an athlete and allowing time for recovery. These allow an athlete to make continued gains throughout a training period.

Specificity

Specificity is the physiological adaptation(s) that associates precisely with the type of training performed. The specific pattern of neuromuscular activation required by a particular exercise or training program will stimulate other systems (e.g., endocrine) in such a way as to provoke a particular response or adaptation. It follows that weight training programs designed for a particular purpose (e.g., sport) should employ the types of muscular actions and velocities encountered in that particular purpose. For example, it is known that exercising at a specific velocity increases strength at that velocity, with smaller effects on strength at other velocities (59). Likewise, training at slow velocities with high resistance results primarily in improvements in maximal force and submaximal forces at slow velocities (59). Power performance (using any appreciable speed) improves less with this type of training. Again, desired outcome dictates training mode.

The specificity principle suggests adaptations can be acquired using a variety of training models. The number of sets, repetitions, and intensity is simply determined by the desired outcome. For instance, one set of a particular exercise can build strength and enlarge musculature (cited in 99). Whether one set promotes the optimal or largest amount of strength and muscle growth is not the issue, if the changes are functional. These data suggest that to build functional strength (defined as the strength needed for normal daily activities), time and resources can be saved by having subjects train using one set of a particular exercise. This is not necessarily pertinent to the world-class powerlifter or bodybuilder, but it is pertinent to rehabilitation programs for the frail elderly, or to sports where large increases in strength and muscle mass are of little concern. Thus, it is important to determine the particular goal of the individual: performance, health, fitness, rehabilitation, and so on. Given the plasticity of the neuromuscular system and the large range of adaptability, a variety of context-dependent models can be envisioned.

Application of these three principles results in increased expression of force-generating capacity and/or velocity of shortening by the neuromuscular system. While improved acuity and mental effort can sometimes explain changes in the neuromuscular system, the changes are beyond the scope of this chapter. For our present purposes, neural refers to changes in higher central command centers, the motor neuron, and the neuromuscular junction.

The primary adaptation of resistance exercise is increased force-generating capacity. The expression of this adaptation can take many forms. Changes in force generation are revealed by upward shifts in isometric torque curves (85, 99). Changes in strength can also be represented by changes in the 1-RM (one-repetition maximum) of a particular muscle group (e.g., squats, bench press, knee extension; 59). Improvements in force-generating capacity may also manifest by increments in the expression of power, reflecting changes in either force-generating capacity or velocity of shortening (8).

The most commonly observed training adaptation coincident with increased strength is increased muscle mass. Muscle enlargement can be considered the predominant consequence of a resistance training program. However, changes in strength have been reported in the absence of muscle mass changes (10, 24, 79), reflecting changes in the way the muscle is activated to produce force. Thus, the adaptations and their mechanisms by which force/strength are increased following resistance exercise training can be divided into two distinct, but not mutually exclusive categories: neural changes and structural changes (26, 58, 72). The balance or predominance of neural and structural adaptations to resistance exercise training is determined by the exercise prescription.

Neural Changes

Neural changes refer to neurally mediated alteration in the pattern by which a motor unit or whole muscle is activated or utilized to express muscular force. Increased motor unit recruitment, increased frequency of stimulation, synchronization, desynchronization, blunted reflexes, cross-education, bilateral deficit, and agonist/antagonist interactions represent neural changes.

Increased Motor Unit Recruitment

Increases in force production seen with resistance exercise training originate from increased recruitment of motor units whether training involves isometric contractions (57) or weightlifting (32, 33, 35, 36, 50, 91). These results are represented by increases in integrated electromyographic (IEMG) activity and are interpreted as indicating that resistance-trained individuals more fully activate the muscles responsible for a particular movement during maximal voluntary contractions. However, some studies have shown no change in motor unit recruitment after resistance training. For instance, voluntary and involuntary training (through electrical stimulation) of the right adductor pollicis muscle, 3 days/week for 5 weeks, resulted in an ~15% increase in MVC but no change in motor unit recruitment (via IEMG; 10). Further, isometric resistance training of the knee extensors of one leg, for 8 weeks in 15 female subjects, resulted in an ~28% increase in MVC but no change in motor unit recruitment (via IEMG; 24). Part of the controversy may reflect technical difficulty in repeated application of EMG surface electrodes over prolonged time. The coefficient of variation for repeated EMG measurements has been reported to be ~20% (110). Variability of EMG measurements has been reviewed on several occasions (6, 53).

Frequency of Stimulation

The mechanism responsible for increased motor unit recruitment is an increased rate of firing after resistance exercise training—that is, increased frequency of stimulation. As the firing rate increases, motor units with higher activation frequencies can be recruited, an extension of the Henneman principle. The more motor units recruited, the more force produced. In addition to recruiting more motor units, an increased firing rate following training also shifts the force-frequency curve. Increased stimulation frequencies (30) result in greater force production by a given motor unit through an upward shift of the force-frequency relationship.

Lastly, changes in firing frequency lead to training-specific changes in the activation pattern of motor units. Resistance exercise training results in greater ability for sustained activation of a given motor unit compared to untrained individuals (30). Sustained activation of a given motor unit leads to greater whole muscle force generation. Training-specific alterations in activation patterns not only impact total force development, but also the rate of force development. Heavy resistance weight training increases strength and motor unit recruitment and causes IEMG activity to occur later in the contraction period (35). Motor unit recruitment is increased by greater frequency of stimulation and a shift of the force-frequency curve. Thus, individuals who participate in heavy resistance training are better able to "summate" and produce a greater force. In contrast, "explosive" jump training leads to increased IEMG activity at the onset of the contraction (34, 114), or a faster *onset* of force. These phenomena play an important role in the specificity of training: slow resistance exercise would improve strength but not necessarily speed of movement.

Additional evidence that motor unit activation and excitability increase during voluntary effort is gleaned from evaluation of reflex potentiation. Evoked potentials are facilitated during maximal voluntary contractions compared to rest (108). Cross-sectional studies have shown that trained weightlifters exhibit greater reflex potentiation than untrained controls (78, 95), indicating greater motor unit activation. The effect has also been observed in longitudinal training studies (93, 96).

Greater neural conduction velocity following resistance training may explain faster onset of stimulation during voluntary contraction. Cross-sectional studies have shown that nerve conduction velocity is greater in power-trained athletes compared to endurance-trained athletes (52) and in weightlifters compared to untrained controls (93). However, the origin of the difference and the mechanism(s) by which nerve conduction velocity is altered remain unknown. In summary, changes in motor unit excitability and neural firing rate following resistance exercise training increase force generation through an interaction of increased motor unit recruitment, force-frequency shifts, enhanced motor unit activation, and altered activation patterns.

Increasing the duration of activation allows for greater synchronization of motor unit firing (79). Indeed, weightlifters show greater synchronization of motor unit firing than untrained individuals (78). Synchronization of motor unit firing also plays an important role in rate of force development (77). During a power movement, when motor units need to be recruited at specific time periods (such as jumping; 35), synchronization is critical to maximize power.

Desynchronization may also be an important training-induced adaptation. Following resistance exercise training, fewer motor units are required to complete a given submaximal task. Desynchronization of motor units would allow fewer motor units to perform the same task (using less muscle to lift the same load). Fatigue would be delayed by now having a greater pool of unrecruited motor units to recruit from during sustained efforts (84).

Blunted Reflexes

As discussed earlier, neuromuscular reflexes modulate force production by skeletal muscles. Neural adaptation to training includes changes that minimize reflexes that normally inhibit force production (termed *disinhibition*). One of the major central neural changes may be increased excitatory postsynaptic potentials from higher brain centers (37, 78). These excitatory potentials counterbalance inhibitory postsynaptic potentials from the muscle spindle, Golgi tendon organ, Renshaw cells, and the cross-extensor reflex, which normally inhibit force production.

Additionally, training-induced reflex disinhibition may include a reduction in postsynaptic inhibitory potentials from peripheral reflexes. Cross-sectional data show that the muscle spindle of endurance-trained athletes is more sensitive to mechanical stimuli than that of power-trained athletes (63). In addition, endurance athletes have a faster monosynaptic reflex recovery time (as measured by a mechanical displacement) (64). However, muscles with more slow-twitch fibers have more muscle spindles. Therefore, the differences in reflexes may simply be due to varying fiber types among the athletes, and not to training per se. Heavy resistance training leads to a significant reduction in reflex amplitude of the patellar tendon reflex (a measure of the muscle spindle reflex system; 32). In this case, resistance exercise training decreases the sensitivity of the muscle spindle. Intrafusal fibers of the muscle spindle do not change in diameter in response to resistance training, even when extrafusal fibers hypertrophy (47). Thus, resistance exercise training alters the sensitivity of the spindle system independent of fiber type (32).

It is generally accepted that the Golgi tendon organ adapts to chronic resistance exercise training. This is related to a change in sensitivity of the Golgi tendon organ secondary to loading associated with resistance exercise. Thus, with less inhibitory input from the Golgi tendon organ, the muscle can produce greater force. Although this mechanism is generally accepted, it is unsupported by experimental evidence (47).

The bilateral deficit of force production is reduced following resistance exercise training. Unlike in untrained individuals, bilateral facilitation occurs in individuals who participate in intense bilateral contractions (12, 45). Comparison of unilateral and bilateral knee extension training shows that both types of training increase the ability to develop tension during bilateral knee extensions, but the increase is greater for bilateral training (90).

The effect of the single-leg training on the untrained leg may be explained by cross-education. Resistance training of a single limb results in increased strength in the contralateral limb, although the increase is always less than in the trained limb (21). For instance, 8 weeks of isometric elbow flexor muscle training (67% of MVC, 10 repetitions, 2/day, 3/week) increased strength by 36.4% in the trained arm and by 24.7% in the untrained arm (79). Several studies have investigated whether this effect is due to postural requirements of the untrained limb during training. However, in this situation, independent activation of the untrained limb was not of sufficient intensity to cause a training effect (15, 21, 80). Further, there are no apparent changes in muscle fiber area or enzyme activities of the untrained limb in association with an increased strength (44). Therefore, it is likely that a centrally mediated neural adaptation, perhaps a blunting of Renshaw cell function and/or cross-extensor reflex, is responsible. This suggests that increased motor unit recruitment following resistance exercise training includes greater activation of synergistic muscles (37).

Co-Contractions

Force production in muscle is facilitated by reduced antagonist co-contractions due to resistance exercise training (6). Over time, the acquisition of skills associated with resistance exercise training reduces the contraction of antagonist muscles, while allowing greater activation of the prime movers.

Structural Changes

Increased muscle size (hypertrophy) is perhaps the most widely recognized response to resistance training. Structural changes also include changes in mitochondrial density, glycolytic enzyme concentration, capillary number, and capillary density (49, 103, 104) (see chapter 3). Less recognized are structural changes that occur in the motor neuron and connective tissue.

Neural Morphometry and Morphology

Little is known about the effects of resistance exercise training on motor neuron morphometry and morphology; however, evidence exists that the neuron can alter metabolic enzyme concentration in an adaptive response to endurance exercise (23). Exercise-trained guinea pigs show enhanced protein synthesis (seen as larger nucleoli and darker staining nucleoplasm) in the motor neuron (20). Motor neuron malic dehydrogenase activity and glucose-6-phosphate-dehydrogenase activity increase in endurance-trained rats (25). In the soleus muscle "trained" by removing synergistic muscles, oxidative enzymes of the innervating motor neurons increase in parallel to muscle oxidative enzyme levels (81).

The neuromuscular junction adapts to resistance training. For instance, the enzyme choline acetyltransferase (involved in the resynthesis of acetylcholine) increases in content following removal of synergistic muscles (98); this increase does not occur in endurance training (13). Fatigue resistance and neuronal terminal mitochondrial density have been noted in chronically stimulated crayfish muscle (23). Adaptations of the neuromuscular junction to resistance training help prevent fatigue. The motor neuron and neuromuscular junction appear plastic and show some adaptation to exercise training paradigms, suggesting that each may adapt in an appropriate manner to resistance exercise.

Muscle Structural Changes

The major structural change to resistance exercise training in the neuromuscular system is muscle enlargement (26). Changes occur within the muscle cell in response to resistance training. Muscles are one of the most "plastic" and adaptable tissues in the human body. While much research has concentrated on hypertrophy and hyperplasia, it must be noted that virtually every structural aspect of muscle can change given the proper stimulus. The increase in size can result from increases in fiber cross-sectional area (hypertrophy), increases in fiber number (hyperplasia), increases in fiber (fascicle) length, increases in connective tissue content, or a combination of these factors.

Hypertrophy.   Myofibrillar content increases in response to resistance exercise due to increased contractile protein (7, 26). One mechanism for hypertrophy is Z-disc (located at the end of the sarcomere) "splits" or "streams," resulting in splitting of the myofibril. The "streaming" is in response to mechanical stress that occurs in the center of the Z-disc during loading of the muscle. This longitudinal splitting of the myofibril results in two or more daughter myofibrils (26, 111). The proliferation of myofibrils increases the cross-sectional area of the muscle fiber. Overload results in an increase in myofibrils and hence an increase in cross-bridge number and force production.

Hyperplasia.   Hyperplasia refers to an increase in actual muscle fiber number; that is, more muscle cells are created. This would again lead to more cross bridges and more force produced by the muscle. The evidence that hyperplasia is an adaptive response comes mainly from animal studies. Heavy weightlifting in cats produces an increase in fiber number (27). Quails who had weights suspended from their wings have also shown muscle enlargement via hyperplasia (4). It is generally accepted that muscle fiber number does not change after puberty; muscle fiber number is largely genetically determined (72, as reviewed by 55). Indirect evidence of hyperplasia in humans exists, but is highly controversial. Bodybuilders have more muscle fibers than untrained subjects (71, 102). However, we cannot be sure that bodybuilders didn't have a higher number of muscle fibers to begin with. Hyperplasia is theoretically the result of many years of high-intensity training and extreme muscle enlargement.

Muscle Fiber Length.   Changes in muscle fiber length (sarcomeres in series) response to resistance exercise has not been studied in great detail. In vivo data from untrained humans suggest a large variability in muscle fascicle lengths among certain muscles, and leave uncertainty about genetic predisposition in determining muscle fascicle length (56). Animal studies have documented increased muscle fiber length following stretching (101) and eccentric exercise (downhill running) training (69).

Fiber-length responses in humans to resistance training are equivocal. In cross-sectional studies, similar fascicle lengths were observed in football players compared to other male and female height-matched athletes (1, 2). The football players had significantly greater lean body mass and a much longer weightlifting history. However, additional cross-sectional data show that resistance-trained males with extreme muscle enlargement (e.g., sumo wrestlers and bodybuilders) have longer muscle fascicle lengths than untrained male controls (56). Further, fascicle length of sumo wrestlers is positively and significantly correlated to isolated muscle thickness (cited in 55). This suggests that, unlike in shorter training studies (54, 61), large amounts of muscle enlargement are necessary to elicit changes in fascicle length.

The implications for increasing fascicle or fiber length or cell number (hyperplasia) on force/cross-sectional area are as follows: Increasing muscle fiber size (hypertrophy) leads to an increase in pennation angle if muscle and fiber length are kept constant (75). Although the pennation angle allows for greater sarcomere packing per cross-sectional area, there is a decrease in force/cross-sectional area of muscle when hypertrophy occurs with increased pennation angle. Increasing fascicle or fiber length or hyperplasia of the muscle would limit the change in pennation angle, and thus reduce the decrease in force/cross-sectional area. Increasing fascicle or fiber length would also increase the number of sarcomeres in series and therefore may increase the velocity of shortening (3, 48, 62). The majority of evidence to support these hypotheses comes from the nonphysiological animal models mentioned above; human data, at least for now, remain largely cross-sectional and equivocal.

Changes in Optimal Length. Optimal length of compound muscle groups might also be affected by changes in muscle fiber length (the number of sarcomeres in series). For instance, training at a shortened or lengthened muscle length may result in addition or loss of sarcomeres in series, which would subsequently shift the optimal length (an apparent increase in force) to reflect the training length (51). Furthermore, differently shaped torque-by-angle relationships have been found for runners, cyclists, and controls (41, 42). Runners produce an ascending torque-by-angle relationship, while cyclists produce a descending torque-by-angle relationship; controls display the typical upside-down U shape. Water-skiers show an extremely altered torque-by-angle curve for the lumbar muscles, producing higher torques at shorter muscle lengths (66). These differences may be due to the different types of contractions required by each sport and, secondary, to differences in the number of sarcomeres in series (66, 88). Muscle length and therefore optimal length, may also change without a change in the number of sarcomeres in series. In pennate muscle, hypertrophy per se results in an increase in muscle length (46). This increase in length could offset the necessity of changing the number of sarcomeres in series, and therefore allow hypertrophy or atrophy of the pennate muscle to shift optimal length. This has been demonstrated in a rat model using immobilization of the hindlimb at a short length (40). The soleus (a fusiform muscle) altered its number of sarcomeres in series to reflect the new optimal length, but the gastrocnemius (a pennate muscle) did not change its number of sarcomeres in series: the gastrocnemius atrophied only to reflect the new optimal length. Human data demonstrating this hypothesis are not yet available. In any event, the shape of the torque-by-angle curve appears to be adaptable in vivo, such that L_O (or optimal angle) appears to change.

Connective Tissue. Connective tissue (of which collagen is the major fiber in all types) is generally thought to change proportionately with muscle tissue in response to resistance training (71, 76). Human (70, 71) and animal studies (105) appear to bear out this relationship. Interestingly, bodybuilders in which steroid use had not been ruled out showed decreases in connective tissue content compared to untrained controls (94). In addition, anabolic steroids have been shown to decrease tensile strength of a tendon or ligament in an animal model (113). These results suggest a negative consequence of steroid use in resistance-training athletes that actually counteracts the natural adaptation to resistance exercise.

Time Course of Adaptation to Resistance Training

The accepted model of time course adaptation to resistance training is that of Moritani and deVries (79), and promoted by Sale (95). In this model, nearly all "strength" gained in the early stages (1-3 weeks) is of "neural" origin, and very little hypertrophy takes place until approximately 4 weeks of training and thereafter. At some later point, hypertrophy plateaus. The initial neural strength changes appear to be improved coordination (95) and/or increased activation of prime mover muscles (33, 79), as previously discussed. It is important to point out, however, that if skeletal muscle responds to a load by increasing cross-sectional area (hypertrophy), then theoretically it should respond immediately in some fashion to loading. Evidence of muscle damage can be found after one intense bout of (typically eccentric) resistance exercise (16). Since the response to eccentric muscle damage is repair/rebuilding (i.e., hypertrophy) (111), hypertrophy is likely occurring at an immeasurable level after the first bout of exercise.

References

1. Abe, T., W.F. Brechue, S. Fujita, and J.B. Brown. 1998. Gender differences in FFM accumulation and architectural characteristics of muscle. *Medicine and Science in Sports and Exercise* 30 (7): 1066-1070.
2. Abe, T., J.B. Brown, and W.F. Brechue. 1998. Architectural characteristics of muscle in black and white college football players. *Medicine and Science in Sports and Exercise* 30 (5): S65.

3. Abe, T., K. Kumagai, and W.F. Brechue. 2000. Fascicle length of leg muscles is greater in sprinters than distance runners. *Medicine and Science in Sports and Exercise* 32: 1125-1129.

4. Alway, S.E., P.K. Winchester, M.E. Davis, and W.J. Gonyea. 1989. Regionalized adaptations and muscle fiber proliferation in stretch-induced enlargement. *Journal of Applied Physiology* 66: 771-781.

5. Balnave, C.D., and D.G. Allen. 1996. The effect of muscle length on intracellular calcium and force in single fibers from mouse skeletal muscle. *Journal of Physiology* 492: 705-713.

6. Basmajian, J.V. 1978. *Muscles alive: Their functions revealed by electromyography.* 4th ed. Baltimore: Williams & Wilkins.

7. Belcastro, A., C. Campbell, A. Bonen, and R. Kirby. 1981. Adaptation of human skeletal muscle myofibril ATPase activity to power training. *Australian Journal of Sports Medicine* 13: 93-97.

8. Bell, G.J., S.R. Petersen, I. MacLean, D.C. Reid, and H.A. Quinney. 1992. Effect of high velocity resistance training on peak torque, cross sectional area and myofibrillar ATPase activity. *Journal of Sports Medicine and Physical Fitness* 32: 10-18.

9. Bodine, S.C., R.R. Roy, D.A. Meadows, R.F. Zemicke, R.D. Sacks, M. Fournier, and V.R. Edgerton. 1982. Architectural, histochemical, and contractile characteristics of a unique biarticular muscle: The cat semitendinosus. *Journal of Neurophysiology* 48: 192-201.

10. Cannon, R.J., and E. Cafarelli. 1987. Neuromuscular adaptations to training. *Journal of Applied Physiology* 63: 2396-2402.

11. Costill, D., E. Coyle, W. Fink, G. Lesmes, and F. Witzman. 1979. Adaptations in skeletal muscle following strength training. *Journal of Applied Physiology* 46 (1): 96-99.

12. Coyle, E.F., D.C. Feiring, and T.C. Rotkis. 1981. Specificity of power improvements through slow and fast isokinetic training. *Journal of Applied Physiology* 46: 96-99.

13. Crockett, J.L., V.R. Edgerton, S.R. Max, and R.J. Barnard. 1976. The neuromuscular junction in response to endurance training. *Experimental Neurology* 51: 207-215.

14. DeLuca, C.J., R.S. LeFever, M.P. McCue, and A.P. Xenakis. 1982. Behavior of human motor units in different muscles during linearly varying contractions. *Journal of Physiology* 329: 113-128.

15. Devine, K.L., B.F. LeVeau, and H.J. Yack. 1981. EMG activity recorded from an unexercised muscle during maximal isometric exercise of the contralateral agonists and antagonists. *Physical Therapy* 61: 898-903.

16. Ebbeling, C.B., and P.M. Clarkson. 1989. Exercise-induced muscle damage and adaptation. *Sports Medicine* 7: 207-234.

17. Edman, K.A.P. 1979. The velocity of unloaded shortening and its relation to sarcomere length and isometric force in vertebrate muscle fibres. *Journal of Physiology* 291: 143-159.

18. Edman, K.A.P., C. Reggiani, S. Schiaffino, and G. te Kronnie. 1988. Maximum velocity of shortening related to myosin isoform composition in frog skeletal muscle fibres. *Journal of Physiology* 395: 679-694.

19. Edman, K.A.P. 1992. Contractile performance of skeletal muscle fibres. In *Strength and power in sport,* edited by P.V. Komi, 96-114. Oxford: Blackwell.

20. Edstrom, J.E. 1957. Effects of increased motor activity on the dimensions and the staining properties of the neuron soma. *Journal of Comparative Neurology* 107: 295-302.

21. Enoka, R.M. 1988. Muscle strength and its development: New perspectives. *Sports Medicine* 6: 146-168.

22. Freund, H.J., and H.J. Budingen. 1978. The relationship between speed and amplitude of the fastest voluntary contractions of human arm muscles. *Experimental Brain Research* 31: 1-12.

23. Gardiner, P.F. 1991. Effects of exercise training on components of the motor unit. *Canadian Journal of Sport Science* 16 (4): 271-288.

24. Garfinkel, S., and E. Cafarelli. 1992. Relative changes in maximal force, EMG, and muscle cross-sectional area after isometric training. *Medicine and Science in Sports and Exercise* 24: 1220-1227.

25. Gerchman, L.B., V.R. Edgerton, and R.E. Carrow. 1975. Effects of physical training on the histochemistry and morphology of ventral motor neurons. *Experimental Neurology* 49: 790-801.

26. Goldspink, G. 1992. Cellular and molecular aspects of adaptation in skeletal muscle. In *Strength and power in sport*, edited by P.V. Komi, 211-229. Oxford: Blackwell.

27. Gonyea, W., G.C. Erickson, and F. Bonde-Peterson. 1977. Skeletal muscle fiber splitting induced by weight lifting exercise in cats. *Acta Physiologica Scandinavia* 99: 105-109.

28. Gordan, A.M., A.F. Huxley, and F.J. Julian. 1966. The variation in isometric tension with sarcomere length in vertebrate muscle fibers. *Journal of Physiology* 184: 170-192.

29. Graves, J.E., C.K. Fix, M.L. Pollock, S.H. Leggett, D.N. Foster, and D.M. Carpenter. 1992. Comparison of two restraint systems for pelvic stabilization during isometric lumbar extension and strength training. *Journal of Orthopaedic and Sports Physical Therapy* 15 (1): 37-42.

30. Grimby, L., J. Hannerz, and B. Hedman. 1981. The fatigue and voluntary discharge properties of single motor units in man. *Journal of Physiology* 316: 545-554.

31. Gydikov, A.A., K.G. Kostov, and P.G. Gatev. 1984. Mechanical properties and discharge frequencies of single motor units in human biceps brachii. In *Neural and mechanical control of movement*, edited by M. Kumamoto, 20-36. Kyoto: Yamaguchi Shoten.

32. Hakkinen, K., and P.V. Komi. 1983. Changes in neuromuscular performance in voluntary and reflex contraction during strength training in man. *International Journal of Sports Medicine* 4: 282-288.

33. Hakkinen, K., and P.V. Komi. 1983. Electromyographic changes during strength training and detraining. *Medicine and Science in Sports and Exercise* 15: 455-460.

34. Hakkinen, K., M. Allen, and P.V. Komi. 1985. Changes in isometric force and relaxation time, electromyographic and muscle fibre characteristics of human skeletal muscle during strength training and detraining. *Acta Physiologica Scandinavica* 125: 573-585.

35. Hakkinen, K., P.V. Komi, and M. Allen. 1985. Effect of explosive type strength training on isometric force and relaxation time, electromyographic and muscle fibre characteristics of leg extensor muscles. *Acta Physiologica Scandinavica* 125: 587-600.

36. Hakkinen, K., and P.V. Komi. 1986. Training-induced changes in neuromuscular performance under voluntary and reflex conditions. *European Journal of Applied Physiology* 55: 147-155.

37. Hakkinen, K. 1994. Neuromuscular adaptation during strength training, aging, detraining, and immobilization. *Critical Reviews in Physical and Rehabilitation Medicine* 6 (3): 161-198.

38. Heckman, C.J., and T.G. Sandercock. 1996. From motor unit to whole muscle properties during locomotor movements. *Exercise and Sport Sciences Reviews* 24: 109-133.

39. Henneman, E. 1957. Relation between size of neurons and their susceptibility to discharge. *Science* 126: 1345-1346.

40. Heslinga, J.W., and P.A. Huijing. 1993. Muscle length force characteristics in relation to muscle architecture: A bilateral study of gastrocnemius medialis muscles of unilaterally immobilized rats. *European Journal of Applied Physiology* 66: 289-298.

41. Herzog, W., and H.E. ter Keurs. 1988. Force-length relation of in-vivo human rectus femoris muscles. *Pflugers Archives* 411: 642-647.

42. Herzog, W., A.C. Guimaraes, M.G. Anton, and K.A. Carter-Erdman. 1991. Moment-length relations of rectus femoris muscles of speed skaters/cyclists and runners. *Medicine and Science in Sports and Exercise* 23: 1289-1296.

43. Hill, A.V. 1938. The heat of shortening and the dynamic constraints of muscle. *Proceedings of the Royal Society, London (Biology)* 126: 136-195.

44. Houston, M.E., E.A. Froese, S.P. Valeriote, H.J. Green, and D.A. Ranney. 1983. Muscle performance, morphology and metabolic capacity during strength training and detraining: A one leg model. *European Journal of Applied Physiology* 51: 25-35.

45. Howard, J.D., and R.M. Enoka. 1987. Interlimb interactions during maximal efforts [abstract]. *Medicine and Science in Sports and Exercise* 19: 53.

46. Huijing. P.A. 1998. Muscle, the motor of movement: Properties in function, experiment and modeling. *Journal of Electromyography and Kinesiology* 8: 61-77.

47. Hutton, R.S., and S.W. Atwater. 1992. Acute and chronic adaptations of muscle proprioceptors in response to increased use. *Sports Medicine* 14 (6): 406-421.

48. Ikai, M., and A.H. Steinhaus. 1961. Some factors modifying the expression of human strength. *Journal of Applied Physiology* 16: 157-163.

49. Jacobs, I., M. Esbjomsson, C. Sylven, I. Holm, and E. Jannson. 1987. Sprint training effects on muscle myoglobin, enzymes, fiber types and blood lactate. *Medicine and Science in Sports and Exercise* 19 (4): 368-374.

50. Jones, D.A., and O.M. Rutherford. 1987. Human muscle strength training: The effects of three different regimes and the nature of the resultant changes. *Journal of Physiology* 391: 1-11.

51. Jones, D.A., O.M. Rutherford, and D.F. Parker. 1989. Physiological changes in skeletal muscle as a result of strength training. *Quarterly Journal of Experimental Physiology* 74: 233-256.

52. Kamen, G., P. Taylor, and P.J. Beehler. 1984. Ulnar and posterior tibial nerve conduction velocities in athletes. *International Journal of Sports Medicine* 5: 26-30.

53. Kamen, G., and G.E. Caldwell. 1996. Physiology and interpretation of the electromyogram. *Journal of Clinical Neurophysiology* 13 (5): 366-384.

54. Kawakami, Y., T. Abe, S. Kuno, and T. Fukunaga. 1995. Training-induced changes in muscle architecture and specific tension. *European Journal of Applied Physiology* 72: 432-437.

55. Kearns, C.F., W.F. Brechue, and T. Abe. 1998. Training-induced changes in fascicle length: A brief review. *Advances in Exercise and Sport Physiology* 4 (3): 77-81.

56. Kearns, C.F., T. Abe, and W.F. Brechue. 2000. Muscle enlargement in sumo wrestlers includes increased muscle fascicle length. *Journal of Applied Physiology* 83 (4/5): 289-296.

57. Komi, P.V., J. Viitasalo, R. Rauramaa, and V. Vihko. 1978. Effect of isometric strength training on mechanical, electrical and metabolic aspects of muscle function. *European Journal of Applied Physiology* 40: 45-55.

58. Kraemer W.J., S.J. Fleck, and W.J. Evans. 1996. Strength and power training: Physiological mechanisms of adaptation. *Exercise and Sport Sciences Reviews* 24: 363-397.

59. Kraemer W.J., N.D. Duncan, and J.S. Volek. 1998. Resistance training and elite athletes: Adaptations and program considerations. *Journal of Orthopaedic and Sports Physical Therapy* 28 (2): 110-119.

60. Kulig, K., J.G. Andrews, and J.G. Hay. 1984. Human strength curves. *Exercise and Sport Sciences Reviews* 12: 417-466.

61. Kumagai, K., T. Abe, and T. Ryushi. 1998. Architectural and functional changes in skeletal muscle by resistance training [abstract]. *Medicine and Science in Sports and Exercise* 30: S206.

62. Kumagai, K., T. Abe, W.F. Brechue, T. Ryushi, S. Takano, and M. Mizuno. 2000. Sprint performance is related to muscle fascicle length in male 100M sprinters. *Journal of Applied Physiology* 88 (3): 811-816.

63. Kyrolainen, H., and P.V. Komi. 1994. Neuromuscular performance of lower limbs during voluntary and reflex activity in power and endurance-trained athletes. *European Journal of Applied Physiology* 69: 233-239.

64. Kyrolainen, H., and P.V. Komi. 1994. Stretch reflex responses following mechanical stimulation in power and endurance trained athletes. *International Journal of Sports Medicine* 15 (6): 290-294.

65. LaGasse, P.P. 1974. Ipsilateral and contralateral effects of superimposed stretch. *Archives of Physical Medicine and Rehabilitation* 55: 305-310.

66. Leggett, S.H., M.N. Fulton, M.L. Pollock, D.M. Carpenter, J.E. Graves, M.B. Shank, A. Engmann, and D. Kaufman. 1994. Physiological evaluation of professional water skiers. *Journal of Strength and Conditioning Research* 8 (1): 20-27.

67. Leiber, R.L. 1992. *Skeletal muscle structure and function*. Baltimore: Williams & Wilkins.
68. Lestienne, F. 1979. Effects of inertial load and velocity on the braking process of voluntary limb movements. *Experimental Brain Research* 35: 407-418.
69. Lynn, R., and D.L. Morgan. 1984. Decline running produces more sarcomeres in rat vastus intermedius fibers than incline running. *Journal of Applied Physiology* 77: 1439-1444.
70. MacDougall, J.D., D.G. Sale, G.C.B. Elder, and J.R. Sutton. 1982. Muscle ultrastructural characteristics of elite power lifters and bodybuilders. *European Journal of Applied Physiology* 48: 117-126.
71. MacDougall, J.D., D.G. Sale, S.E. Alway, and J.R. Sutton. 1984. Muscle fiber number in biceps brachii in bodybuilders and control subjects. *Journal of Applied Physiology* 57: 1399-1403.
72. MacDougall, J.D. 1992. Hypertrophy or hyperplasia. In *Strength and power in sport*, edited by P.V. Komi, 230-238. Oxford: Blackwell.
73. Maganaris, C.N., V. Baltzopoulos, and A.J. Sargeant. 1998. In vivo measurements of the triceps surae complex architecture in man: Implications for muscle function. *Journal of Physiology* 512 (pt. 2): 603-614.
74. Marsden, C.D., J.A. Obeso, and J.C. Rothwell. 1983. The function of the antagonist muscle during fast limb movement in man. *Journal of Physiology* 335: 1-13.
75. Maxwell, L.C., J.A. Faulkner, and G.J. Hyatt. 1974. Estimation of number of fibers in guinea pig skeletal muscles. *Journal of Applied Physiology* 37: 259-264.
76. Mikesky, A.E., C.J. Giddings, W. Matthews, and W.J. Gonyea. 1991. Changes in muscle fiber size and composition in response to heavy-resistance exercise. *Medicine and Science in Sports and Exercise* 23 (9): 1042-1049.
77. Miller, R.G., A. Mirka, and M. Maxfield. 1981. Rate of tension development in isometric contractions of a human hand muscle. *Experimental Neurology* 73: 267-285.
78. Milner-Brown, H.S., R.B. Stein, and R.G. Lee. 1975. Synchronization of human motor units: Possible roles of exercise and supraspinal reflexes. *Electroencephalography and Clinical Neurophysiology* 38: 245-254.
79. Moritani, T., and H.A. deVries. 1979. Neural factors vs. hypertrophy in time course of muscle strength gain. *American Journal of Physical Medicine and Rehabilitation* 58: 115-130.
80. Panin, N., H.J. Lindenhauer, A.A. Weiss, and A. Ebel. 1961. EMG evaluation of the "cross exercise" effect. *Archives of Physical Medicine and Rehabilitation* 42: 47-53.
81. Pearson, J.K., and D.W. Sickles. 1987. Enzyme activity changes in rat soleus motor neurons and muscle after synergist ablation. *Journal of Applied Physiology* 63: 2301-2308.
82. Person, R.S. 1958. An electromyographic investigation of co-ordination of the activity of antagonist muscles in man during development of a motor habit. *Pavlov Journal of Higher Nerve Activity* 8: 13-23.
83. Peters, S.E. Structure and function in vertebrate skeletal muscle. 1989. *American Zoology* 29: 221-234.
84. Ploutz, L.L., P.A. Tesch, R.L. Biro, and G.A. Dudley. 1994. Effect of resistance training on muscle use during exercise. *Journal of Applied Physiology* 76 (4): 1675-1681.
85. Pollock, M.L., J.E. Graves, M.M. Bamman, S.H. Leggett, D.M. Carpenter, C. Carr, J. Cirulli, J. Matkozich, and M. Fulton. 1993. Frequency and volume of resistance training: Effect on cervical extension strength. *Archives of Physical Medicine and Rehabilitation* 74: 1080-1086.
86. Prietto, C.A., and V.J. Caizzo. 1989. The in vivo force-velocity relationship of the knee flexors and extensors. *American Journal of Sports Medicine* 17 (5): 607-611.
87. Rack, P.M.H., and D.R. Westbury. 1969. The effects of length and stimulus rate on tension in the isometric cat soleus muscle. *Journal of Physiology* 204: 443-460.
88. Rassier, D.E., B.R. MacIntosh, and W. Herzog. 1999. Length dependence of active force production in skeletal muscle. *Journal of Applied Physiology* 86 (5): 1445-1457.

89. Roy, R.R., and V.R. Edgerton. 1992. Skeletal muscle architecture and performance. In *Strength and power in sport,* edited by P.V. Komi, 115-129. Oxford: Blackwell.

90. Rube, N., and N.H. Secher. 1990. Effect of training on central factors in fatigue following two- and one-leg static exercise in man. *Acta Physiologica Scandinavica* 141: 87-95.

91. Rutherford, O.M., and D.A. Jones. 1986. The role of learning and coordination in strength training. *European Journal of Applied Physiology* 55: 100-105.

92. Sacks, R.D., and R.R. Roy. 1982. Architecture of the hindlimb of muscle of cats: Functional significance. *Journal of Morphology* 173: 185-195.

93. Sale, D.G., J.D. MacDougall, A.R.M. Upton, and A.J. McComas. 1983. Effect of strength training upon motor neuron excitability in man. *Medicine and Science in Sports and Exercise* 15: 57-62.

94. Sale, D.G., J.D. MacDougall, S.E. Alway, and J.R. Sutton. 1987. Voluntary strength and muscle characteristics in untrained men and women and male bodybuilders. *Journal of Applied Physiology* 62: 1786-1793.

95. Sale, D.G. 1988. Neural adaptation to resistance training. *Medicine and Science in Sports and Exercise* 20 (suppl. 5): S135-S145.

96. Sale, D.G. 1992. Neural adaptation to strength training. In *Strength and power in sport,* edited by P.V. Komi, 249-265. Oxford: Blackwell.

97. Smith, A.M. 1981. The coactivation of antagonist muscles. *Canadian Journal of Physiology and Pharmacology* 59: 733-747.

98. Snyder, D.H., D.H. Rifenberick, and S.R. Max. 1973. Effects of neuromuscular activity on choline acetyltransferase and acetylcholinesterase. *Experimental Neurology* 40: 36-42.

99. Starkey, D.B., M.L. Pollock, Y. Ishida, M.A. Welsch, W.F. Brechue, J.E. Graves, and M.S. Feigenbaum. 1996. Effects of resistance training volume on strength and muscle thickness. *Medicine and Science in Sports and Exercise* 28 (10): 1311-1320.

100. Stephenson, D.G., and I.R. Wendt. 1984. Length dependence of changes in sarcoplasmic calcium concentration and myofibrillar calcium sensitivity in striated muscle fibers. *Journal of Muscle Research and Cell Motility* 5: 243-272.

101. Tarbary, J.C., C. Tarbary, C. Tardieu, G. Tardieu, and G. Goldspink. 1972. Physiological and structural changes in the cat's soleus muscle due to immobilization at different lengths by plaster casts. *Journal of Physiology* 224: 231-244.

102. Tesch, P.A., and L. Larsson. 1982. Muscle hypertrophy in bodybuilders. *European Journal of Applied Physiology* 49: 301-306.

103. Tesch, P.A. 1992. Short and long term histochemical and biochemical adaptations in muscle. In *Strength and power in sport,* edited by P.V. Komi, 239-248. Oxford: Blackwell.

104. Thorstensson, A., B. Sjodin, and J. Karlsson. 1975. Enzyme activities and muscle strength after "sprint training" in man. *Acta Physiologica Scandinavica* 94: 313-318.

105. Tomanek, R.J., and Y.K. Woo. 1970. Compensatory hypertrophy of the plantaris muscle in relation to age. *Journal of Gerontology* 25: 23-29.

106. Trotter, J.A., F.J.R. Richmond, and P.P. Purslow. 1995. Functional morphology and motor control of series-fibered muscles. *Exercise and Sport Sciences Reviews* 23: 167-213.

107. Tyler, A.E., and R.S. Hutton. 1986. Was Sherrington right about co-contractions? *Brain Research* 370: 171-175.

108. Upton, A.R.M., A.J. McComas, and R.E.P. Sica. 1971. Potentiation of "late" responses evoked in muscles during effort. *Journal of Neurology, Neurosurgery, and Psychiatry* 34: 699-711.

109. Vandervoort, A.A., D.G. Sale, and J. Moroz. 1984. Comparison of motor unit activation during unilateral and bilateral leg extension. *Journal of Applied Physiology* 56: 46-51.

110. Veiersted, K.B. 1991. The reproducibility of test contractions for calibration of electromyographic measurements. *European Journal of Applied Physiology* 62: 91-98.

111. Waterman-Storer, C.M. 1991. The cytoskeleton of skeletal muscle: Is it affected by exercise? A brief review. *Medicine and Science in Sports and Exercise* 23 (11): 1240-1249.

112. Wickiewicz, T.L., R.R. Roy, P.L. Powell, J.J. Perrine, and V.R. Edgerton. 1984. Muscle architecture and force-velocity relationships in humans. *Journal of Applied Physiology* 57 (2): 435-443.

113. Wood, T.O., P.H. Cooke, and A.E. Goodship. 1988. The effect of exercise and anabolic steroids on the mechanical properties and crimp morphology of the rat tendon. *American Journal of Sports Medicine* 16: 153-158.

114. Zehr, E.P., and D.G. Sale. 1994. Ballistic movement: Muscle activation and neuromuscular adaptation. *Canadian Journal of Applied Physiology* 19 (4): 363-378.

115. Zurbier, C.J., and Huijing, P.A. 1992. Influence of muscle geometry on shortening speed of fiber, aponeurosis, and muscle. *Journal of Biomechanics* 25: 1017-1025.

5

The Safety of Resistance Training: Hemodynamic Factors and Cardiovascular Incidents

Neil McCartney, PhD
McMaster University

There has been considerable investigation of the changes in arterial blood pressure and left-ventricular performance during both static (isometric) and dynamic exercise, but the acute responses to weightlifting, or resistance exercise, have been characterized for little more than the past decade. Studies have been conducted on healthy young (19, 20) and older individuals (9, 21), relatively low-risk postmyocardial infarction patients (4, 6, 7, 13, 36), as well as those with congestive heart failure (22) and after orthotopic heart transplantation (26). A number of factors have been identified as contributing to the circulatory responses to resistance exercise, and the effects of resistance training have also been documented. The present chapter will evaluate the current state of knowledge in this area and will also address the subject of cardiovascular risk.

Dynamic, Static, and Resistance Exercise

Dynamic exercise (e.g., cycling) involves a brief static muscular contraction followed by concentric shortening and almost immediate eccentric lengthening. This pattern of movement results in large increases in venous return as a result of the muscle "pump." Together with reductions in peripheral vascular resistance and an increased heart rate and stroke volume, there are significant increases in cardiac output—that is, a "volume load" on the heart (24). In contrast, static contractions above 20% of the maximum voluntary contraction strength result in a substantial rise in mean arterial pressure, and only a modest increase in cardiac output, primarily due to an increased heart rate; this pattern of response reflects a "pressure load" on the heart (24).

Depending on the magnitude of the load lifted, resistance exercise produces a circulatory response that reflects either a volume load or a pressure load. The lifting and lowering of a weight is achieved by a combination of static and dynamic contractions. Before any lifting takes place, there is a static contraction until the muscle force exceeds the weight of the object to be lifted. This is followed by concentric shortening to raise the weight, a variable period of muscle "unloading" when the limb joint(s) reaches the end of its range of motion (may be extended or flexed), and then eccentric lengthening to lower the weight to its starting position. During lifting of light-to-moderate weights, both the duration and magnitude of the static contraction are very brief, and the circulatory response should be more of a volume load. In contrast, during very heavy lifting and when lifting successively to failure, there is a longer and more pronounced static contraction that may evoke a response more typical of a pressure load. There is now considerable evidence that this is in fact the case; the circulatory responses to resistance exercise vary throughout the various lifting stages according to the degree of effort required to do the maneuver.

Acute Circulatory Responses to Resistance Exercise

The first observation of large, pulsatile swings in intra-arterial pressure throughout each repetition of resistance exercise was by MacDougall et al. (19). Young subjects did single-arm and single- and double-leg exercises to failure (i.e., volitional fatigue) with loads corresponding to 80-100% of the one-repetition maximum (1-RM, the heaviest load that can be lifted once only throughout a complete range of motion); intra-arterial pressures were monitored continuously via a catheter inserted into the brachial artery of the nonexercising arm. Both systolic and diastolic pressures showed large fluctuations throughout each lift, becoming more pronounced over repetitions as the subjects began to fatigue; in one individual the peak values were 480/350 mmHg. The investigators' explanation for the extremely high levels cited the contribution of the Valsalva maneuver, mechanical compression of the exercising musculature, and a significant pressor response. More recent studies have extended these initial observations and also examined how the circulatory responses are affected by such factors as the load lifted and the degree of effort required to lift it, the number of repetitions performed, the size of the active muscle mass, and the variations in joint angle throughout the movement. As will be discussed, these factors influence the circulatory responses in predictable ways and account for much of the variability both within a given individual and between different individuals.

The Effects of Load and Repetitions

When a person lifts weights, the heart rate and arterial pressure responses increase in proportion to the absolute load lifted. The greatest response during a single lift occurs while completing a 1-RM, but the values attained are still less than those observed during a set of heavy lifting to failure (20). When one compares individuals with different lifting capacities, however, the variation in absolute load lifted seems to have little effect on the heart rate and arterial pressure as long as it represents a similar relative challenge (20). For example, a strong person lifting a very heavy load at 70% of the 1-RM will generate much the same circulatory response as a weaker individual lifting a light load that also corresponds to 70% of their maximum capacity. In a study by MacDougall et al., the peak systolic and diastolic pressures were similar among a group of subjects performing a 10-RM of leg press exercise with loads that ranged from 190 kg to almost 300 kg (20). Thus, it is the relative effort, rather than the absolute load, that dictates the circulatory response to resistance exercise, an important concept for practitioners who design these training programs. This lends support to the hypothesis (19, 20, 29, 30) that the major influence on the circulatory response during resistance exercise is a feed-forward, central command mechanism, reflecting the central activity for the recruitment of motor units (25).

The arterial pressures in the first repetition of a set of lifts are greater than during the subsequent 2 to 3 lifts; thereafter the values rise progressively, and the slope of the increase is much greater once the intensity of lifting exceeds approximately 80% of the 1-RM (20). During a set of lifts with such heavy loads (and with the onset of fatigue), there is an obligatory use of the Valsalva maneuver to stabilize the trunk and to facilitate the requisite force generation; the intrathoracic pressure may rise above 100 mmHg (equal to 60% of the pressure generated during a maximum voluntary Valsalva maneuver), and this contributes directly to the increase in arterial pressure (11). For this reason, and also because of a potential reduction in venous return, individuals doing static exercise and those engaged in resistance training are often advised not to perform a Valsalva (1, 2, 6). A counterview is that an initial, brief Valsalva may be an inherent protective mechanism, by increasing intrathoracic pressure and thus effecting a lower left-ventricular transmural pressure (hence afterload) than would be predicted from the arterial pressure at the beginning of systole (18). As any increases in intrathoracic pressure are also relayed directly to the cerebrospinal fluid (11), the Valsalva may offer similar protection to cerebral vessels by reducing their transmural pressure.

After the final repetition in a set, the arterial pressures drop almost immediately to resting levels or below; in a postmyocardial infarction patient performing an overhead military press at 60% of the 1-RM, the systolic and diastolic pressures decreased by 105 and 66 mmHg, respectively, within 2 s of the final lift (36). Indirect measures, such as auscultation and sphygmomanometry, may be reflective of the exercising pressures only if they are taken from a nonexercising limb during the actual lifting phase. Even then, it must be appreciated that such indirect methods are likely to underestimate the true intra-arterial systolic pressure by approximately 13% (36).

The variability in arterial pressure throughout a set of repetitions may be attributed to the following. In the initial lift, the concentric contraction is not preceded by an eccentric contraction (as it is in subsequent lifts) and therefore receives no benefit from the potentiating effects of the stretch-shortening cycle described by Komi (16); this would mean a greater relative effort in the first lift and thus a greater arterial pressure response. In subsequent repetitions the stretch-shortening cycle is active, the voluntary effort is reduced (thus the motor unit activation is similarly reduced), and the arterial pressure is attenuated (29, 30). In the later phases of a set of lifts, the muscles become fatigued and the arterial pressure rises. It is likely that several factors contribute to this increase: a greater use of the Valsalva maneuver; greater voluntary effort may be needed to drive tired muscles to generate the same level of force; increased feedback from muscle afferents to the cardiovascular control center in the medulla (25); and an increased recruitment of accessory muscles. MacDougall et al. have postulated that the rapid drop in pressure immediately after the final lift is likely due to a rapid reperfusion of the exercising musculature, which had previously been subjected to high compressive forces, and a temporary, baroreceptor-mediated pressure undershoot as a consequence of the very high pressures in the final lift (19).

The circulatory responses over a number of sets has not been investigated in any great detail. In a study of postmyocardial infarction patients doing 2 sets of 10 repetitions at 60% of the 1-RM interspersed with 2 min of rest, there was no difference in the heart rate and arterial pressure responses between the sets. It seems likely that the responses would be higher during a training session after the onset of fatigue, when more conscious effort would be needed to generate the necessary muscular force. It might also be expected that training sessions that utilize brief rest periods between sets would also provoke a heightened circulatory response, but this has not been investigated using direct measurements of blood pressure.

The Effects of Muscle Mass

Within a given individual, the relation between the circulatory responses to lifting and the size of the active muscle mass is not entirely clear. In general, it appears that the greater the muscle mass, the more pronounced the rise in heart rate and blood pressure; but the relation is clearly not linear. For example, bilateral leg press may elicit a greater response than the same exercise done with only one leg, but nowhere near double (20). Also, in one study of postmyocardial infarction patients, we noted higher pressures during single-arm curl and military press exercises than during either single- or double-leg press, despite the smaller muscle mass engaged (36).

When the circulatory responses among different individuals are compared, variations in muscle mass seem to have little effect. In the study by MacDougall et al., the peak arterial pressures during a 10-RM of double-leg press lifting were similar among a group of young subjects despite quadriceps muscle cross-sectional areas that varied from approximately 155 to 345 cm^2 (20). This lends further credence to the hypothesis that relative effort is the major influence on the circulatory responses to resistance exercise, as the effort to complete a 10-RM would have been similar for each individual.

The Effects of Joint Angle

If it is indeed the relative intensity of effort that dominates the circulatory response to resistance exercise, then one would expect variations throughout a range of motion in accordance with the strength curve of the engaged muscles. At the beginning of a lift, the joint(s) may be either in extension or flexion depending on the particular movement, and either way the muscles will be at a weak point on their strength curve, thus requiring a high degree of initial effort to move the weight. This being the case, the highest arterial pressures in a single lift should occur when the muscles are working in their inner and outer range. This has been investigated in studies of double-leg press exercises (18, 20). At the initiation of the movement, the knee joint angle is 90°, and the leg extensors are at their weakest point on the strength curve; it is in this very early phase that the rise in arterial pressure is the greatest. As the movement proceeds, the pressure decreases, reaching almost resting levels at the time of lockout when the knee joint angle is 170°, the strongest position for the leg extensors. During the eccentric lowering of the weight, the arterial pressures rise again, but not to the same level as in the initial concentric phase. Once again, this can be explained by the relative effort required in the two types of contraction. Muscles can generate significantly more force during an eccentric contraction than in a concentric contraction (17); so lowering a given weight will require a reduced relative effort compared with raising it, and this will be associated with a reduced circulatory response (19-21, 29, 30).

Acute Left-Ventricular Responses to Resistance Exercise

The first study of the acute left-ventricular responses to resistance exercise was done by Miles et al. in 1987, who used impedance cardiography to assess left-ventricular function in young men doing 12 repetitions of leg extension exercise to fatigue over 90 s (23). There were decreases in stroke volume in both the concentric (~35 ml) and eccentric phases (~24 ml), but an increased heart rate and an apparent increase in myocardial contractility resulted in an unchanged cardiac output.

A more recent study by Lentini et al. extended these observations by using intrabrachial artery catheterization simultaneously with 2-D echocardiography to provide a more detailed analysis of the arterial pressure and left-ventricular volume changes throughout the various phases of bilateral leg-press exercise, done at 95% of the 1-RM to failure (18). In the early phase of the concentric contraction, the circulatory response resembled the changes in a static contraction. Mean arterial pressure increased from 114 ± 3 to 212 ± 19 mmHg, total peripheral resistance rose by a mean value of 4 mmHg · L · min^{-1}, whereas end-diastolic volume and end-systolic volume declined by 30% and 50%, respectively. Although the stroke volume decreased by 17 ml, it was not significantly different from that at rest; a fourfold increase in the peak systolic pressure to end-systolic volume ratio confirmed a notable augmentation of myocardial contractility. By the time the legs had straightened in the lockout phase, all volumes had returned to near resting values. During the eccentric lowering of the weight, the responses were qualitatively similar to those in the concentric lifting but of a lesser magnitude. The researchers attributed these rapid circulatory changes during the course of a single lift to the varying degrees of effort required in each phase of the movement, being greatest in the concentric (weakest) phase and least at the point of lockout (strongest phase).

These findings are in contrast to those recorded during a prolonged isometric dead lift, when the end-systolic volume increased (32) and there was no apparent improvement in myocardial contractility (28, 32,

35). Except when lifting is at almost maximum capacity, it is probably incorrect to equate resistance exercise with isometric exercise, although this has often been done (3, 12, 25).

The Effects of Resistance Training

Given the evidence that the acute circulatory responses to resistance exercise are predominantly influenced by the degree of relative effort required to lift the load, stronger muscles after training should lift a given weight more easily and evoke a less pronounced increase in heart rate and blood pressure. This hypothesis has been tested in a group of young subjects (30) and in two cohorts of older men (9, 21). After 12 (21) and 19 (30) weeks of training, the double-leg press 1-RM increased by 24% (21) and 26% (30); and during 10-20 repetitions of lifting with heavy submaximal loads, there were reductions in systolic pressure, diastolic pressure, and the rate-pressure product of 17-20%. The other study (9) found similar increases in the 1-RM and similar decreases in heart rate and blood pressure during heavy lifting, but also measured the responses in tasks such as treadmill walking with and without weight carrying, and during stair-climbing ergometry. The responses during stair climbing were unchanged after the training period, but in the treadmill walking there were significant reductions in diastolic pressure, mean arterial pressure, and the rate-pressure product while walking at 2.5 mph, and in the systolic pressure while walking and carrying a 30 lb (13.61 kg) shopping bag. Although the improved 1-RM strength resulted in an attenuated circulatory response during weightlifting, there was only a modest transfer of this effect to the simulated activities of daily living.

Because there is a high degree of specificity associated with many of the adaptations to resistance training (27), it would not be surprising if reductions in the circulatory response were greatest when the trained muscles were engaged in weightlifting training movements. There is a single report that highly trained weightlifters have a blunted circulatory response to resistance exercise compared with controls (8), but more research is needed to confirm this observation.

Safety of Resistance Training and Cardiovascular Incidents

It would appear that resistance training has a remarkable record of safety with respect to cardiovascular incidents. Researchers at the Cooper Clinic and the University of Florida have conducted over 26,000 assessments of maximum dynamic strength without one single cardiovascular event (10); in preparation for this chapter, an extensive MEDLINE search also failed to locate any such reports. This is in marked contrast to the well-established increased risk of cardiac problems, and sudden death, associated with aerobic exercise such as jogging (31). Nevertheless, despite a higher incidence of cardiovascular events during aerobic exercise, the data are insufficient to infer an increased relative risk. More complications during these activities may simply reflect the greater relative participation in these types of exercise. The reason(s) for this difference between the two types of exercise may also be explained by the contrasting hemodynamic stresses that they induce and the time over which they are sustained.

Aerobic exercise training is usually performed for sustained periods of 20 min or more, whereas resistance training is done in sets, each of which may be completed within 1 or 2 min and is then followed by a variable period of rest. Any increases in blood pressure, heart rate, and cardiac output are thus borne over a longer period during aerobic exercise training, and this alone is likely associated with increased cardiovascular risk.

The best indirect indicator of myocardial oxygen requirements, and hence the demand for increased coronary artery blood flow, is the rate-pressure product (15). In a study of postmyocardial infarction patients (13), the largest contributor to the rate-pressure product during resistance exercise was the systolic pressure, whereas in cycling it was the heart rate. Diastolic pressure was also much higher during the resistance exercise, and this, coupled with the reduced heart rate, theoretically should have facilitated more prolonged coronary artery filling at a higher perfusion pressure. Similar results were obtained in a study of patients with congestive heart failure who completed 10 repetitions of single-leg press resistance exercise at 70% of the 1-RM and 4 min of steady-state cycling at 70% of the peak power output (22). The heart rate, stroke volume, cardiac output, and rate-pressure product were significantly higher, and the total peripheral resistance was lower, during cycling compared with the leg press. There were no significant differences in left-ventricular volumes or the ejection fraction, but the diastolic pressure was notably higher in the resistance training by a mean value of 12 mmHg. The results suggested a reduced myocardial oxygen demand during the resistance exercise and a comparable left-ventricular response.

The myocardial oxygen supply to demand balance may be estimated from the ratio of the diastolic pressure-time index to rate-pressure product (DPTI:RPP). In a study of 12 postmyocardial infarction patients, Featherstone et al. compared this ratio during arm and leg resistance exercises to failure at 40, 60, 80, and 100% of the 1-RM with the response during maximal treadmill exercise testing (7). With resistance exercise there was a reduced heart rate, a similar systolic pressure, and a higher diastolic pressure, combining to produce a significantly increased

DPTI:RPP and thus a more favorable myocardial oxygen supply to demand balance. In support of this assertion, none of the patients demonstrated any ECG evidence of myocardial ischemia during the resistance training, whereas 5 of the 12 had greater than 1 mm of ST-segment depression while on the treadmill.

If resistance exercise were a potential stimulus for untoward cardiovascular events, one would expect patients with coronary artery disease to be the most vulnerable. However, there are many reports of reduced ischemic signs or symptoms during resistance training (4, 13, 34), and this form of exercise is now widely recommended as part of the cardiac rehabilitation process (1, 2). As far as this author is aware, there are no reports of cardiac patients suffering an acute event while engaged in resistance training; in one study a single patient suffered a myocardial infarction, but apparently it was unrelated to the training itself (5). We have recently completed a 12-month aerobic and resistance training study in patients with stage II and III congestive heart failure, with no untoward cardiac events (33).

Although the evidence suggests that resistance training is extremely safe for the majority of the population, Haykowsky et al. reported three cases of nonfatal subarachnoid hemorrhage apparently precipitated by this form of exercise (14). The authors suggested that the individuals perhaps harbored an unidentified intracranial aneurysm, which ruptured because of a sharp increase in cerebral arterial transmural pressure associated with the lifting. It is estimated that 1% of the population may have an undetected intracranial aneurysm, and thus be at increased risk with resistance training, but routine detection of this defect is not readily available (14).

In general, it appears that appropriately prescribed resistance training is a safe form of exercise for the majority of the population and is associated with minimal risk of cardiovascular events, even in those with previous myocardial infarction or chronic congestive heart failure. Nevertheless, practitioners should recognize that the acute circulatory responses are influenced in predictable ways by such factors as the number of repetitions, the absolute and relative load, the engaged muscle mass, the changing joint angle(s), and the Valsalva maneuver, and should consider these factors when designing training programs.

References

1. American Association of Cardiovascular and Pulmonary Rehabilitation. 1995. *Guidelines for cardiac rehabilitation programs*, 44-50. Champaign, IL: Human Kinetics.
2. American College of Sports Medicine. 2000. *ACSM's guidelines for exercise testing and prescription*. 6th ed., 176-181. Baltimore: Lippincott Williams & Wilkins.
3. Balady, G.J. 1993. Types of exercise: Arm-leg and static-dynamic. *Cardiology Clinics* 11: 297-308.

4. Butler, R.M., W.H. Beierwaltes, and F.J. Rogers. 1987. The cardiovascular response to circuit weight training in patients with cardiac disease. *Journal of Cardiopulmonary Rehabilitation* 7: 402-409.

5. Crozier Ghilarducci, L.E., R.G. Holly, and E.A. Amsterdam. 1989. Effects of high resistance training in coronary artery disease. *American Journal of Cardiology* 64: 866-870.

6. Effron, M.B. 1989. Effects of resistive training on left ventricular function. *Medicine and Science in Sports and Exercise* 21: 694-697.

7. Featherstone, J.F., R.G. Jolly, and E.A. Amsterdam. 1993. Physiologic responses to weight lifting in coronary artery disease. *American Journal of Cardiology* 71: 287-292.

8. Fleck, S.J., and L.S. Dean. 1987. Resistance-training experience and pressor response during resistance exercise. *Journal of Applied Physiology* 63:116-120.

9. Gibson, S.J. 1991. Weightlifting training: Effects on circulatory responses during weightlifting and activities of daily living in older men. MS thesis, McMaster University, Ontario.

10. Gordon, N.F., H.W. Kohl, M.L. Pollock, H. Vaandrager, L.S. Gibbons, and S.N. Blair. 1995. Cardiovascular safety of maximal strength testing in healthy adults. *American Journal of Cardiology* 76: 851-853.

11. Hamilton, W.F., R.A. Woodbury, and H. T. Harper Jr. 1944. Arterial, cerebrospinal, and venous pressures in man during cough and strain. *American Journal of Physiology* 141: 42-50.

12. Hanson, P., and F. Nagle. 1987. Isometric exercise: Cardiovascular responses in normal and cardiac populations. *Cardiology Clinics* 5: 157-170.

13. Haslam, D.R.S., N. McCartney, R.S. McKelvie, and J.D. MacDougall. 1988. Direct measurements of arterial blood pressure during formal weightlifting in cardiac patients. *Journal of Cardiopulmonary Rehabilitation* 8: 213-225.

14. Haykowsky, M.J., J.M. Findlay, and A.P. Ignaszewski. 1996. Aneurysmal subarachnoid hemorrhage associated with weight training: Three case reports. *Clinical Journal of Sports Medicine* 6: 52-55.

15. Kitamura, K., C.R. Jorgensen, F.L. Gobel, H.L. Taylor, and H. Wang. 1972. Hemodynamic correlates of myocardial oxygen consumption during upright exercise. *Journal of Applied Physiology* 32: 516-522.

16. Komi, P.V. 1973. Relationship between muscle tension, EMG and velocity of contraction under concentric and eccentric work. In *New developments in electromyography and clinical neurophysiology*, 596-606. Basel: Karger.

17. Komi, P.V. 1992. Stretch-shortening cycle. In *Strength and power in sport*, edited by P.V. Komi, 169-179. London: Blackwell.

18. Lentini, A.C., R.S. McKelvie, N. McCartney, C.W. Tomlinson, and J.D. MacDougall, 1993. Left-ventricular response in healthy young men during heavy-intensity weightlifting exercise. *Journal of Applied Physiology* 75: 2703-2710.

19. MacDougall, J.D., D. Tuxen, D.G. Sale, J.R. Moroz, and J.R. Sutton, 1985. Arterial blood pressure response to heavy resistance exercise. *Journal of Applied Physiology* 58: 785-790.

20. MacDougall, J.D., R.S. McKelvie, D.E. Moroz, D.G. Sale, N. McCartney, and F. Buick. 1992. Factors affecting blood pressure during heavy weightlifting and static contractions. *Journal of Applied Physiology* 73: 1590-1597.

21. McCartney, N., R.S. McKelvie, J. Martin, D.G. Sale, and J.D. MacDougall. 1993. Weight-training induced attenuation of the circulatory response to weightlifting in older males. *Journal of Applied Physiology* 74: 1056-1060.

22. McKelvie, R.S., N. McCartney, C.W. Tomlinson, R. Bauer, and J.D. MacDougall. 1995. Comparison of hemodynamic responses to cycling and resistance exercise in congestive heart failure secondary to ischemic cardiomyopathy. *American Journal of Cardiology* 76: 977-979.

23. Miles, D.S., J.J. Owens, J.C. Golden, and W.R. Gotshall. 1987. Central and peripheral hemodynamics during maximal leg extension exercise. *European Journal of Applied Physiology* 56: 12-17.

24. Mitchell, J.H., and K. Wildenthal. 1974. Static (isometric) exercise and the heart: Physiological and clinical considerations. *Annual Review of Medicine* 24: 369-381.
25. Mitchell, J.H. 1985. Cardiovascular control during exercise; central and reflex neural mechanisms. *American Journal of Cardiology* 55: 34D-41D.
26. Oliver, D., P.W. Pflugfelder, N. McCartney, R.S. McKelvie, C. James, and W.J. Kostuk. 1998. Acute cardiovascular responses to resistance exercise in heart transplant patients. *Canadian Journal of Cardiology* 14 (suppl. F): 132F.
27. Rutherford, O.M., and D.A. Jones. 1986. The role of learning and coordination in strength training. *European Journal of Applied Physiology* 55: 100-105.
28. Sagiv, M., P. Hanson, M. Besozzi, and F. Nagle. 1985. Left ventricular responses to upright isometric handgrip and deadlift in men with coronary artery disease. *American Journal of Cardiology* 55: 1298-1302.
29. Sale, D.G., D.E. Moroz, R.S. McKelvie, J.D. MacDougall, and N. McCartney. 1993. Comparison of blood pressure response to isokinetic and weight-lifting exercise. *European Journal of Applied Physiology* 67: 115-120.
30. Sale, D.G., D.E. Moroz, R.S. McKelvie, J.D. MacDougall, and N. McCartney. 1994. Effect of training on the blood pressure response to weight lifting. *Canadian Journal of Applied Physiology* 19: 60-74.
31. Siscovick, D.S. 1997. Exercise and its role in sudden death. *Cardiology Clinics* 15: 467-472.
32. Sullivan, J.P., P. Hanson, S. Rahko, and J.D. Folts. 1992. Continuous measurement of left ventricular performance during and after maximal isometric deadlift exercise. *Circulation* 85: 1406-1413.
33. Teo, K., R.S. McKelvie, S. Yusuf, N. McCartney, G. Guyatt, R. Roberts, D. Humen, and T. Montague. 1995. Randomized controlled trial of aerobic plus resistance exercise training in patients with congestive heart failure. *Controlled Clinical Trials* 16: 99S.
34. Vander, L.B., B.A. Franklin, D. Wrisley, and M. Rubenfire. 1986. Acute cardiovascular responses to Nautilus exercise in cardiac patients: Implications for exercise training. *Annals of Sports Medicine* 2: 165-169.
35. Vitcenda, M.S., P. Hanson, J.D. Folts, and M. Besozzi. 1990. Impairment of left ventricular function during maximal isometric deadlifting. *Journal of Applied Physiology* 69: 2062-2066.
36. Wiecek, E.M., N. McCartney, and R.S. McKelvie. 1990. Comparison of direct and indirect measures of systemic arterial pressure during weightlifting in coronary artery disease. *American Journal of Cardiology* 66: 1065-1069.

CHAPTER 6

Resistance Training: Reduced Training and Long-Term Adherence

James E. Graves, PhD
Syracuse University

The physiological adaptations to resistance training that promote the health and fitness benefits discussed by Feigenbaum in chapters 2 and 7 are reversible. Training cessation (detraining) leads to a substantial decline of physiological function in recently trained individuals and highly trained athletes. Thus, the adage "use it or lose it" definitely applies to the benefits associated with resistance training.

Fortunately, the overall volume of activity required to maintain the benefits of resistance training is relatively small compared to the stimulus required to promote initial gains, at least for a short period of time (up to 3 months). Recently trained persons and highly trained athletes can reduce training volume (primarily through the manipulation of training frequency) without detriment, as long as the quality (intensity) of training is not compromised. This means individuals who are forced to reduce training volume, for whatever reason, have the opportunity to retain training benefits.

That's the good news; and it is a welcome message for those individuals who are committed to participating in a well-rounded exercise program on a regular basis. Unfortunately, regular participants in physical activity are a minority. Data summarized in the 1996 *Physical Activity and Health: A Report of the Surgeon General* (43) indicate that only one-quarter of the U.S. population meets the recommended guidelines for physical activity. One-half of us are inadequately active, and another quarter lead a completely sedentary lifestyle. Further, only 20% of men and 8.8% of women surveyed report participation in weightlifting or other exercises to increase muscle strength (32). These percentages are lowest in the elderly, uneducated, and certain minority ethnic populations (32). We are just beginning to understand the factors that motivate individuals to participate in physical activity programs. Critical to this understanding is the identification of factors that motivate people to adhere to programs they have started. The typical dropout rate from supervised exercise programs is approximately 50% (4).

Our understanding of the maintenance of physiological function and program adherence with respect to resistance training is further limited by the fact that most research has considered only aerobic modes of conditioning. While there is a significant body of literature on detraining from resistance exercise programs, data on reduced resistance training and resistance training program adherence are lacking. This chapter reviews the existing literature on the maintenance of muscle strength during reduced training and makes recommendations based on the limited information available for resistance training program maintenance and adherence. The information presented should serve to stimulate research in these critical areas of health-related physical fitness.

Maintenance of Muscular Strength and Endurance

Adaptations to resistance training include improvements in muscular strength, power, and muscular endurance (7). These adaptations are associated with a greater ability to recruit skeletal muscle fibers (30, 34, 38), increased muscle size (16, 28), and metabolic adaptations that enhance anaerobic energy production (27, 41). Resistance training adaptations are under hormonal control (24-26) and depend on the amount of muscle mass recruited, the intensity of the workout, the amount of rest between sets and exercises, the total volume of work, and the training status of the individual (7). Morphological adaptations to resistance training include the development of muscle mass (9, 44) and increased density and strength of bone (3) and connective tissues (45). Increases in muscle mass improve body composition (percent fat) independent of changes in fat weight, although several studies have reported decreases in fat weight as well as increases in muscle mass following strength training programs (e.g., 44). Bone has a tendency to adapt more slowly to physiological stress than muscle, and therefore changes occur over longer periods of time (3). Presumably, these morphological adaptations to resistance training reduce the risk of orthopedic injury (7) and may have a favorable influence on resting metabolic rate (2, 35). Other benefits of resistance training that have been reported, but are somewhat inconsistent, include modest improvements in cardiorespiratory fitness (8), slight reductions in blood pressure (10), reduced glucose-stimulated plasma insulin concentrations (23), and improved blood lipid-lipoprotein profiles (23).

Cessation of resistance training results in relatively rapid but variable declines in muscular strength. Hakkinen et al. (17) and Hortobagyi et al. (22) observed little change in functional capacity (maximal volume isometric knee extension strength and one-repetition maximum [1-RM] squat and bench press strength, respectively) following 2 weeks of detraining in strength-trained athletes. Narici et al. (31) and Dudley et al. (6) found significant reductions in strength following 3-6 weeks of detraining in males that had been previously trained for less than 20 weeks. Studies with longer detraining periods (8-12 weeks) have observed that approximately half of the strength gained during the training period is lost within 12 weeks (13, 14). Graves et al. (11) reported a 68% loss in isometric knee extension strength in men and women following 12 weeks of detraining in men and women that had been training for 10-18 weeks. Staron et al. (40) also reported significant decreases in 1-RM squat, leg press, and knee extension strength following 30-32 weeks of detraining in trained females. However, strength values observed even after this lengthy period of detraining were significantly higher than pretraining values. These studies suggest that muscular strength is rapidly lost during the cessation of training, but this loss appears to level off above pretraining values, and most subjects are able to retain at least some of the initial strength gains for up to 32 weeks of detraining.

Few studies have examined the influence of detraining on variables other than muscular strength. Short periods of detraining result in nonsignificant changes in lean body mass and percent body fat (15, 18, 22, 40). Narici et al., however, found a significant decrease in muscle cross-sectional area following short-duration detraining, indicating that the lack of changes in overall body composition observed in other studies may be due to the gross nature and variability of the body composition measurement (31). As with early strength gains from resistance training, early losses in functional capacity during detraining appear to be mediated, at least in part, by neural mechanisms, with muscle atrophy contributing to further strength losses as detraining continues (13, 14).

The hormonal response to detraining is varied (7). Short-term detraining has been shown to increase growth hormone and testosterone and reduce cortisol in strength-trained athletes (22). Long-term (12 weeks) detraining decreases serum testosterone and testosterone-cortisol ratios (12).

Studies by Hickson and others have shown that aerobic capacity ($\dot{V}O_2$max) can be maintained in previously trained individuals when training frequency (21) or training duration (20) is reduced by as much as two-thirds, as long as training intensity is maintained. When training intensity drops by as little as one-third, however, $\dot{V}O_2$max declines dramatically (19). The magnitude of decline in $\dot{V}O_2$max during reduced training is related to the degree to which intensity is compromised. A one-third reduction in training intensity resulted in a 4.2-5.8% decline in $\dot{V}O_2$max, whereas a two-thirds reduction in intensity resulted in a 9.5-25.8% decline (19). Interestingly, most of the decrease in $\dot{V}O_2$max occurs during the first 5 weeks of reduced training, regardless of the magnitude to which intensity is changed (19).

Although few studies have been conducted on the physiological consequences of reduced resistance training, as with aerobic training, muscular strength can be maintained for up to 3 months with reduced training volume as long as intensity is not compromised. Graves et al. studied the influence of dynamic, variable-resistance strength training, followed by 12 weeks of reduced training, on isometric strength of the knee extensor muscles (11). College-aged men and women trained either 2 times per week or 3 times per week for 10-18 weeks. Training consisted of 1 set of 7-10 bilateral knee extensions performed with a 7-10 RM load. After the training period, subjects reduced their training frequency from 3 to 2 days per week, 3 to 1 day per week, 2 to 1 day per week, or they stopped training completely. Increases in isometric strength following 12 weeks of training were 25.8% for the group that trained 3 days per week and 16.7% for the group that trained 2 days per week. Subjects who reduced training frequency to 2 days per week or 1 day per week were able to maintain essentially all of the strength gained during the initial training period. This finding was somewhat surprising in light of the fact that training 3 days per week elicited greater strength gains than training 2 days per week. The investigators felt that if increases in muscular strength were dependent on training frequency, then maintenance of muscular strength would be dependent on training frequency as well. This was not the case. Training intensity may be a more important factor than training frequency for the maintenance of muscular strength. Whether longer periods of reduced training or reduced training in more highly trained athletes would produce different results is not known.

Tucci et al. completed a reduced training frequency study on the lumbar extensor muscles (42). These muscles are interesting because they show unusually large adaptations to resistance training. Pollock et al. reported improvements in isometric lumbar extension strength in excess of 100% following just 10 weeks of resistance training with a frequency of only one exercise session per week (37). The subjects in the study by Tucci et al. trained initially 1 to 3 times per week for up to 12 weeks (42). After the initial training, subjects reduced training frequency to once every 2 weeks or once every 4 weeks for 12 weeks. Only the frequency of training was changed; the mode, volume, and intensity of exercise remained constant for both reduced frequency training groups. An additional 10 subjects stopped training completely and served as controls. After 12 weeks of reduced training, the once every 2 weeks and once every 4 weeks groups showed no significant reduction in lumbar extension strength. The detraining group, however, demonstrated an average 55% reduction in strength. These findings indicate that strength of the lumbar musculature can be maintained for up to 12 weeks with a reduced training frequency as low as once per month when intensity and volume of exercise per training session are maintained. Careful observation of the data reported for the group that reduced training to once per month reveals a strong and potentially physiologically meaningful reduction in strength, even though it was not statistically significant. Thus, reducing the frequency of training to as low as once per month is not recommended. Whether reduced resistance training influences the neural, morphological, metabolic, and/or hormonal adaptations to resistance training is not known.

Adherence to Resistance Training Programs

The determinants of participation in physical activity are complex and not completely understood (5). The primary determinants have been identified as past and present personal attributes (demographic variables, behaviors, beliefs, etc.), past and present environments, and the nature of the physical activity itself (5). Table 6.1 summarizes some of the factors in each of the determinants. It is beyond the scope of this chapter to discuss the current state of knowledge for each of these factors. Program adherence is especially difficult to address for resistance training because most studies have focused on aerobic activities or "overall" levels of activity. In addition, the factors identified depend in part on the extent of program supervision and interact with many other variables.

Pollock and coworkers (36) evaluated the effects of 26 weeks of aerobic and resistance training on the incidence of injury and program adherence in 57 healthy men and women 70-79 years of age. Subjects were randomly assigned to walk/jog, strength training, or control groups. Adherence to training was 87% for the strength group and 81% for the walk/joggers. This level of adherence is greater than the overall 50%

TABLE 6.1   Known Determinants of Participation in Physical Activity*

PERSONAL ATTRIBUTES

Demographic variables	Activity history
Biomedical status	Psychological traits and states
Past and present behaviors	

ENVIRONMENTAL FACTORS

Facility convenience	Climate or region
Time	

PHYSICAL ACTIVITY CHARACTERISTICS

Intensity/perception of effort

* Summarized from Dishman et al. 1990 (5).

adherence rates reported in the 1996 *Physical Activity and Health: A Report of the Surgeon General* (43) and may be related to the level of commitment demonstrated (or exhibited) by individuals who volunteer for research projects in a university setting.

It is interesting that the adherence rates to both training programs in the Pollock et al. study were so high, considering the injury rates reported (36). Of the subjects who started to jog in the walk/jog group, 57% (8 of 14) were injured. Strength testing resulted in a 19.3% (11 of 57) injury rate (only two injuries were observed during strength training). Only one dropout occurred due to injury, and just one dropout was due to poor program adherence.

Sidney and Jette compared the characteristics of dropouts with continuing program participants in a group of 122 women who volunteered for a 7-week program of heavy resistance training (39). Regular attendees (attendance greater than 80%) represented 72% of the sample and were physically smaller but had greater strength per kilogram per body mass compared with participants who were classified as either infrequent attendees (24-76% attendance) or dropouts (less than 20% attendance). Irregular attendees and dropouts were more likely to smoke tobacco, drink coffee, and skip meals than regular attendees. Most dropouts quit during the first week of training, and among those that continued, adherence was unrelated to assigned training intensity, strength gains, anthropometric adaptations, or injury. These data are interesting considering the attributes described by Dishman as being the most strongly related to program adherence (5). Cross-sectional correlational studies show little association between participation in physical activity and other health-related behaviors (1). It is difficult to draw conclusions regarding long-term adherence from a 7-week training program. It is interesting that the injuries observed in the study by Sidney and Jette were also not associated with any reduction in program adherence (39).

Mikesky et al. investigated the effectiveness of adherence to a 12-week home-based progressive resistance training program for older adults (29). Sixty-two men and women (71 years of age) were assigned to either an exercise group ($n = 31$) that trained with elastic tubing, or to a nonexercise control group ($n = 31$). Within the exercise group, 25 of the 31 subjects (80.6%) completed the study. Of those subjects that completed the study, adherence to the 3 times per week training schedule was 90%. The relatively high adherence reported in the aforementioned studies is attributed, at least in part, to the relatively short-term nature of the training.

To determine the influence of resistance training on program adherence in physically active older women, Nichols et al. recruited 18 women (mean age = 67 years) to participate in a resistance training program 3 times per week for 24 weeks (33). All subjects had already participated in regular aerobic exercise for at least 6 months. Monthly attendance averaged almost 90%, and overall program adherence was 83% (15/18). Adherence to a control group was identical (15/18). There were no injuries reported during the training sessions.

Collectively, these studies suggest that resistance training is safe and enjoyable for all individuals, including older men and women. Whether the positive outcomes related to program adherence in the supervised programs carry over to "free-living" physical activity is not known. It is likely that volunteers for resistance training research have personal attributes that predispose them to program adherence.

Summary

Resistance training is an important component of a well-rounded exercise program. Benefits of resistance training include increased levels of muscular strength, muscular endurance, and a favorable effect on body composition. Several studies have also reported positive health benefits associated with resistance training, such as reduced blood pressure, improved insulin sensitivity, and an increase in bone mass. Cessation of resistance training results in a rapid and significant reversal of these physiological adaptations. A reduction in functional capacity (muscular strength) occurs within 2-4 weeks of detraining. Declines continue to occur during the length of the detraining period; however, there is some evidence to suggest that levels of strength will plateau above pretraining values even when detraining occurs for up to 32 weeks. The influence of detraining for more than 32 weeks has not been reported.

The benefits of resistance training may be maintained for up to 12 weeks with a reduced training volume (brought about by a reduction in training frequency). Training frequency can be reduced to 1 time per week and in some cases (such as the lumbar extensors, for example) as low as 1 time every other week, as long as the intensity of training is maintained. The maintenance of functional capacity with reduced training may offer individuals the opportunity to retain their training benefit under a variety of circumstances.

Adherence to physical activity programs is a complex issue determined by the interaction of a variety of factors related to personal attributes, the environment, and the nature of the activity. Few data are available on the adherence to resistance training programs, and the existing information has been obtained largely from relatively short-term training studies. Factors that are important for participation in aerobic and overall activity are likely also relevant to resistance training. These factors include a high self-efficacy, previous participation in physical activity, and an understanding of health benefits. Programs should encourage individuals to participate at a level that will promote favorable adaptation and improvement. The few studies that exist on adherence to resistance training programs suggest that supervised resistance training is safe and enjoyable for all individuals, including the elderly. There is a critical need to identify strategies to motivate more individuals to participate in well-rounded exercise programs to meet our society's health objectives.

References

1. Blair, S.N., D.R. Jacobs Jr., and K.E. Powell. 1985. Relationships between exercise or physical activity and other health behaviors. *Public Health Report* 100: 172-180.
2. Campbell, W.W., M.C. Crim, V.R. Young, and W.J. Evans. 1994. Increased energy requirements and changes in body composition with resistance training in older adults. *American Journal of Clinical Nutrition* 60 (2): 167-175.
3. Conroy, B.P., W.J. Kraemer, C.M. Maresh, and G.P. Dalsky, 1992. Adaptive responses of bone to physical activity. *Medicine, Exercise, Nutrition, and Health* 1: 64-74.
4. Dishman, R., ed. 1988. *Exercise adherence: Its impact on public health.* Champaign, IL: Human Kinetics.
5. Dishman, R.K. 1990. Determinants of participation in physical activity. In *Exercise, fitness, and health,* edited by C. Bouchard, R.J. Shephard, T. Stephens, J.R. Sutton, and B.D. McPherson, 75-102. Champaign, IL: Human Kinetics.
6. Dudley, G.A., P.A. Tesch, B.J. Miller, and P. Buchanan. 1991. Importance of eccentric actions in performance adaptations to resistance training. *Aviation, Space, and Environmental Medicine* 62: 543-550.
7. Fleck, S., and W. Kraemer. 1997. *Designing resistance training programs.* Champaign, IL: Human Kinetics.
8. Fleck, S.J. 1988. Cardiovascular adaptations to resistance training. *Medicine and Science in Sports and Exercise* 20: S146-S151.
9. Gettman, L.R., and J.J. Ayres. 1978. Aerobic changes through 10 weeks of slow and fast speed isokinetic training [abstract]. *Medicine and Science in Sports* 10: 47.

10. Goldberg, L., D.L. Elliot, and K.S. Kuehl. 1994. A comparison of the cardiovascular effects of running and weight training. *Journal of Strength and Conditioning Research* 8: 219-224.

11. Graves, J.E., M.L. Pollock, S.H. Leggett, R.W. Braith, D.M. Carpenter, and L.E. Bishop. 1988. Effect of reduced training frequency on muscular strength. *International Journal of Sports Medicine* 9: 316-318.

12. Hakkinen, K., M. Alen, and P.V. Komi. 1985. Changes in isometric force- and relaxation-time, electromyographic and muscle fibre characteristics of human skeletal muscle during strength training and detraining. *Acta Physiologica Scandinavica* 125: 573-585.

13. Hakkinen, K., and P.V. Komi. 1985. Changes in electrical and mechanical behavior of leg extensor muscles during heavy resistance strength training. *Scandinavian Journal of Sports Science* 7: 55-64.

14. Hakkinen, K., and P.V. Komi. 1985. The effect of explosive type strength training on electromyographic and force production characteristics of leg extensor muscles during concentric and various stretch-shortening cycle exercises. *Scandinavian Journal of Sports Science* 7: 65-76.

15. Hakkinen, K., P.V. Komi, and P.A. Tesch. 1981. Effect of combined concentric and eccentric strength training and detraining on force-time, muscle fiber and metabolic characteristics of leg extensor muscles. *Scandinavian Journal of Sports Science* 3 (2): 50-58.

16. Hakkinen, K., A. Pakarinen, M. Alen, H. Kauhanen, and P.V. Komi. 1988. Neuromuscular and hormonal adaptations in athletes to strength training in two years. *Journal of Applied Physiology* 65: 2406-2412.

17. Hakkinen, K., A. Pakarinen, P.V. Komi, T. Ryushi, and H. Kauhanen. 1989. Neuromuscular adaptations and hormone balance in strength athletes, physically active males, and females during intensive strength training. Paper presented at the Proceedings of the XII International Congress of Biomechanics, Champaign, IL.

18. Hakkinen, K., A. Pakarinen, H. Kyrolainen, S. Cheng, D.H. Kim, and P.V. Komi. 1990. Neuromuscular adaptations and serum hormones in females during prolonged training. *International Journal of Sports Medicine* 11: 91-98.

19. Hickson, R.C., C. Foster, M.L. Pollock, T.M. Galassi, and S. Rich. 1985. Reduced training intensities and loss of aerobic power, endurance, and cardiac growth. *Journal of Applied Physiology* 58 (2): 492-499.

20. Hickson, R.C., C. Kanakis Jr., J.R. Davis, A.M. Moore, and S. Rich. 1982. Reduced training duration effects on aerobic power, endurance, and cardiac growth. *Journal of Applied Physiology* 53: 225-229.

21. Hickson, R.C., and M.A. Rosenkoetter. 1981. Reduced training frequencies and maintenance of increased aerobic power. *Medicine and Science in Sports and Exercise* 13: 13-16.

22. Hortobagyi, T., J.A. Houmard, J.R. Stevenson, D.D. Fraser, R.A. Johns, and R.G. Israel. 1993. The effects of detraining on power athletes. *Medicine and Science in Sports and Exercise* 25: 929-935.

23. Hurley, B.F., J.M. Hagberg, A.P. Goldberg, D.R. Seals, A.A. Ehsani, R.E. Brennan, and J.O. Holloszy. 1988. Resistive training can reduce coronary risk factors without altering VO_2max or percent body fat. *Medicine and Science in Sports and Exercise* 20 (2): 150-154.

24. Kraemer, W.J. 1988. Endocrine responses to resistance exercise. *Medicine and Science in Sports and Exercise* 20: S152-S157.

25. Kraemer, W.J. 1992. Endocrine responses and adaptations to strength training. In *Strength and power in sport,* edited by P.V. Komi, 291-304. Oxford: Blackwell.

26. Kraemer, W.J. 1992. Hormonal mechanisms related to the expression of muscular strength and power. In *Strength and power in sport,* edited by P.V. Komi, 64-76. Oxford: Blackwell.

27. MacDougall, J.D., G.R. Ward, D.G. Sale, and J.R. Sutton. 1977. Biochemical adaptation of human skeletal muscle to heavy resistance training and immobilization. *Journal of Applied Physiology* 43: 700-703.

28. McDonagh, M.J., and C.T. Davies. 1984. Adaptive responses of mammalian skeletal muscle to exercise with high loads. *European Journal of Applied Physiology* 52: 139-155.
29. Mikesky, A.E., R. Topp, J.K. Wigglesworth, D.M. Harsha, and J.E. Edwards. 1994. Efficacy of a home-based training program for older adults using elastic tubing. *European Journal of Applied Physiology* 69 (4): 316-320.
30. Moritani, T. 1992. Time course of adaptations during strength and power training. In *Strength and power in sport*, edited by P.V. Komi, 266-278. Oxford: Blackwell.
31. Narici, M.V., G.S. Roi, L. Landoni, A.E. Minetti, and P. Cerretelli. 1989. Changes in force, cross-sectional area and neural activation during strength training and detraining of the human quadriceps. *European Journal of Applied Physiology and Occupational Physiology* 59: 310-319.
32. National Center for Health Statistics Behavior. 1991. Current estimates from the National Health Interview Survey, 1990. Hyattsville, MD: U.S. Department of Health and Human Service, Public Health Service, Centers for Disease Control, National Center for Health Statistics.
33. Nichols, J.F., D.K. Omizo, K.K. Peterson, and K.P. Nelson. 1993. Efficacy of heavy-resistance training for active women over sixty: Muscular strength, body composition, and program adherence. *Journal of the American Geriatrics Society* 41 (3): 205-210.
34. Ploutz, L.L., P.A. Tesch, R.L. Biro, and G.A. Dudley. 1994. Effect of resistance training on muscle use during exercise. *Journal of Applied Physiology* 76: 1675-1681.
35. Poehlman, E.T., and C. Melby. 1998. Resistance training and energy balance. *International Journal of Sport Nutrition* 8 (2): 143-159.
36. Pollock, M.L., J.F. Carroll, J.E. Graves, S.H. Leggett, R.W. Braith, M. Limacher, and J.M. Hagberg. 1991. Injuries and adherence to walk/jog and resistance training programs in the elderly. *Medicine and Science in Sports and Exercise* 23 (10): 1194-1200.
37. Pollock, M.L., S.H. Leggett, J.E. Graves, A. Jones, M. Fulton, and J. Cirulli. 1989. Effect of resistance training on lumbar extension strength. *American Journal of Sports Medicine* 17 (5): 624-629.
38. Sale, D.G. 1992. Neural adaptations to strength training. In *Strength and power in sport*, edited by P.V. Komi, 249-265. Oxford: Blackwell.
39. Sidney, K., and M. Jette. 1992. Characteristics of women performing strength training: Comparison of participants and dropouts. *Journal of Sports Medicine and Physical Fitness* 32 (1): 84-95.
40. Staron, R.S., M.J. Leonardi, D.L. Karapondo, E.S. Malicky, J.E. Falkel, F.C. Hagerman, and R.S. Hikida. 1991. Strength and skeletal muscle adaptations in heavy-resistance-trained women after detraining and retraining. *Journal of Applied Physiology* 70: 631-640.
41. Tesch, P.A. 1992. Short- and long-term histochemical and biochemical adaptations in muscle. In *Strength and power in sport*, edited by P.V. Komi, 239-248. Oxford: Blackwell.
42. Tucci, J.T., D.M. Carpenter, M.L. Pollock, J.E. Graves, and S.H. Leggett. 1992. Effect of reduced frequency of training and detraining on lumbar extension strength. *Spine* 17 (12): 1497-1501.
43. U.S. Department of Health and Human Services. 1996. Physical activity and health: A report of the surgeon general. Atlanta: Centers for Disease Control and Prevention, National Center for Chronic Disease Prevention and Health Promotion.
44. Wilmore, J.G. 1974. Alterations in strength, body composition, and anthropometric measurements consequent to a 10-week weight training program. *Medicine and Science in Sports* 6: 133-138.
45. Zernicke, R.F., and B.J. Loitz. 1992. Exercise-related adaptations in connective tissue. In *Strength and power in sport*, edited by P.V. Komi, 77-95. Oxford: Blackwell.

7

CHAPTER

Exercise Prescription for Healthy Adults

Matthew S. Feigenbaum, PhD
Furman University

Introduction

Participation in a comprehensive exercise program that incorporates aerobic activity, resistance training, and exercises to develop flexibility reduces the risk of several chronic diseases (e.g., coronary heart disease [CHD], hypertension, obesity, diabetes, osteoporosis). These diseases are expected to remain the leading causes of morbidity and mortality in the United States well into the 21st century. It has been estimated that, at present, as many as 250,000 deaths per year in the United States can be attributed to a lack of regular physical activity (61, 100). Although epidemiological studies and clinical trials conducted throughout the past 50 years have indicated a significant relationship between physical activity patterns, caloric expenditure, and the development of CHD, only within the past decade have medical organizations formally acknowledged the role of physical activity in chronic disease prevention (40, 109, 139). For example, it was not until 1992 that the American Heart Association identified physical inactivity, or lack of exercise, as the fourth primary controllable risk factor for the development of CHD, along with cigarette smoking, hypertension, and hyperlipidemia (40).

Despite the documented protective health benefits resulting from regular participation in physical activity, the majority of Americans are not physically active (139). The 1996 *Physical Activity and Health: A Report of the Surgeon General* reported that only 22% of the adult population in the United States exercise on a regular basis and that 25% lead an essentially sedentary lifestyle. Among American children and youth aged 6-17 years, 22% are overweight and only 50% exercise at a level considered vigorous enough to obtain health and fitness benefits. Approximately one-half of males and two-thirds of females between 12 and 21 years of age do not participate regularly in resistance training activities (i.e., push-ups, curl-ups, weight training), which may, in part, contribute to the report that approximately 50% of today's youth cannot perform a single pull-up (139). A 1997 survey by the Centers for Disease Control and Prevention also indicated that as many as 60% of American adolescents already have two or more major risk factors for chronic disease (15). Consequently, the general perception among the major health organizations is that the majority of Americans are less active than required for optimal protection against chronic disease development. Not surprisingly, a major public health goal is to improve the collective health and fitness levels of all Americans. Within the past decade, the American College of Sports Medicine (ACSM) and the Surgeon General's Office have established guidelines for exercise programs as an intervention strategy designed to positively affect the health status in the predominantly sedentary U.S. population (table 7.1).

Resistance training is well established as an effective method for developing musculoskeletal strength and is currently prescribed by many major health organizations for improving health and fitness levels, athletic performance, and/or for the prevention and rehabilitation of orthopedic injuries (3, 5, 6, 30, 39, 41, 116). Until recently, however, the effects of resistance training on long-term health status and the role resistance training may play in preventing many of the leading chronic diseases have been largely overlooked. The physiological responses to resistance training traditionally described in the literature include improvements in muscular strength and endurance associated with increases in muscle mass (hypertrophy), bone mass, and connective tissue thickness (21, 133, 136). Adaptations contributing to muscle hypertrophy include alterations in stored levels of intramuscular metabolites and enzymes, an accelerated rate of protein synthesis, and enhanced motor unit recruitment (28, 122). With the recognition that these benefits had a direct application to athletic performance, resistance training became synonymous with strength, power, and athletic prowess. For these reasons, the majority of studies conducted prior to the 1980s experimented with training regimens that would develop "bigger, faster, and stronger" athletes. Only within the past decade have we

TABLE 7.1 Physical Activity Recommendations for Healthy/Sedentary Adults

	1998 ACSM Position Stand [a]	*1995 ACSM Guidelines* [b]	*1996 Surgeon General's Report* [c]
CARDIORESPIRATORY FITNESS			
Frequency	3-5 days/week	3-5 days/week	Daily
Intensity	55/65-90% HRmax or 40/50-85% $\dot{V}O_2$max or HRmax reserve	50/60-90% HRmax or 40/50-85% $\dot{V}O_2$max or HRmax reserve	Moderate
Duration	20-60 min continuous; 10 min bouts minimum	20-60 min continuous; 20-30 min minimum	Accumulate 30 min/day
Mode	Aerobic activities	Aerobic activities	Health promotion activities
RESISTANCE TRAINING			
Frequency	2-3 days/week	2 days/week minimum	2 days/week minimum
Intensity	1 set; multiple sets may provide greater benefits if time allows; <50 years old: 8-12 RM or >50-60 years old: 10-15 reps	1 set; 8-12 RM	1-2 sets; 8-12 reps
Duration	8-10 exercises; major muscle groups[d]	8-10 exercises; major muscle groups	8-10 exercises; major muscle groups
Mode	Machines/free weights	Machines/free weights	Machines/free weights
FLEXIBILITY TRAINING			
Frequency	2-3 days/week	3 days/week minimum	Addressed; not specified
Intensity	Point of mild discomfort	Position of mild discomfort	
Mode/ duration	Static stretches: 10-30 s; 4 reps/stretch for major muscle/tendon groups; PNF: 6 s contraction followed by a 10-30 s assisted stretch	Static stretches: 10-30 s; 3-5 reps/stretch with emphasis on low back and thigh muscles	

Note. ACSM = American College of Sports Medicine; HRmax = maximum heart rate; $\dot{V}O_2$max = maximum oxygen consumption; min = minutes; RM = repetition maximum; reps = repetitions; s = seconds; PNF = proprioceptive neuromuscular facilitation. [a] ACSM (5): guidelines developed for healthy adults. [b] ACSM (6): guidelines developed for healthy, sedentary, and low-risk diseased populations. [c] Surgeon General's Report (139): guidelines developed for healthy and sedentary adults (see U.S. Department of Health and Human Services). [d] Minimum one exercise per major muscle group: e.g., chest press, pull-down (upper back), shoulder press, biceps curl, triceps extension, abdominal crunch/curl-up, lower back extension, leg press, quadriceps extension, leg curls (hamstrings).

explored the potential health benefits of resistance training for the nonathletic adult.

Although the fitness-related benefits had been established, there was very little evidence that resistance training-induced physiological adaptations could also provide direct health benefits against debilitating diseases, including cardiovascular disease, cancer, and osteoporosis. There is increasing evidence that resistance training plays a significant role in improving many health factors associated with chronic diseases (see table 7.2) (78, 113, 117, 134). Resistance training, particularly when incorporated into a comprehensive exercise program, significantly reduces the risk of CHD (53, 66, 76) and type 2 diabetes (42, 103, 125), prevents osteoporosis (58, 94), reduces the risk of colon cancer (83), improves body composition (13, 73, 81, 140, 143), preserves functional capacity (50, 82, 126, 129, 130), and fosters psychological well-being (31, 32, 129). These benefits can be safely obtained by most segments of the population when prescribed appropriate resistance exercise programs, especially when program variables (e.g., frequency, volume, and modality of training), are manipulated to meet the needs of the individual. Participation in resistance training programs may also reduce the risk of fall-related fractures in older adults by improving their leg strength, neuromuscular function, and gait stability and velocity (35, 36, 37, 57).

The current recommendation for untrained adults is 1 set of 8-12 repetitions to volitional fatigue of 8-10 exercises performed 2-3 times per week for persons under 50 years of age, and the same regimen using 10-15 repetitions for persons older than 50 years of age. The research suggests that 80% or more of the potential strength gains can be elicited using this regimen during the initial training period (e.g., up to the first 4 months). The rationale for the current recommendations regarding resistance training program guidelines is presented in chapter 2 and has been reviewed previously (5, 34). For healthy untrained adults, the existing research literature indicates that multiple-set programs provide little, if any, additional stimulus for improving the rate of physiological adaptations during the initial training period compared to single-set programs. For serious weightlifters whose goals are to maximize muscle size and strength, there is evidence to support a multiple-set program using periodization protocols (39). However, because the amount of time required to participate in exercise is an important factor in program compliance, participants are more likely to adhere to the current ACSM recommendations (59, 112).

Muscular Strength and Function

Inadequate muscular strength and flexibility lead to serious musculoskeletal disorders (e.g., lower back problems) that result in considerable

TABLE 7.2 Comparison of the Effects of Aerobic Endurance Training to Resistance Training on Health and Fitness Variables

Variable	Aerobic exercise	Resistance exercise
Bone mineral density	↑↑	↑↑
Body composition		
% fat	↓↓	↓
LBM	↔	↑↑
Strength	↔	↑↑↑
Glucose metabolism		
Insulin response to glucose challenge	↓↓	↓↓
Basal insulin levels	↓	↓
Insulin sensitivity	↑↑	↑↑
Serum lipids		
HDL	↑↑	↑↔
LDL	↓↓	↓↔
Resting heart rate	↓↓	↔
Stroke volume	↑↑	↔
Blood pressure at rest		
Systolic	↓↓	↔
Diastolic	↓↓	↓↔
$\dot{V}O_2$max	↑↑↑	↑
Endurance time	↑↑↑	↑↑
Physical function	↑↑	↑↑↑
Basal metabolism	↑	↑↑

Note. % fat = percent body fat; LBM = lean body mass; HDL = high-density lipoprotein; LDL = low-density lipoprotein; $\dot{V}O_2$max = maximum oxygen consumption.

Reprinted from Pollock and Vincent 1996 (117).

pain and discomfort, loss in income, increased disability, and premature retirement (14, 127). Although very few people die from a lack of muscular strength or flexibility, the overwhelming majority of adults experience sarcopenia, and a substantial number suffer from chronic lower back problems and disease/disability-related decreases in muscle mass. In addition to contributing to a reduction in basal metabolic rate due to reduced muscle mass, inactivity, bed rest, and immobilization are accompanied by loss of bone matrix and minerals and often result in osteopenia and osteoporosis-related fractures. Resistance training can offset the age- and disease/disability-related declines in strength and musculoskeletal mass and improve functional capacity, which in turn can enhance one's quality of life (14, 120). This benefit alone provides a strong rationale for incorporating resistance training into exercise programs for healthy persons as well as for those with chronic diseases.

Strength development depends on neural and morphological factors. Neural factors account for most of the strength gains during the initial stages (first 3-5 weeks) of a resistance training program (104, 122). Electromyographic studies indicate that resistance training induces several adaptations in the nervous system that allow greater coordination between primary movers, synergists, and antagonists in order to develop a greater net force in the intended direction of movement (122). Moritani and deVries (104) indicated that muscle hypertrophy becomes the dominant factor influencing strength gains after the first 3-5 weeks; however, the increase in motor unit coactivation and the resultant improvements in coordinated movement continue to influence strength gains throughout the duration of the training program.

While neural factors are believed to contribute to most of the strength gains during the first month of a resistance training program, muscle hypertrophy (morphological adaptation) accounts for the majority of subsequent strength gains (104). The genetically determined fiber-type composition of a muscle significantly influences how much the overall functional capacity of the muscle can be improved through resistance training. The functional characteristics of skeletal muscle largely depend on the relative distribution of fiber types within the muscle: muscles with a greater relative distribution of slow-twitch oxidative (type I) fibers exhibit a longer capacity to sustain aerobic activities; muscles with fast-twitch glycolytic (type IIb) fibers exhibit a longer capacity to sustain anaerobic work; and muscles with fast-twitch oxidative-glycolytic (type IIa) fibers adapt toward either extreme depending on the training stimulus. Skeletal muscle tissue comprising predominantly fast-twitch fibers possess greater potential for improvements in muscular strength and hypertrophy, whereas slow-twitch muscle fibers are generally characterized by their ability to improve muscular endurance capacity. Although regular exercise training can significantly influence skeletal muscle fiber morphology, genetic components governing motor unit stimulation frequency, protein metabolism, and general somatotyping ultimately limit skeletal muscle phenotype (39).

As described in chapter 2, the extent of improvement in strength from resistance training in healthy nonathletic adults is difficult to assess because increases in muscular strength are affected by a multitude of factors including the participant's initial level of fitness, their potential and desire for improvement, the intensity and volume of their training regimen, their genetic potential, and dietary and other lifestyle habits (39, 63, 68). Although the current literature reflects a wide range of improvement (2% to 200%+) in strength with traditional resistance training programs, untrained men and women following the 1998 ACSM recommendations can expect to see strength gains averaging 25-30% in each exercise performed after training consistently for 4-6 months (39). After the initial training period, healthy adults who want optimal gains in strength and muscle mass could pursue higher-volume training programs (i.e., periodization format), which incorporate multiple-set (3-6) regimens with relatively high training intensities (1-6 RM range) performed more frequently (3-5 days/week). When compared to lower-volume resistance training programs, higher-volume regimens provide a stronger stimulus for activating several neuroendocrines, which induce long-term cellular adaptations in skeletal muscle and connective tissue (88, 133). Research studies consistently report that higher-volume resistance training programs evoke significantly greater serum concentrations of hormones with anabolic properties (e.g., testosterone, growth hormone, insulin-like growth factors), which stimulate protein synthesis resulting in tissue hypertrophy (22, 88, 89, 90, 105). However, the benefits in gains in musculoskeletal mass and strength obtained from high-volume training regimens must be carefully weighed against the increased risk of injury and program compliance issues such as the time required to complete multiple sets.

Bone Mineral Density

During the 1990s, resistance training gained considerable attention as a therapeutic modality to improve bone health by increasing bone mineral density (BMD). Several review articles on this topic have been published (58, 94). The fastest growing segment of the population in the United States is the elderly, who are susceptible to many degenerative diseases, particularly osteoporosis, and it is prudent to advocate weight-bearing exercise for all healthy adults as a preventive medicine strategy. Osteoporosis is a degenerative disease characterized by a decrease in BMD, which in turn increases the susceptibility of bones to fractures. Consequently, osteoporotic-related fractures, which occur most often in the vertebrae, hip, or wrist, generally lead to a decreased level of mobility and are often accompanied by additional debilitating diseases (e.g., CHD) and premature mortality. Osteoporosis is a degenerative process that often begins in the second decade of life, and numerous studies have been conducted to evaluate the role of progressive resistance training on bone formation and remodeling in both young and older adults. Although some studies have examined BMD differences among athletes, the majority of studies conducted have involved postmenopausal women (58, 94).

Wolff's law states that stress or mechanical loading applied to the bone via the muscle and tendons has a direct effect on bone formation and remodeling (16). Applying this principle, researchers evaluating the effect of resistance training and/or weight-bearing aerobic endurance exercise on bone formation have demonstrated that both forms of exercise increase BMD, with the increase being sport- and/or site-specific to the joints involved (58, 94, 121). For example, Hamdy et al. reported an increased BMD in the upper arm in male weightlifters and crosstrainers (who included upper-body resistance training exercises as part of their program) when compared to runners, but that vertebral and lower-body BMD were not significantly different between groups as each group performed some type of weight-bearing exercise (64). Studies involving female athletes also indicate that increases in BMD are sport- and/or site-specific (23, 67, 95). For example, Heinonen et al. reported that female weightlifters had increased BMD in the lumbar spine, distal femur, patella, and distal radius when compared to cyclists, cross-country skiers, and orienteers (67). Although most weight-bearing activities appear to increase BMD, the majority of cross-sectional and longitudinal studies conducted to date suggest that high-intensity resistance training increases BMD more than other forms of exercise (58, 94, 115). Further, studies suggest that resistance training-induced increases in BMD are retained even after exercise program compliance ceases (80). For example, Karlsson et al. reported that both active and retired weightlifters had increased BMD for the spine, hip, tibia, and radius when compared to a control group (80).

Collectively, these studies indicate that, although aerobic endurance exercise and participation in traditional weight-bearing physical activities are important in maintaining or improving overall health and fitness, resistance training is more positively associated with increases in BMD (58, 94, 115). The most significant increases in BMD have been demonstrated by randomized clinical trials using progressive high-intensity resistance training protocols. The results from these studies indicate that resistance training may have significant clinical applications as a preventive treatment strategy for osteoporosis and other degenerative bone diseases. Incorporating resistance training into a comprehensive fitness program may help women achieve the highest possible peak bone mass prior to menopause and may increase or at least offset losses in BMD postmenopause. Healthy middle-aged and elderly men as well as women can benefit substantially from resistance training-induced increases in BMD and muscle function, which in turn improve balance, agility, and mobility (101, 107). Regardless of gender, these improvements are essential in maintaining functional independence and reducing the risk associated with falls and fractures. The prescription of resistance training for the prevention of osteoporosis is discussed in detail in chapter 20 by Jennifer Layne and Dr. Miriam Nelson.

Aerobic Capacity

In contrast to the 15-30% increase in maximum oxygen consumption ($\dot{V}O_2$max) typically elicited by aerobic endurance exercise programs following the ACSM recommendations (5, 6), the contribution of resistance training to improvements in cardiorespiratory fitness are comparatively modest (3-12%) in healthy adults. The improvements in $\dot{V}O_2$max —corresponding to training-induced adaptations in myofibrillar protein content, mitochondrial volume density, capillary density, and in enzymes reflecting aerobic/anaerobic energy production—differ significantly between resistance training and aerobic endurance exercise programs (27, 28, 91).

Traditional resistance training programs emphasize heavy resistance (60-100% of 1-RM), few repetitions (3-10/set), multiple sets (3-5), and frequent rest periods of 1-2 min between sets (39). Available evidence indicates that an acute bout of resistance training elicits an increase in the rate of oxygen uptake to approximately 50% $\dot{V}O_2$max, which, depending on pretraining fitness level, is generally lower than loading and duration limits of the training threshold necessary to facilitate improvements in aerobic capacity. Oxygen consumption of approximately 50% of $\dot{V}O_2$max has been measured during programs incorporating multiple sets of squat, leg press, and leg extension exercises with 6-12 repetitions/set lasting approximately 30 s and followed by 1 min rest periods (124) and with 26-28 repetitions/set (26). Similarly, high-intensity circuit weight training (CWT) on variable-resistance equipment (e.g., Nautilus) elicits a $\dot{V}O_2$ of about 45% of $\dot{V}O_2$max (74, 76).

Nagle and Irwin (106) conducted one of the earliest studies on cardiorespiratory adaptations to traditional resistance training and reported no change in cardiorespiratory fitness responses to cycle ergometer exercise following 8 weeks of low-repetition–high-resistance (5) and high-repetition–low-resistance (15) training programs. Additional studies involving 3-5 sets (~5 repetitions/set with 3 min of rest between sets) of high resistance (80-90% of 1-RM) for 10 weeks showed no change in aerobic power (69, 70). More recently, Goldberg et al. (54) and McCarthy et al. (99) have reported small or nonsignificant increases in $\dot{V}O_2$max with resistance training. The results from these studies indicated that 10-16 weeks of high-intensity exercise results in negligible changes (4.9-6.0% increases) in $\dot{V}O_2$max. Perhaps the most clinically applicable data reported are those of Swenson et al. (135) and Harris and Holly (66) who found 13.4% and 21% increases in $\dot{V}O_2$peak for the arms with 4 weeks of traditional resistance training and 9 weeks of CWT, respectively. These results have important implications particularly for healthy elderly persons and/or those with chronic diseases and disabilities who benefit from the improved ability to perform daily activities that require arm/upper-body endurance.

The results of cross-sectional studies evaluating aerobic power indicate that competitive Olympic-style weightlifters, powerlifters, and bodybuilders present values for $\dot{V}O_2$max (40-55 ml $\cdot$ kg^{-1} $\cdot$ min^{-1}) similar to or just slightly greater than those of sedentary persons (33, 62, 87, 123). Stone et al. reported that a 7-week Olympic-style weightlifting program consisting of 2 training sessions/day, 3 days/week, with 3-5 sets of 10 repetitions/set interspersed with long rest periods (3.5-4 min) produced moderate gains (8%) in $\dot{V}O_2$max (132). The data from the studies involving competitive athletes suggest that these types of regimens may induce moderate increases in $\dot{V}O_2$max.

The CWT format that was recommended by Nautilus Sports/Medical Industries and gained popularity during the 1970s has also been reported to induce modest increases in cardiorespiratory fitness in healthy initially untrained adults (48). The 20 min CWT regimen consists of a circuit of 10-12 exercises (4-6 lower body and 6-8 upper body) and involves the use of 8-15 repetitions/set performed to fatigue with 15-30 s rest between sets or exercises. During the late 1970s and early 1980s, several investigators reported that CWT regimens increased $\dot{V}O_2$max 5-8%, with the magnitude of gain depending largely on the subjects' pretraining fitness status (2, 44, 46, 47, 48, 49, 74, 102, 144). However, a few investigators have suggested that an increase in lean body mass rather than improved cardiorespiratory function may account for most of the increase in $\dot{V}O_2$max reported in CWT studies (47, 51).

Longer rest periods (60 s) and lower repetitions/set (8) result in nonsignificant changes in $\dot{V}O_2$max, cardiac output, stroke volume, or arteriovenous oxygen content difference measured on a combined arm and cycle ergometer (2). When rest periods between sets are kept to a minimum (15 s) and subjects perform as many repetitions as possible, $\dot{V}O_2$max improved 11% in women but not in men after 10 weeks of training (3 days/week). The investigators reasoned that the men, who had a greater initial $\dot{V}O_2$max than the women, trained at a lower relative intensity (41.1% $\dot{V}O_2$max) than the women (46.8% $\dot{V}O_2$max) and subsequently did not reach the training threshold level necessary to induce the physiological adaptations associated with improved cardiorespiratory fitness (2).

The majority of studies investigating the effect of traditional resistance training and CWT programs on aerobic capacity have focused on the number of sets and repetitions and/or the intensity of training; however, the speed at which each repetition is performed may also affect the cardiorespiratory response (45). Following 10 weeks of isokinetic training conducted at slow (60°/s) and fast (120°/s) speeds, the slow-speed group improved 10% in $\dot{V}O_2$max compared to a 3% improvement in the fast-speed group. The number of repetitions was the same for both groups, progressing from 10 to 12 to 15 per set with 30 s of recovery between sets (45). A subsequent study compared slow-speed isokinetic training with isotonic CWT in a 20-week, 3 days/week program, with 12 repetitions/set at 50% 1-RM and 30 s rest periods between sets (48). Both groups improved significantly in $\dot{V}O_2$max, 8% in the isokinetic group and 7% in the CWT group. These studies suggest that improvements in $\dot{V}O_2$max depend on the amount of work performed and not on the speed of contraction or type of equipment used.

Although resistance training has only a modest effect on $\dot{V}O_2$max, it elicits dramatic improvements in walking gait and endurance (1, 47, 70). Hickson et al. demonstrated that despite only modest gains in $\dot{V}O_2$max (4%), 10 weeks of heavy resistance leg exercises increased thigh muscle strength (40%) and improved performance time on both the treadmill (12%) and stationary cycle (47%) (70). Ades et al. also reported that 12 weeks of resistance training improved submaximal treadmill walking time by 38% (1). These improvements translate into increased mobility and endurance, which are required to perform tasks associated with daily living.

Several investigators have evaluated the interaction of resistance training and aerobic endurance exercise on cardiorespiratory performance (11, 46, 69). Gettman et al. compared CWT to jogging and evaluated responses to CWT after training by jogging (47). For the 16 men enrolled in the study, the initial 8 weeks of CWT (3 days/week, 10-15 repetitions/set) improved $\dot{V}O_2$max by 3%. The subsequent 8-week jogging program at 85% HRmax improved $\dot{V}O_2$max by an additional 8%. At the conclusion of the jogging program, 8 men returned to the CWT program, and the other 8 men continued their jogging program. Both groups maintained cardiorespiratory fitness levels equally well for the final 8 weeks. These findings have important implications for training and rehabilitation, in that persons with injuries or orthopedic limitations could participate in a CWT program to help maintain cardiorespiratory fitness during convalescence. The ability to maintain cardiorespiratory fitness with CWT is probably related to the fact that once fitness is attained, less effort is required to maintain it. Additional studies report that subjects who reduce their jogging mileage by as much as 50% may maintain their cardiorespiratory endurance for 5-15 weeks (11, 69).

In conclusion, resistance training has been reported to increase $\dot{V}O_2$max 3-12%. The magnitude of improvement is determined by several factors, which include

1. the subjects' pretraining fitness level (e.g., aerobic capacity, muscle mass),
2. the volume of training,

3. the rest interval between sets, and
4. the duration of training. (Most studies were conducted for periods less than 20 weeks and longer duration studies may show greater improvements in muscle mass and $\dot{V}O_2$max.)

The reported 3-12% increase in $\dot{V}O_2$max with resistance training, while not substantial when compared to increases from aerobic training, is significant from a health perspective for the largely sedentary U.S. population. Considering the low health and fitness levels of the average American and of those with chronic diseases or disabilities, resistance training should be considered a training modality for improving $\dot{V}O_2$max and walking endurance as well as for increasing musculoskeletal mass and strength. For healthy persons, resistance training should be incorporated into a comprehensive exercise program that includes cardiorespiratory fitness-specific exercises if improvements in $\dot{V}O_2$max are desired.

Body Composition and Insulin Resistance

Data from the third National Health and Nutrition Examination Survey (NHANES III) indicate that the prevalence of obese adults in the United States is increasing and has an estimated economic cost of over $39.3 billion (19, 93). Obesity exacerbates many chronic conditions, including hypertension, dyslipidemia, type 2 diabetes, osteoarthritis, and other musculoskeletal-related disabilities (12, 24, 145). An excessive deposition of visceral adipose tissue relative to gluteal or femoral adipose tissue is associated with several metabolic complications, particularly glucose intolerance, hyperinsulinemia, and hyperlipidemia. Although it is generally agreed that obesity occurs when energy intake exceeds energy expenditure, the issue of obesity is complex, and genetics, overeating, inactivity, and/or metabolic disorders are contributing factors (128, 145).

A gradual weight management program including caloric restriction and a prescribed exercise regimen is recommended for overweight yet otherwise healthy individuals because it promotes numerous health benefits secondary to maintainable weight loss (112, 117). Regular physical activity may offset the reduction in basal metabolic rate (BMR) associated with caloric deprivation, but the increased level of energy expenditure depends on the type, duration, and intensity of the activity. Aerobic exercise has been widely prescribed as a nonpharmacological tool in the treatment of abdominal obesity and associated metabolic disorders, and short-term aerobic endurance training studies indicate that it attenuates or prevents the reduction in BMR (12, 128). However, the effect of aerobic endurance exercise on fat-free mass (FFM) and subsequently long-term BMR remains controversial, as some training studies have demonstrated a loss in FFM (60), preservation of FFM (65, 71, 110, 111), or gain in FFM (147). Despite the increased reliance on lipolysis and subsequent reduction in adiposity, the loss of FFM from a combination of diet and an aerobic endurance exercise program may decrease BMR and result in additional weight gain if exercise program compliance deteriorates (112, 141).

Incorporating resistance training is also recommended when developing a long-term weight management program. Walberg (141) and Kreitzman (92) suggested that resistance training, although less likely than aerobic endurance exercise to acutely increase energy and lipid utilization, may be more effective in maintaining or increasing FFM and BMR and thus indirectly improve body composition and aid in weight reduction. The increases in FFM and BMR associated with resistance training are, in part, related to the rate of protein synthesis, which is increased up to 24 h postresistance exercise (18). However, a review of the literature indicates that the effect of resistance training on FFM, BMR, and overall body mass remains unresolved. Donnelly et al. (25) and Pronk et al. (119) reported that adding aerobic endurance exercise and/or resistance training to a very-low-calorie liquid diet resulted in similar decreases in fat and FFM as well as overall body mass. In contrast, Ballor et al. (7) and Marks et al. (97) reported that women who added a resistance training regimen to a moderate calorie-restricted diet had an increase in FFM compared to women who dieted only. Despite the increase in FFM, a lack of significant change in body weight has been reported for college-aged adults (73, 98, 108, 143, 144), middle-aged adults (13, 49), and the elderly (17). A meta-analysis conducted by Garrow and Summerbell (43) on the effect of exercise with or without dieting on the body composition of overweight subjects indicated that resistance training had little effect on weight loss, but consistently increases FFM by approximately 2 kg in men and 1 kg in women.

The relationship between obesity and type 2 diabetes is well established, with the majority of type 2 diabetics classified as clinically obese (BMI [kg/m^2] > 30) when diagnosed. Although the pathogenesis of type 2 diabetes is complex, multiple organ systems are involved, including abnormalities of insulin secretion and hepatic and peripheral insulin resistance. In obese type 2 diabetics, resistance training may improve insulin sensitivity, glucose metabolism, and plasma lipid profiles and reduce the risk of developing hypertension, CHD, and/or peripheral vascular disease (142, 146). Although the exact sequence of cellular mechanisms is not fully understood, resistance training-induced muscle contractions elicit an insulin-like effect on glucose uptake (72). In the few longitudinal studies involving healthy untrained adults, resistance training has been shown to reduce basal insulin levels in response to a glucose challenge (76, 103). Studies conducted by Miller et al. (103) and

Hurley et al. (76) demonstrated that the insulin response to glucose ingestion was significantly reduced following resistance training for 10 and 16 weeks, respectively. In a more recent study, Smutok et al. compared the effect of aerobic endurance exercise and resistance training on insulin response to a glucose tolerance test and reported that the two exercise modalities equally decreased glucose levels and insulin response (125).

Questions remain as to the optimal mode and minimal volume of resistance training to be included with aerobic endurance exercise and caloric restriction to induce substantial fat-weight loss and increase FFM and BMR. The 1998 ACSM guidelines to incorporate regular physical activity, which promotes a daily energy expenditure in excess of 300 kcal, remain the best recommendations to date. However, exercise program compliance is closely related to exercise prescription and remains a critical issue, particularly for sedentary overweight individuals (24, 112). Further, the quantity and quality of energy nutrients (e.g., proteins, carbohydrates) in the calorie-restricted diets may interact with the prescribed exercise regimen and influence the effects of the exercise program on the body composition and physical performance of obese individuals. Additional longitudinal studies (>20 weeks) combining resistance training and/or aerobic endurance exercise with restricted caloric intake are clearly warranted to resolve these issues. A detailed description of the prescription of resistance training for weight control is given by Dr. William Evans in chapter 9.

Serum Lipid-Lipoprotein Profiles

Hyperlipidemia is an alterable risk factor for many chronic diseases (61, 100). While aerobic endurance exercise has been well established as a means for favorably altering serum lipid-lipoprotein concentrations, the results from cross-sectional and longitudinal studies regarding specific changes in serum lipid profiles have provided inconsistent information (29, 77, 84, 86). This inconsistency has resulted from the majority of studies failing to use appropriate experimental designs to account for factors that affect lipoprotein metabolism or techniques that would accurately reflect serum lipid-lipoprotein concentrations. The limitations of the earlier studies were reviewed by Kokkinos et al. (86) and include major methodological and design limitations that preclude conclusions about using resistance training as a therapeutic modality to favorably alter serum lipid concentrations. Most studies, for example, have not monitored subjects' dietary habits prior to blood sampling or have not attempted to control subjects' dietary habits throughout the training program, usually not considered feasible due to the inconvenience and expense. Further, the possibility that the results reported in these studies are only representative of acute exercise responses cannot be ruled out, as only one blood sample was obtained after the final training session and thus would not be indicative of a chronic training adaptation (86).

Several investigators have reported favorable improvements in serum lipid-lipoprotein profiles (e.g., increased high-density lipoprotein cholesterol [HDL-C]) in healthy nonathletic adults using traditional resistance training regimens (52, 75, 76, 79). For example, a recently published study by Prabhakaran et al. reported that healthy premenopausal women who participated in a 14-week resistance training program significantly improved serum lipid profiles (9% decrease in total cholesterol, 14% decrease in low-density lipoprotein cholesterol [LDL-C], and 14.3% decrease in total cholesterol/HDL-C) independent of changes in body fat (118). Significant improvements in lipid profiles have also been reported for training regimens associated with bodybuilding, powerlifting, and Olympic-style weightlifting (74, 131, 138). The results from the majority of these studies suggest that regular participation in competition-oriented resistance training programs may induce modest improvements in plasma HDL-C concentrations but not plasma triglycerides, total cholesterol, LDL-C, or apolipoproteins (29).

In contrast to the studies indicating favorable changes in serum lipid profiles following resistance training, several investigators have reported that traditional resistance training regimens do not significantly alter serum lipid-lipoprotein concentrations (29, 86). Studies by Conley et al. (20) and Blumenthal et al. (9) reported no significant changes in serum lipid profiles in healthy premenopausal women following 8 and 12 weeks of resistance training, respectively. Similar findings have been reported by several other investigators (8, 85, 96, 125).

Although the reports that resistance training may favorably alter serum lipid profiles are intriguing, additional well-controlled prospective randomized trials need to be conducted. Considering the inconsistencies in the results of the studies reported to date, healthy adults with elevated serum lipid-lipoprotein profiles are encouraged to incorporate aerobic endurance exercise into their training regimen and to consult their personal physician for advice on dietary modifications and pharmacological treatment strategies.

Fitness Maintenance

Fleck stated that two training sessions a week are needed to maintain strength increases in conditioned athletes (38). Normal resistance training with an eccentric as well as concentric component may maintain strength gains and muscle hypertrophy to a greater extent during reduced training periods. Furthermore, similar to with aerobic endurance training, the intensity of resistance training must be maintained when the frequency is reduced. In healthy nonathletes, as long as the training intensity is maintained, reduced training to even 1 day per week has been shown to maintain muscle strength (55).

As described in chapter 2, research studies indicate that adaptations to resistance training may vary between specific muscle groups. For example, Graves et al. reported that training the lumbar extensor muscles 1 time per week elicited maximal gains in isometric strength compared to programs of 2 and 3 days per week after 12 and 20 weeks of training (56). In a follow-up study measuring the effect of reduced training on lumbar extensor muscle strength, Tucci et al. demonstrated that groups of healthy adults that reduced their low back training regimen to once every 2-4 weeks were able to maintain their lumbar extensor strength for up to 12 weeks (137). Recognizing that isolated muscle groups demonstrate different response rates, which may be dependent on various neural, morphological, or biochemical adaptation capabilities, further research is needed to gain a better understanding of the implications of the reduced frequency of training on the development and maintenance of lean body mass, as well as for long-term chronic disease prevention and rehabilitation. Although the preceding studies have provided insights into the minimal level of exercise needed to increase or maintain musculoskeletal mass and function, further investigations are needed to determine the rate of increase and decrease in musculoskeletal mass and function in relation to the level of fitness, age, health status, and resistance training program parameters.

Safety Considerations and Practical Application

To reduce the risk of injury and overtraining in beginning participants, intensity should start low and progress slowly, allowing time for adaptation. If a 1-RM test is administered for the purposes of assessing muscular strength at the beginning of a resistance training program, 30-40% of the 1-RM for the upper body and 50-60% of the 1-RM for the hips and legs should be used as the starting weight for the first exercise training session. When the participant can comfortably lift the weight 12 repetitions using good form and perceive it to be light to somewhat hard (12-13 on the Borg RPE scale) (10), 5% can be added to the next training session. Although completing one set of 8-12 repetitions at a comfortably hard level (RPE = 12-13) is the initial goal, the participant should strive to progress to a higher intensity (RPE = 15-16, hard). Since the level of fatigue (intensity) is an important factor for attaining a maximal benefit, exercising to a maximal effort gives the best results (RPE = 19-20; cannot complete another repetition using good form). At this level of training, progression to a heavier weight should occur every 1-2 weeks. If a subject cannot lift the weight a minimum of 8 times, the weight should be reduced for the next training session.

Variable-resistance machines with selectorized weight stacks are generally recommended for several reasons:

1. the initial weight can be applied at a low level and increased in small increments (1 kg or less);
2. the equipment is usually designed to protect the lower back, thus reducing the risk of injury;
3. many machines are designed to avoid handgripping, thus reducing the risk of exercise-induced hypertension;
4. the machines are usually designed to allow the resistance to be applied evenly through the participant's full range of motion;
5. many types of equipment can be double pinned to allow the subject to exercise through their pain-free range of motion; and
6. many resistance machines do not require the participant to balance or control the weight, as do dumbbells and barbells, which may reduce the likelihood of injury.

Besides being safer, variable-resistance machines generally require less time to use when compared to free-weight exercises, allowing the participant more opportunity to pursue and obtain the benefits from aerobic endurance activities and flexibility exercises. The ability to complete a comprehensive exercise program within 45-60 min, 2-3 days/week, should translate into improved program compliance.

Future Directions

The amount of emphasis to be placed on performing resistance training exercises compared to aerobic endurance training in daily regimens has received considerable attention in recent years. Whether this emphasis should be different among the young, middle-aged, elderly, or diseased populations remains to be determined. As the evidence mounts for the importance of resistance training for both health and fitness, a more balanced approach to the comprehensive exercise program model will be incorporated for all age groups. The total time available for training will continue to be a major consideration because of adherence and injury problems related to programs of greater frequency or volume of training (59, 112, 114). Health and fitness professionals, as well as the participants, will have to make value judgments about the time available to accomplish their goals. Whether there is enough evidence available now to warrant a shift to a 50-50 balance or to recommend a minimum 60% aerobic endurance training and 40% resistance training remains questionable.

While most of the studies conducted to date have addressed gains in muscular strength, future studies manipulating exercise program variables need to be designed to address the role of resistance exercise on improving health factors associated with the development or progression of chronic diseases. The majority of the reported data contributing to our current understanding of how resistance training may affect clinical outcomes were obtained from relatively short-term training studies, and there is a lack of prospective randomized long-term trials in the literature. Although the importance and emphasis of resistance training is debatable, it seems prudent to increase the emphasis on resistance training in programs prescribed for the healthy middle-aged and elderly populations. Resistance training should be emphasized for these groups because of its impact on the attenuation of sarcopenia and osteoporosis and the related risks associated with falling and reduced functional capacity.

Conclusion

Participation in a resistance training program has been shown to be beneficial in improving many health factors to include increases or maintenance of muscle mass and basal metabolic rate, increased bone mineral density, improved walking gait and prevention of falls, decreased pain in persons with chronic lower back problems, improved glucose tolerance and insulin sensitivity, and, most importantly, improved functionality and quality of life. There is also increasing evidence to indicate that resistance training programs may favorably alter risk factors associated with chronic diseases, including diseases of the cardiovascular system and certain types of cancer. Additional longitudinal epidemiological studies are clearly warranted to address these issues. Although higher-volume resistance training regimens may elicit greater gains, the available evidence indicates that the 1998 ACSM Position Stand resistance training guidelines for healthy adults provides the minimal stimulus necessary to induce the physiological adaptations that translate into improved health status. Recognizing the benefits associated with resistance training, most of the major health organizations have included resistance training guidelines as an important component of a comprehensive exercise program.

References

1. Ades, P.A., D.L. Ballor, T. Ashikaga, J.L. Utton, and K.S. Nair. 1996. Weight training improves walking endurance in healthy sedentary persons. *Annals of Internal Medicine* 124: 568-572.
2. Allen, T.E., R.J. Byrd, and D.P. Smith. 1976. Hemodynamic consequences of circuit weight training. *Research Quarterly* 47: 299-306.

3. American Association of Cardiovascular and Pulmonary Rehabilitation. 1999. *Guidelines for cardiac rehabilitation programs*. 3d ed., 110-115. Champaign, IL: Human Kinetics.
4. American College of Sports Medicine. 1990. The recommended quantity and quality of exercise for developing and maintaining cardiorespiratory and muscular fitness in healthy adults. *Medicine and Science in Sports and Exercise* 22: 265-274.
5. American College of Sports Medicine. 1998. The recommended quantity and quality of exercise for developing and maintaining cardiorespiratory and muscular fitness, and flexibility in healthy adults. *Medicine and Science in Sports and Exercise* 30: 975-991.
6. American College of Sports Medicine. 1995. *ACSM's resource manual for guidelines for exercise testing and prescription*. 3d ed., 448-455. Baltimore: Williams & Wilkins.
7. Ballor, D.L., V.L. Katch, M.D. Becque, and C.R. Marks. 1988. Resistance weight training during caloric restriction enhances lean body maintenance. *American Journal of Clinical Nutrition* 47: 19-25.
8. Blessing, D.L., H.N. Willford, J.M. Barksdale, and F.H. Smith. 1988. Alterations in lipids and cardiorespiratory function after weight training. *Journal of Human Movement Studies* 14: 75-83.
9. Blumenthal, J.A., C.F. Emery, D.J. Madden, R.E. Coleman, M.W. Riddle, S. Schniebolk, F.R. Cobb, M.J. Sullivan, and M.H. Higganbotham. 1991. Effects of exercise training on cardiorespiratory function in men and women older than 60 years of age. *American Journal of Cardiology* 67: 633-639.
10. Borg, G.A.V. 1982. Psychophysical bases of perceived exertion. *Medicine and Science in Sports and Exercise* 14: 377-381.
11. Brynteson, P., and W.E. Sinning. 1973. The effects of training frequencies on the retention of cardiovascular fitness. *Medicine and Science in Sports* 5: 29-33.
12. Buemann, B., and A. Tremblay. 1996. Effects of exercise training on abdominal obesity and related metabolic complications. *Sports Medicine* 21: 191-212.
13. Butts, N.K., and S. Price. 1994. Effects of a 12-week weight training program on the body composition of women over 30 years of age. *Journal of Strength and Conditioning Research* 8: 265-269.
14. Carpenter, D., and B. Nelson. 1999. Low back strengthening for health, rehabilitation, and injury prevention. *Medicine and Science in Sports and Exercise* 31: 18-24.
15. Centers for Disease Control and Prevention. 1997. Guidelines for school and community programs to promote lifelong physical activity among young people. *Morbidity and Mortality Weekly Report* 46 (No. RR-6): 1-35.
16. Chamay, A., and P. Tschantz. 1972. Mechanical influences in bone remodeling. Experimental research on Wolff's law. *Journal of Biomechanics* 5: 173-180.
17. Charlette, S.L., L. McEvoy, G. Pyka, C. Snow-Harter, D. Guideo, R.A. Wiswell, and R. Marcus. 1991. Muscle hypertrophy responses to resistance training in older women. *Journal of Applied Physiology* 70: 1912-1916.
18. Chesley, A., J. MacDougall, M. Tamopolsky, S. Atkinson, and K. Smith. 1992. Changes in human muscle protein synthesis after resistance exercise. *Journal of Applied Physiology* 73: 1383-1388.
19. Colditz, G.A. 1992. Economic cost of obesity. *American Journal of Clinical Nutrition* 55: 503S-507S.
20. Conley, D.S., K.L. Hill, S.C. Glass, M.A. Collins, K.K. Estes, and R.R. Holcomb. 1995. Short term resistance training does not alter lipoprotein-lipids in young women. *Medicine and Science in Sports and Exercise* 27: S20.
21. Costill, D.L., E.F. Coyle, W.F. Fink, G.R. Lesmes, and F.A. Witzmann. 1979. Adaptations in skeletal muscle following strength training. *Journal of Applied Physiology* 46: 96-99.
22. Craig, B.W., and H.Y. Kang. 1994. Growth hormone release following single versus multiple sets of back squats: Total work versus power. *Journal of Strength and Conditioning Research* 8: 270-275.
23. Davee, A.M., C.J. Rosen, and R.A. Adler. 1990. Exercise patterns and trabecular bone density in college women. *Journal of Bone Mineral Research* 5: 245-250.

24. Dipietro, L. 1995. Physical activity, body weight, and adiposity: An epidemiological perspective. In *Exercise and Sport Sciences Reviews,* edited by J.O. Holloszy, 275-303. Baltimore: Williams & Wilkins.

25. Donnelly, J.E., N.P. Pronk, D.J. Jacobson, and J.M. Jackic. 1991. Effects of very-low calorie diet and physical training regimens on body composition and resting metabolic rate in obese females. *American Journal of Clinical Nutrition* 54: 56-61.

26. Dudley, G.A., and R. Djamil. 1985. Incompatibility of endurance and strength-training modes of exercise. *Journal of Applied Physiology* 59: 1446-1451.

27. Dudley, G.A., and S.J. Fleck. 1987. Strength and endurance training: Are they mutually exclusive? *Sports Medicine* 4: 79-85.

28. Dudley, G.A. 1988. Metabolic consequences of resistive-type exercise. *Medicine and Science in Sports and Exercise* 20: S158-S161.

29. Durstine, J.L., and W.L. Haskell. 1994. Effects of exercise training on plasma lipids and lipoproteins. In *Exercise and Sport Sciences Reviews,* edited by J.O. Holloszy, 477-520. Baltimore: Williams & Wilkins.

30. Evans, W.J. 1999. Exercise training guidelines for the elderly. *Medicine and Science in Sports and Exercise* 31: 12-17.

31. Ewart, C.K., K.J. Stewart, R.E. Gillian, and M.H. Kelemen. 1986. Self-efficacy mediates strength gains during circuit weight training in men with coronary artery disease. *Medicine and Science in Sports and Exercise* 18: 531-540.

32. Ewart, C.K. 1989. Psychological effects of resistive weight training: Implications for cardiac patients. *Medicine and Science in Sports and Exercise* 21: 683-688.

33. Fahey, T.D., L. Akka, and R. Rolph. 1975. Body composition and VO_2max of exceptional weight-trained athletes. *Journal of Applied Physiology* 39: 559-561.

34. Feigenbaum, M.S., and M.L. Pollock. 1999. Prescription of resistance training for health and disease. *Medicine and Science in Sports and Exercise* 31: 38-45.

35. Fiatarone, M.A., E.C. Marks, N.D. Ryan, C.N. Meredith, L.A. Lipsitz, and W.J. Evans. 1990. High-intensity strength training in nonagenarians: Effects on skeletal muscle. *Journal of the American Medical Association* 263: 3029-3034.

36. Fiatarone, M.A., and W.J. Evans. 1993. The etiology and reversibility of muscle dysfunction in the aged. *Journal of Gerontology* 48: 77-83.

37. Fiatarone, M.A., E.F. O'Neil, N.D. Ryan, K.M. Clements, G.R. Solares, M.E. Nelson, S.B. Roberts, J.J. Kehayias, L.A. Lipsitz, and W.J. Evans. 1994. Exercise training and nutritional supplementation for physical frailty in very elderly people. *New England Journal of Medicine* 330: 1769-1775.

38. Fleck, S.J. 1994. Detraining: Its effects on endurance and strength. *Strength and Conditioning Journal* 16: 22-28.

39. Fleck, S.J., and W.J. Kraemer. 1997. *Designing resistance training programs.* 2d ed., 1-115. Champaign, IL: Human Kinetics.

40. Fletcher, G.F., S.N. Blair, J. Blumenthal, C. Caspersen, B. Chaitman, S. Epstein, H. Falls, E.S. Sivarajan Froelicher, V.F. Froelicher, and I.L. Pina. 1992. Statement on exercise: Benefits and recommendations for physical activity programs for all Americans. A statement for health professionals by the committee on exercise and cardiac rehabilitation of the council of cardiology, American Heart Association. *Circulation* 86: 340-344.

41. Fletcher, G.F., G. Balady, V.F. Froelicher, L.H. Hartley, W.L. Haskell, and M.L. Pollock. 1995. Exercise Standards: A statement for healthcare professionals from the American Heart Association. *Circulation* 91: 580-615.

42. Fluckey, J.D., M. Hickey, J.K. Brambrink, K.K. Hart, K. Alexander, and B.W. Craig. 1994. Effects of resistance exercise on glucose tolerance in normal and glucose-intolerant subjects. *Journal of Applied Physiology* 77: 1087-1092.

43. Garrow, J.S., and C.D. Summerbell. 1995. Meta-analysis: Effects of exercise, with or without dieting on the body composition of overweight subjects. *European Journal of Clinical Nutrition* 49: 1-10.

44. Gettman, L.R., J.J. Ayres, M.L. Pollock, and A. Jackson. 1978. The effect of circuit weight training on strength, cardiorespiratory function, and body composition of adult men. *Medicine and Science in Sports* 10: 171-176.

45. Gettman, L.R., and J.J. Ayres. 1978. Aerobic changes through 10 weeks of slow and fast speed isokinetic training. *Medicine and Science in Sports* 10: 47.

46. Gettman, L.R., J.J. Ayres, M.L. Pollock, J.L. Durstine, and W. Grantham. 1979. Physiological effects on adult men of circuit strength training and jogging. *Archives of Physical Medicine and Rehabilitation* 60: 115-120.

47. Gettman, L.R., L.A. Culter, and T.A. Strathman. 1980. Physiologic changes after 20 weeks of isotonic vs. isokinetic circuit training. *Journal of Sports Medicine and Physical Fitness* 20: 265-274.

48. Gettman, L.R., and M.L. Pollock. 1981. Circuit weight training: A critical review of its physiological benefits. *Physician and Sportsmedicine* 9: 44-60.

49. Gettman, L.R., P. Ward, and R. Hagan. 1982. A comparison of combined running and weight training with circuit weight training. *Medicine and Science in Sports and Exercise* 14: 229-234.

50. Ghilarducci, L.E., R.G. Holly, and E.A. Amsterdam. 1989. Effects of high resistance training in coronary artery disease. *American Journal of Cardiology* 64: 866-870.

51. Girandola, R.N., and V. Katch. 1973. Effects of nine weeks of physical training on aerobic capacity and body composition in college men. *Archives of Physical Medicine and Rehabilitation* 54: 521-524.

52. Goldberg, L., D.L. Elliott, R.W. Schutz, and F.E. Kloster. 1984. Changes in lipid and lipoprotein levels after weight training. *Journal of the American Medical Association* 252: 504-506.

53. Goldberg, A.P. 1989. Aerobic and resistive exercise modify risk factors for coronary heart disease. *Medicine and Science in Sports and Exercise* 21: 669-674.

54. Goldberg, L., D.L. Elliot, and K.S. Kuehl. 1994. A comparison of the cardiovascular effects of running and weight training. *Journal of Strength and Conditioning Research* 8: 219-224.

55. Graves, J.E., M.L. Pollock, S.H. Leggett, R.W. Braith, D.M. Carpenter, and L.E. Bishop. 1988. Effect of reduced training frequency on muscular strength. *International Journal of Sports Medicine* 5: 316-319.

56. Graves, J.E., M.L. Pollock, D. Foster, S.H. Leggett, D.M. Carpenter, R. Vuoso, and A. Jones. 1990. Effect of training frequency and specificity on isometric lumbar extension strength. *Spine* 15: 504-509.

57. Greenspan, S.L., E.R. Myers, L.A. Maitland, N.M. Resnick, and W.C. Hayes. 1994. Fall severity and bone mineral density as risk factors for hip fracture in ambulatory elderly. *Journal of the American Medical Association* 271: 128-133.

58. Gutin, B., and M.J. Kasper. 1992. Can exercise play a role in osteoporosis prevention? A review. *Osteoporosis International* 2: 55-69.

59. Haas, C.J., L. Garzarella, D. Dehoyas, and M.L. Pollock. 1999. Single versus multiple sets and long-term recreational weightlifters. *Medicine and Science in Sports and Exercise* 32: 235-242.

60. Hagan, R.D., S.J. Upton, L. Wong, and J. Whittam. 1986. The effects of aerobic conditioning and/or caloric restriction in overweight men and women. *Medicine and Science in Sports and Exercise* 18: 87-94.

61. Hahn, R.A., S.M. Teutsch, R.B. Rothenberg, and J.S. Marks. 1986. Excess deaths from nine chronic diseases in the United States. *Journal of the American Medical Association* 262: 2654-2659.

62. Hakkinen, K., M. Allen, and P.V. Komi. 1984. Neuromuscular, anaerobic, and aerobic performance characteristics of elite power athletes. *European Journal of Applied Physiology (Occupational Physiology)* 53: 97-105.

63. Hakkinen, K. 1989. Neuromuscular and hormonal adaptations during strength and power training. A review. *Journal of Sports Medicine and Physical Fitness* 29: 9-26.

64. Hamdy, R., J. Anderson, K. Whalen, and L. Harvill. 1994. Regional differences in bone density of young men involved in different exercises. *Medicine and Science in Sports and Exercise* 26: 884-888.
65. Hammer, R.L., C.A. Barrier, E.S. Roundy, J. Bradford, and A.G. Fisher. 1989. Calorie-restricted low-fat diet and exercise in obese women. *American Journal of Clinical Nutrition* 49: 77-85.
66. Harris, K.A., and R.G. Holly. 1987. Responses to circuit weight training in hypertensive subjects. *Medicine and Science in Sports and Exercise* 19: 246-252.
67. Heinonen, A., P. Oja, P. Kannus, H. Sievanen, A. Manttari, and I. Vuori. 1993. Bone mineral density of female athletes in different sports. *Calcification Tissue International* 23: 1-14.
68. Hettinger, R. 1961. *Physiology of strength,* 18-40. Springfield, IL: C. Thomas.
69. Hickson, R.C. 1980. Interference of strength development by simultaneously training for strength and endurance. *European Journal of Applied Physiology (Occupational Physiology)* 45: 255-269.
70. Hickson, R.C., M.A. Rosenkoetter, and M.M. Brown. 1980. Strength training effects on aerobic power and short term endurance. *Medicine and Science in Sports and Exercise* 12: 336-339.
71. Hill. J.O., P.B. Sparling, T.W. Shields, and P.A. Heller. 1987. Effects of exercise and food restriction on body composition and metabolic rate in obese women. *American Journal of Clinical Nutrition* 46: 622-630.
72. Holloszy, J.O., C.H. Constable, and D.A. Young. 1986. Activation of glucose transport in muscle by exercise. *Diabetes/Metabolism Review* 1: 409-423.
73. Hunter, G.R. 1985. Changes in body composition, body build, and performance associated with different weight training frequencies in males and females. *Strength and Conditioning Journal* 1: 26-28.
74. Hurley, B.F., D.R. Seals, A.A. Ehsani, L.J. Cartier, G.P. Dalsky, J.M. Hagberg, and J.O. Holloszy. 1984. Effects of high-intensity strength training on cardiovascular function. *Medicine and Science in Sports and Exercise* 16: 483-488.
75. Hurley, B.F., and P.F. Kokkinos. 1987. Effects of weight training on risk factors for coronary heart disease. *Sports Medicine* 4: 231-238.
76. Hurley, B.F., J.M. Hagberg, A.P. Goldberg, D.R. Seals, A.A. Ehsani, R.E. Brennan, and J.O. Holloszy. 1988. Resistive training can reduce coronary risk factors without altering VO_2max or percent body fat. *Medicine and Science in Sports and Exercise* 20: 150-154.
77. Hurley, B.F. 1989. Effects of resistive training on lipoprotein-lipid profiles: A comparison to aerobic exercise training. *Medicine and Science in Sports and Exercise* 21: 689-693.
78. Hurley, B. 1994. Does strength training improve health status? *Journal of Strength and Conditioning Research* 2: 7-13.
79. Johnson, C.C., M.H. Stone, and S.A. Lopez. 1982. Diet and exercise in middle-aged men. *Journal of the Dietetic Association* 81: 695-701.
80. Karlsson, M., O. Johnell, and K. Obrant. 1993. Bone mineral density in weight lifters. *Calcification Tissue International* 52: 212-215.
81. Katch, F.I., and S.S. Drum. 1986. Effects of different modes of strength training on body composition and anthropometry. *Clinical Sports Medicine* 4: 413-459.
82. Keleman, M.H., K.J. Stewart, R.E. Gillian, C.K. Ewart, S.A. Valenti, J.D. Manley, and M.D. Keleman. 1986. Circuit weight training in cardiac patients. *Journal of the American College of Cardiology* 7: 38-42.
83. Koffler, K.H., A. Menkes, R.A. Redmond, W.E. Whitehead, R.E. Pratley, and B.F. Hurley. 1992. Strength training accelerates gastrointestinal transit in middle-aged and older men. *Medicine and Science in Sports and Exercise* 24: 415-419.
84. Kohl, H.W., N.F. Gordon, C.B. Scott, H. Vaandrager, and S.N. Blair. 1992. Musculoskeletal strength and serum lipid levels in men and women. *Medicine and Science in Sports and Exercise* 24: 1080-1087.

85. Kokkinos, P.F., B.F. Hurley, P. Vaccaro, J.C. Patterson, L.B. Gardner, S.M. Ostrove, and A.P. Goldberg. 1987. Effects of low- and high-repetition resistance training on lipoprotein-lipid profiles *Medicine and Science in Sports and Exercise* 20: 50-54.

86. Kokkinos, P.F., B.F. Hurley, M.A. Smutok, C. Fanner, C. Reece, R. Shulman, C. Charabogos, J. Patterson, S. Will, J. Devane-Bell, and A.P. Goldberg. 1991. Strength training does not improve lipoprotein-lipid profiles in men at risk for CHD. *Medicine and Science in Sports and Exercise* 23: 1134-1139.

87. Kraemer, W.J., S.J. Fleck, and M. Deschenes. 1988. A review: Factors in exercise prescription of resistance training. *Strength and Conditioning* 10: 36-41.

88. Kraemer, W.J. 1988. Endocrine responses to resistance exercise. *Medicine and Science in Sports and Exercise* 20: S152-S157.

89. Kraemer, W.J., L. Marchitelli, S. Gordon, E. Harman, J. Dziados, R. Mells, P. Frykman, D. McMurry, and S. Fleck. 1990. Hormonal and growth factor responses to heavy resistance exercise protocols. *Journal of Applied Physiology* 69: 1442-1450.

90. Kraemer, W.J., S.E. Gordon, S.J. Fleck, L.J. Marchitelli, R. Mello, J.E. Dziados, K. Friedl, E. Harman, C. Maresh, and A.C. Fry. 1991. Endogenous anabolic hormonal and growth factor responses to heavy resistance exercise in males and females. *International Journal of Sports Medicine* 12: 228-235.

91. Kraemer, W.J., S.J. Fleck, and W.J. Evans. 1996. Strength and power training: Physiological mechanisms of adaptation. In *Exercise and Sport Sciences Reviews*, edited by J.O. Holloszy, 363-397. Baltimore: Williams & Wilkins.

92. Kreitzman, S.N. 1986. Lean body mass, exercise and VLCD. *International Journal of Obesity* 10: 331-341.

93. Kuczmarski, R.J., K.M. Flegal, S.M. Campbell, and C.L. Johnson. 1994. The increasing prevalence of overweight among U.S. adults. The National Health and Nutrition Examination Surveys, 1960 to 1991. *Journal of the American Medical Association* 272: 205-211.

94. Layne, J.E., and M.E. Nelson. 1999. The effect of progressive resistance training on bone density: A review. *Medicine and Science in Sports and Exercise* 31: 25-30.

95. Lohman, T., S. Going, R. Pamenter, M. Hall, T. Boyden, L. Houtkepper, C. Ritenbaugh, L. Bare, A. Hill, and M. Aickin. 1995. Effects of resistance training on regional and total bone mineral density in premenopausal women: A randomized prospective study. *Journal of Bone Mineral Research* 10: 1015-1024.

96. Manning, J.M., C.R. Dooly-Manning, K. White, I. Kampa, S. Silas, M. Kesselhaut, and M. Ruoff. 1991. Effects of resistive training program on lipoprotein-lipid levels in obese women. *Medicine and Science in Sports and Exercise* 23: 1222-1226.

97. Marks, B.L., A. Ward, D.H. Morris, J. Castellani, and J.M. Rippe. 1995. Fat-free mass is maintained in women following a moderate diet and exercise program. *Medicine and Science in Sports and Exercise* 27: 1243-1251.

98. Mayhem, J., and P. Gross. 1974. Body composition changes in young women with high resistance weight training. *Research Quarterly* 45: 433-440.

99. McCarthy, J.P., J.C. Agre, B.K. Graf, M.A. Pozniak, and A.C. Vailas. 1995. Compatibility of adaptive responses with combined strength and endurance training. *Medicine and Science in Sports and Exercise* 27: 429-436.

100. McGinnis, J.M., and W.H. Foege. 1993. Actual causes of death in the United States. *Journal of the American Medical Association* 270: 2207-2212.

101. Menkes, A., S. Mazel, R. Redmond, K. Koffler, C.R. Libanati, C.M. Gundberg, T.M. Zizic, J.M. Hagberg, R. E. Pratley, and B.F. Hurley. 1993. Strength training increases regional bone mineral density and bone remodeling in middle-aged and older men. *Journal of Applied Physiology* 74: 2478-2484.

102. Messier, S.P., and M.E. Dill. 1985. Alterations in strength and maximal oxygen uptake consequent to Nautilus circuit weight training. *Research Quarterly* 56: 345-351.

103. Miller, W.J., W.M. Sherman, and J.L. Ivy. 1984. Effect of strength training on glucose tolerance and post-glucose insulin response. *Medicine and Science in Sports and Exercise* 16: 539-543.

104. Moritani, T., and H.A. deVries. 1979. Neural factors versus hypertrophy in the time course of muscle strength gains. *American Journal of Physical Medicine and Rehabilitation* 58: 115-130.

105. Mulligan, S.E., S.J. Fleck, S.E. Gordon, L.P. Koziris, N.T. Triplett-McBride, and W.J. Kraemer. 1996. Influence of resistance exercise volume on serum growth hormone and cortisol concentrations in women. *Journal of Strength and Conditioning Research* 10: 256-262.

106. Nagle, F.J., and L.W. Irwin. 1960. Effects of two systems of weight training on cardiorespiratory endurance and related physiological factors. *Research Quarterly* 31: 607-615.

107. Nevitt, M.C., S.R. Cummings, and E.S. Hudes. 1991. Risk factors for injurious falls: A prospective study. *Journal of Gerontology* 46: M164-M170.

108. Oyster, N. 1979. Effects of a heavy-resistance weight training program on college women athletes. *Journal of Sports Medicine and Physical Fitness* 19: 79-83.

109. Pate, R.R., M. Pratt, S.N. Blair, W.L. Haskell, C.A. Macera, C. Bouchard, D. Buchner, W. Effinger, G.W. Heath, A.C. King, A. Krista, A.S. Leon, B.H. Marcus, J. Morris, R.S. Paffenbarger, K. Patrick, M.L. Pollock, J.M. Rippe, J. Sallis, and J.H. Wilmore. 1995. Physical activity and public health: A recommendation from the Centers for Disease Control and Prevention and the American College of Sports Medicine. *Journal of the American Medical Association* 273: 402-407.

110. Pavlou, K.N., W.P. Steffee, R.H. Lertnan, and B.A. Burrows. 1985. Effects of dieting and exercise on lean body mass, oxygen uptake, and strength. *Medicine and Science in Sports and Exercise* 17: 466-471.

111. Pavlou, K.N., J.E. Whatley, P.W. Jannace, J.J. DiBartolomeo, B.A. Burrows, E.A. Duthie, and R.H. Lerman. 1989. Physical activity as a supplement to a weight-loss dietary regimen. *American Journal of Clinical Nutrition* 49: 1110-1114.

112. Pollock, M.L. 1988. Prescribing exercise for fitness and adherence. In *Exercise adherence: Its impact on public health,* edited by R.K. Dishman, 259-282. Champaign, IL: Human Kinetics.

113. Pollock, M.L., and J.H. Wilmore. 1990. *Exercise in health and disease: Evaluation and prescription for prevention and rehabilitation.* 2d ed., 202-231. Philadelphia: Saunders.

114. Pollock, M.L., J.F. Carroll, J.E. Graves, S.H. Leggett, R.W. Braith, M. Limacher, and J.M. Hagberg. 1991. Physical fitness and performance: Injuries and adherence to walk/jog and resistance training programs in the elderly. *Medicine and Science in Sports and Exercise* 23: 1194-1200.

115. Pollock, M., L. Garzarella, J. Graves, D.M. Carpenter, S.H. Leggett, D. Lowenthal, M.N. Fulton, D. Foster, J. Tucci, and R. Mananquil. 1992. Effects of isolated lumbar extension resistance training on bone mineral density of the elderly. *Medicine and Science in Sports and Exercise* 24: S66.

116. Pollock, M.L., J.E. Graves, D.L. Swart, and D.T. Lowenthal. 1994. Exercise training and prescription for the elderly. *Southern Medical Journal* 87: S88-S95.

117. Pollock, M.L., and K.R. Vincent. 1996. Resistance training for health. *The President's Council on Physical Fitness and Sports Research Digest,* series 2, no. 8 (December).

118. Prabhakaran, B., E.A. Dowling, J.D. Branch, D.P. Swain, and B.C. Leutholtz. 1999. Effect of 14 weeks of resistance training on lipid profile and body fat percentage in premenopausal women. *British Journal of Sports Medicine* 33: 190-195.

119. Pronk, N.P., J.E. Donnelly, and S.J. Pronk. 1992. Strength changes induced by extreme dieting and exercise in severely obese females. *Journal of the American College of Nutrition* 11: 152-158.

120. Risch, S., N. Norvell, M. Pollock, E.V. Risch, H. Langer, M. Fulton, J.E. Graves, and S.H. Leggett. 1993. Lumbar strengthening in chronic low back pain patients: Physiologic and psychological benefits. *Spine* 18: 232-238.

121. Rubin, C.T., and L.E. Lanyon. 1984. Regulation of bone formation by applied dynamic loads. *Journal of Bone and Strength* 66: 397-402.

122. Sale, D.G. 1988. Neural adaptation to resistance training. *Medicine and Science in Sports and Exercise* 20: S135-S145.

123. Saltin, B., and P.O. Astrand. 1967. Maximal oxygen uptake in athletes. *Journal of Applied Physiology* 23: 353-368.

124. Seals, D.R., and J.M. Hagberg. 1984. The effect of exercise training on human hypertension. *Medicine and Science in Sports and Exercise* 16: 207-215.

125. Smutok, M.A., C. Reece, P.F. Kokkinos, C. Farmer, P. Dawson, D. Shulman, J. DeVane-Bell, J. Patterson, S. Charabogos, and A.P. Goldberg. 1993. Aerobic versus strength training for risk factor intervention in middle-aged men at high risk for coronary heart disease. *Metabolism* 42: 177-184.

126. Sparling, P.B., J.D. Cantwell, C.M. Dolan, and R.K. Niederman. 1990. Strength training in a cardiac rehabilitation program: A six-month follow-up. *Archives of Physical Medicine and Rehabilitation* 71: 148-152.

127. Spengler, D., S. Bigos, N. Martin, J. Zeh, L. Fisher, and A. Nachemson. 1986. Back injuries in industry: A retrospective study. 1. Overview and cost analysis. *Spine* 11: 241-246.

128. Stefanick, M.L. 1993. Exercise and weight control. In *Exercise and Sport Sciences Reviews*, edited by J.O. Holloszy, 363-396. Baltimore: Williams & Wilkins.

129. Stewart, K.J., M. Mason, and M.H. Kelemen. 1988. Three-year participation in circuit weight training improves muscular strength and self-efficacy in cardiac patients. *Journal of Cardiopulmonary Rehabilitation* 8: 292-296.

130. Stewart, K.J. 1989. Resistive training effects on strength and cardiovascular endurance in cardiac and coronary prone patients. *Medicine and Science in Sports and Exercise* 21: 678-682.

131. Stone, M.H., D. Blessing, R. Byrd, J. Tew, and D. Boatwright. 1982. Physiological effects of a short term resistive training program on middle-aged untrained men. *Strength and Conditioning*, October/November: 16-20.

132. Stone, M.H., G.D. Wilson, D. Blessing, and R. Rozenek. 1983. Cardiovascular responses to short-term Olympic-style weight training in young men. *Canadian Journal of Applied Sport Science* 8: 134-139.

133. Stone, M.H. 1988. Implications for connective tissue and bone alterations resulting from resistance exercise training. *Medicine and Science in Sports and Exercise* 20: S162-S168.

134. Stone, M.H., S.J. Fleck, N.T. Triplett, and W.J. Kraemer. 1991. Health-and performance-related potential of resistance training. *Sports Medicine* 11: 210-231.

135. Swenson, T., P. Mancuso, and E.T. Howley. 1993. The effect of resistance weight training on peak aerobic power. *International Journal of Sports Medicine* 14: 43-47.

136. Tesch, P.A. 1988. Skeletal muscle adaptations consequent to long-term heavy resistance exercise. *Medicine and Science in Sports and Exercise* 20: S132-S134.

137. Tucci, J.T., D.M. Carpenter, M.L. Pollock, J.E. Graves, and S.H. Leggett. 1993. Effect of reduced training frequency and detraining on lumbar extensor strength. *Spine* 17: 1497-1501.

138. Ullrich, I.H., C.M. Reid, and R.A. Yeater. 1987. Increased HDL-cholesterol levels with a weight lifting program. *Southern Medical Journal* 80: 328-331.

139. U.S. Department of Health and Human Services. 1996. *Physical activity and health: A report of the surgeon general*, 22-29. Atlanta: U.S. Department of Health and Human Services, Centers for Disease Control and Prevention, National Center for Chronic Disease Prevention and Health Promotion.

140. Van Etten, L.M.L.A., F.T.J. Verstappen, and K.R. Westerterp. 1994. Effect of body build on weight-training-induced adaptations in body composition and muscular strength. *Medicine and Science in Sports and Exercise* 26: 515-521.

141. Walberg, J.L. 1989. Aerobic exercise and resistance weight-training during weight reduction: Implications for obese persons and athletes. *Sports Medicine* 47: 343-346.

142. Wallberg-Henriksson, H. 1992. Exercise and diabetes mellitus. In *Exercise and Sport Sciences Reviews*, edited by J.O. Holloszy, 339-368. Baltimore: Williams & Wilkins.

143. Wilmore, J. 1974. Alterations in strength, body composition, and anthropometric measurements consequent to a 10-week weight training program. *Medicine and Science in Sports* 6: 133-138.

144. Wilmore, J.H., R.B. Parr, R.N. Girandola, P. Ward, P.A. Vodak, T.J. Barstow, T.V. Pipes, G.T. Romero, and P. Leslie. 1978. Physiological alterations consequent to circuit weight training. *Medicine and Science in Sports* 10: 79-84.

145. Zachwieja, J.J. 1996. Exercise as treatment for obesity. *Endocrinology and Metabolism Clinics of North America* 25: 965-988.

146. Zierath, J.R., and H. Wallberg-Henriksson. 1992. Exercise training in obese diabetic patients. Special considerations. *Sports Medicine* 14: 171-189.

147. Zuti, W.B., and L.A. Golding. 1976. Comparing diet and exercise as weight reduction tools. *Physician and Sportsmedicine* 4: 49-53.

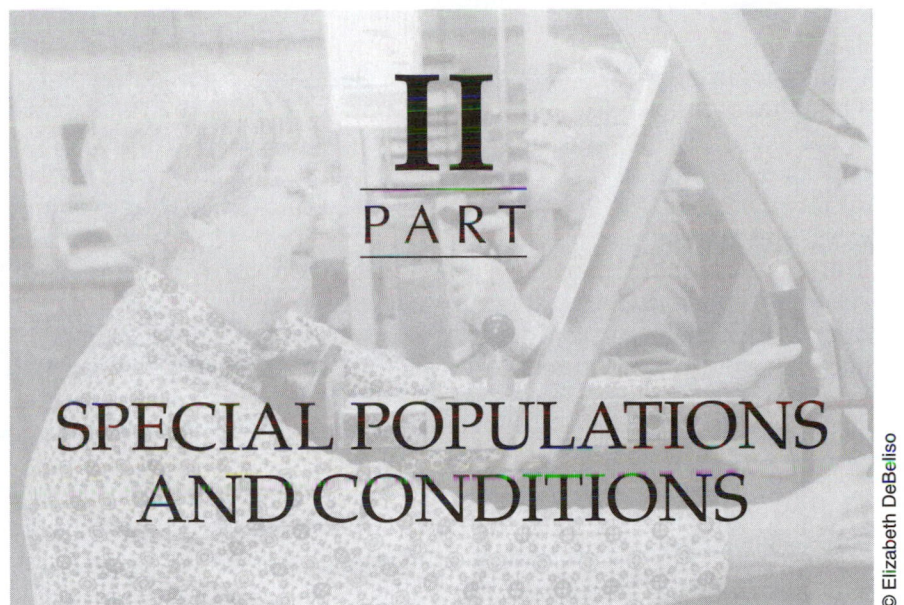

II PART

SPECIAL POPULATIONS AND CONDITIONS

Although regular endurance exercise in healthy women has been shown to yield significant improvements in aerobic capacity and reductions in body weight and fat stores, the health and fitness benefits of resistance training have been less well studied. More than half of all deaths from coronary artery disease now occur in women, and mortality after myocardial infarction is higher among women than among men. Because women are also more likely to experience decreased muscle mass and bone mineral density, the potential for comprehensive exercise regimens to attenuate these conditions is a critical issue.

In sedentary persons, the primary determinant of energy expenditure is lean body tissue (fat-free mass), which declines by about 15% between the third and eighth decades of life. Unfortunately, it appears that the associated declining caloric needs are often not matched by an appropriate reduction in caloric intake, with the ultimate result being an increase in adiposity with advancing age. This may be camouflaged by our "scale weight," which may remain largely unchanged over time, reflecting decreases in fat-free mass and increases in fat mass.

The associated sarcopenia, or loss of skeletal muscle mass that accompanies aging, may be partially compensated for by increasing the strength of the remaining muscle cells. Researchers have shown that men and women who do some form of progressive resistance exercise, or weight training, can improve their strength by at least 25%. Moreover, some of the greatest improvements have been reported in very old and frail people. This is especially noteworthy since the Framingham Heart Study found that about half of women over age 65 could not lift 10 pounds!

The proportion of U.S. adults who are classified as obese (defined as a body mass index >30 kg/m^2) rose dramatically over the last decade, with the greatest increases among the youngest age group, the college-educated, and those of Hispanic ethnicity. During this time period, obesity increased in every state, in both sexes, and across all age groups, races, educational levels, and smoking statuses. Indeed, the latest figures show that more than half of all Americans are overweight or obese.

For most persons, the optimal approach to weight loss combines mild caloric restriction (energy intake of not lower than 1200 kcal/day), a negative caloric balance (not to exceed 500 to 1000 kcal/day), and an exercise program that promotes a daily caloric expenditure of more than 300 kcal. Multiple short bouts of aerobic exercise have been shown to be as effective, or more effective, than longer continuous sessions in promoting reductions in body weight and fat stores, if the total caloric expenditure is comparable. However, endurance exercise should be complemented with resistance training, which also assists in the maintenance of basal metabolic rate. The goal should be a gradual weight loss (i.e., not more than 1 kg/week) without metabolic derangements such as ketosis.

Finally, it should be recognized that injuries (e.g., ligament sprains, muscle strains, and fractures) can occur while using either free weights or weight machines, especially during higher-level competitive sports and in the recreational setting. To achieve a balanced increase in both muscular strength and endurance, resistance training regimens should include 8 to 10 different exercises at a load that permits 8 to 12 repetitions/set for healthy, sedentary adults or 10 to 15 repetitions/set for participants older than 50 to 60 years of age. The increased repetition range at a lower relative effort for older or frailer patients is designed for injury prevention.

Orientation to a weight training program should be done individually and include instruction and demonstration on setting the resistance, proper body mechanics, optimal range of motion, and avoiding the hemodynamic consequences of expiratory strain. The single greatest cause of musculoskeletal injury in resistance training is a previous injury. Also, higher-intensity lifting (fewer repetitions with heavier weights) can have adverse effects on the knee (leg extension) and shoulder (rotator cuff) joints.

8
CHAPTER

Resistance Training in Women

Lori Ploutz-Snyder, PhD
Syracuse University

Women are increasingly participating in resistance exercises. This participation spans the age range from adolescents and young adults seeking to improve athletic performance to the elderly seeking to maintain independent living. Increasingly, resistance exercises are being prescribed for women as adjunct therapies for various diseases and conditions such as diabetes, obesity, and osteoporosis prevention. This chapter discusses some of the major issues related specifically to women and resistance exercise.

Basic Physiological Responses

These issues can be divided into basic physiological responses such as cellular morphology and fiber type, protein synthesis, neuromuscular adaptation, and hormonal responses unique to females or applied physiological related issues. The first section will discuss basic physiological responses of women to resistance training; the second section will discuss the more applied issues.

Cellular Responses

The plasticity of skeletal muscle is most evident in its response to resistance training. It is generally believed that female and male muscle have the same capacity to adapt to heavy resistance training. However, there are relatively fewer resistance training studies conducted using female subjects. Generally women have a smaller total muscle mass due to smaller cross-sectional area of all fibers. Gender differences have not been reported for fiber-type composition (42). However, gender differences have been reported with respect to the hierarchy of fiber size in the vastus lateralis. In females, the fiber-size order is I > IIa > IIb, in contrast to males where type IIa fibers are the largest and type I the smallest (33, 36, 37). This may help to explain some reports suggesting that women have greater relative muscular endurance than men. One of the most comprehensive cellular studies to assess the effect of heavy resistance training in women utilized 18 weeks of lower-body training at approximately 85% of one-repetition maximum (1-RM) (42). Training was conducted 2 times/week using 3 sets of 6-8 RM (heaviest weight that can be lifted 6-8 times) for squats, leg press, leg extension, and leg curl. The results generally showed that the intracellular components of all fiber types increased with fiber size and that the muscle as a whole became slightly more oxidative. Specific adaptations are shown in table 8.1.

Protein Synthesis

Few studies have evaluated protein synthesis in response to weightlifting specifically in women. One notable study used radioactively labeled phenylalanine to measure fractional synthetic rate of protein synthesis and protein breakdown in the anterior deltoid of trained female swimmers (39). The combination of resistance training and swim exercise induced the greatest increase in fractional synthetic rate (81% increase above resting) compared with either swim training or resistance exercise alone. Resistance exercise alone did not induce a significant increase in the fractional rate of protein synthesis (FSR) above resting values. This is in contrast to the 100% increase in FSR found in both trained and untrained males (4, 6). It is unknown whether this is indeed a significant gender effect or whether the discrepancy is due to methodological issues (different muscle groups and exercise intensities among the studies).

Neuromuscular Responses

It is well known that the early phases of resistance training are associated with rapid increases in muscle strength in the absence of hypertrophy. These changes are typically attributed to neural adaptations—specifically, increases in maximal integrated electromyographic (IEMG) activity and improvements in neural efficiency as measured by the ratio of

TABLE 8.1   Metabolic Parameters Evaluated During Resistance Training in Women

Changes
  Increased cross-sectional area of all fiber types
  Transformation of IIb to IIa fibers
  Increased absolute volume of myofibrils in type I and IIa fibers
  Increased intermyofibrillar space
  Increased mitochondrial size and number
  Increased cytochrome oxidase activity
  Increased hexokinase activity
  Increased absolute volume of lipid droplets in type IIa and IIb fibers

No changes
  Citrate synthase activity
  Creatine kinase activity
  Phosphofructokinase activity
  Glyceraldehyde-phosphate-dehydrogenase activity
  Hydroxyacyl-CoA-dehydrogenase activity
  Capillary density or capillaries per fiber
  Relative volume percent of myofibrils
  Intermyofibrillar space
  Volume percent of mitochondria

IEMG to force production. The magnitude of these changes is similar in men and women (21).

The neuromuscular changes associated with acute resistance exercise have also been studied in women. These changes are related to neuromuscular fatigue and rate of recovery, which are relevant to prescribing exercise for women. Hakkinen evaluated young, middle-aged, and elderly women's neuromuscular fatigue and recovery in response to 5 sets of 10 repetitions to failure using bilateral leg-press exercise (14). Three minutes of rest was allowed between sets. Considerable acute neuromuscular fatigue, as evidenced by decreases in maximal force, force-time characteristics, and maximal voluntary neural activation (IEMG), was observed in all age groups. The fatigue was more pronounced in the young and middle-aged women compared with the elderly. The time needed for recovery varied with the pretraining history of the women and their age. Athletes recovered faster than their sedentary counterparts (who still exhibited reduced force after 2 days of recovery). Young and middle-aged women recovered faster than the elderly. This study highlights the need for individual exercise prescription for resistance training to optimize the frequency of sessions based on activity history and age of adult women.

Hormonal Responses

It is well known that strength training is an effective stimulus for both strength increase and fiber hypertrophy, and it is widely believed that the hormonal milieu is important in regulating the muscle adaptations to resistance training. Testosterone, growth hormone, and other growth factors have been implicated in the hypertrophy response to strength training. A limited number of studies have evaluated the hormonal responses to resistance exercise in women, and gender differences have been reported. Most notable is either a blunted or complete lack of testosterone increase in response to resistance exercise in females compared to males (12, 23, 43). This is not surprising considering the gender differences associated with testosterone production and metabolism. Although most studies do not demonstrate marked testosterone responses to resistance exercise, some studies do show moderate increases. For example, Cumming et al. have shown that women who have performed isokinetic resistance training for 2 months have higher testosterone levels than sedentary controls (8). They also observed acute anticipatory increases in testosterone in the minutes before exercise, which were not associated with changes in luteinizing horomone (LH) or cortisol, suggesting an adrenal response. Late in the exercise bout, elevations were observed in testosterone, LH, follicle-stimulating hormone (FSH), and cortisol. The concentrations of these hormones all correlated significantly with peak lactate and with each other.

A comprehensive study by Kraemer et al. investigated the hormonal responses to varying resistance exercise protocols (24), since the intensity of resistance and rest period length have been suggested as important factors influencing hormonal responses in women. Six different protocols were tested; three were primarily strength workouts (heavier weights and longer rest periods), and three were primarily hypertrophy workouts (lighter weights and shorter rest periods). All protocols were performed for eight different muscle groups. Generally, the greatest changes in hormones were associated with the hypertrophy workouts, in particular, the one that required lifting a 10-RM load with 1 min rest periods. Increases in serum growth hormone, cortisol, and plasma ammonia were observed during and after exercise. No changes were observed in any protocol for serum testosterone or insulin-like growth factor (IGF-1). Decreases in plasma glucose were found for most protocols.

When studying hormone concentrations in response to acute resistance exercise, it is important to consider the marked hemoconcentration that occurs following weightlifting exercises. Because plasma volume can be reduced by 22% immediately following resistance exercise (29), it is important to consider possible dilution effects and correct values for changes in plasma volume.

Regarding exercise prescription, the hypertrophy workouts, which consisted of a whole-body workout lifting a load of 10 RM with 1 min rest, followed by either 10 RM with 3 min rest or 5 RM with 1 min rest, tended to provide the greatest hormonal stimuli in women. It could be suggested that these types of protocols provide the greatest stimulus for hypertrophy in women.

Applied Physiological Responses

The applied physiological responses such as muscle strength and hypertrophy, weight loss and body composition, functional tasks, and issues related to menopause, amenorrhea, and pregnancy will be discussed in the next section.

Muscle Strength and Hypertrophy

Gender differences in absolute strength are well documented. For example, it has been reported that on average, considering whole-body strength, women's strength is only 63.5% that of the average man (25). When lean body mass and muscle group are taken into consideration, these differences are altered. Women's upper-body strength is less than men's regardless of how compared, but women's lower-body strength is comparable to that of their male counterparts. For example, considering 1-RM bench press strength corrected for lean body mass, women are 55% as strong as men are. When leg press strength is corrected for lean body mass, women are actually stronger than men (106%) (44).

Previously it was believed that resistance training could not induce comparable increases in strength in men and women. However, more recent research indicates that in a relative sense resistance training is as beneficial for women as men. Several studies have shown that women can improve their strength at least as rapidly as men can when performing identical resistance training programs (9, 44). Some women may be hesitant to become involved in high-intensity resistance training for fear of becoming "muscle bound." This term refers to a lack of flexibility around the joints, and results only from improperly designed training programs. In fact, several studies have shown that well-designed resistance training programs actually enhance flexibility (45), making this an unnecessary concern. It is widely believed that the resistance exercise prescription for health and fitness should not vary with gender (13).

Weight Loss and Body Composition

Many women may be interested in resistance training to augment weight loss or improve body composition. Hypocaloric dieting is the most potent method of achieving short-term weight loss (34). The greater the caloric restriction, the greater and more rapid the weight loss.

Such dieting has been shown to decrease fat mass, with concomitant adverse reductions in lean body mass, muscle strength (10), and immune function (7, 22). This often has the result of decreasing resting metabolic rate, which makes long-term weight maintenance more difficult. These undesirable consequences are particularly deleterious in middle-aged and elderly women who are already vulnerable to muscle atrophy and decreases in bone mineral density associated with aging. Fortunately, several studies have shown that moderate resistance training is effective for maintaining lean body mass even during severe caloric restriction (5, 10, 34). Furthermore, resistance training is preferable to aerobic type training for maintenance of lean body mass during dieting (5). Moreover, muscle hypertrophy and increased resting metabolic rate can be achieved during hypocaloric dieting (10). Immune function can also be maintained with resistance training. One study has demonstrated that the combination of aerobic and resistance training (resistance exercise alone has not been evaluated) during dieting attenuates some of the immune system impairments usually associated with caloric restriction in obese women (32). Typically, the resistance training prescriptions in these studies used 3 sets of 8-12 repetitions at 70-80% of 1-RM, exercising 6-8 upper- and lower-body muscle groups for about 45 min 3 days/week.

Some women self-report that one of their goals is "spot reduction" of body fat, referring to loss of fat from a specific area of the body, such as the abdominal area. It is important to note that resistance training alone is not effective for reducing skinfold measurements or body girth. For example, a study by Thomas and Ridder demonstrated that abdominal resistance exercises on a variety of different machines were effective in increasing abdominal muscle strength and power, but not effective in altering abdominal skinfold or girth in young women or men (38).

Functional Tasks

Not surprisingly, resistance training has been shown to improve the performance of functional tasks in women of all ages. For example, 14 weeks of resistance training resulted in increases in manual material handling (maximal mass lifted from floor to knuckle height) in young adult women (20). These findings are becoming more important as women move into military and other manual labor-type occupations. Resistance training of the neck muscles for 8 weeks has been shown to be effective in relieving occupational neck pain in middle-aged female office workers (3). Additionally, resistance training has been shown to be useful in maintaining and improving activities of daily living in older women (11). Even in the healthy elderly female population, weight training has been shown to improve walking endurance and other everyday tasks (1).

Menopause

Resistance training in combination with estrogen therapy can have benefits for menopausal women. For example, a study by Notelovitz et al. demonstrated that surgically menopausal women can increase their regional and overall bone mineral density in both the axial and appendicular skeleton using a combination of isotonic resistance training and estrogen replacement (28). Estrogen replacement alone was not sufficient to increase bone mineral density (BMD) and tended to elicit small decreases in bone density over one year. This is important because surgical menopause, usually due to hysterectomy, typically occurs at a younger age than natural menopause and renders such women more vulnerable to osteoporosis and muscle atrophy in later life.

In older (> age 50) naturally postmenopausal women, resistance exercise has also been shown to maintain BMD. Regarding exercise prescription, peak load has been shown to be more important than number of repetitions in influencing BMD (19). Furthermore, resistance training can increase and maintain BMD in younger and middle-aged women, respectively, potentially preventing osteoporosis in later years. Resistance training, even in elderly women, has been shown to have a positive effect on multiple-risk factors for osteoporotic fractures (11).

Resistance training alone, or in combination with weight loss, has been shown to increase insulin action and reduce hyperinsulinemia in naturally postmenopausal women (17, 30). This is especially important in the prevention and treatment of type 2 diabetes, which is prevalent in postmenopausal women, especially those who are obese.

Secondary Amenorrhea

Secondary amenorrhea is the condition in which menstruation ceases in previously menstruating women. This is different from primary amenorrhea in which menstruation has never previously occurred. Secondary amenorrhea has been reported in female athletes engaged in strenuous training. There is evidence that women who participate in resistance exercise are more vulnerable to menstrual irregularities compared with sedentary controls. The prevalence, however, varies with the intensity of resistance exercise. For example, 25% of competitive female Olympic-style weightlifters report irregular menses (26) compared with 14% of those who had competed in only one bodybuilding contest, 2% of recreational lifters, and 4% of sedentary controls (41). It is not known whether this is a result of the resistance exercise per se or of caloric restriction, psychological stress, or other factors associated with competitive resistance exercise. Nevertheless, resistance exercise is associated with fewer menstrual irregularities than aerobic-type exercises, as it has been reported that 50% of competitive runners experience amenorrhea (31).

Pregnancy

Despite the fact that 15-20 million women in the United States are involved in organized exercise programs (15), there is little research related to the physiological effects of exercise during pregnancy. There is even less research specifically related to exercise prescription and resistance training during pregnancy. This is probably due to difficulties with experimental controls, self-selection biases, and ethical concerns of exposing pregnant women to unknown health risks. There is theoretical reason to believe that strength training may be beneficial for pregnant women. For example, development of muscular strength and flexibility may help compensate for the progressive biomechanical changes that occur during pregnancy, specifically related to abdominal muscle weakness and back pain. Furthermore, adequate levels of strength and flexibility likely contribute to an enhanced ability to minimize exaggerations in posture such as thoracic kyphosis and lumbar lordosis, which often accompany pregnancy. Additionally, resistance exercise has been shown to transiently improve glucose control in female type 2 diabetic subjects (18), and may be useful in controlling gestational diabetes. Two studies have evaluated maternal hemodynamic effects of isometric exercise. As expected, both studies showed elevated maternal mean arterial blood pressure and heart rate with acute isometric exercise (27, 40). One of the studies also demonstrated that the increased mean arterial pressure was due to increased total peripheral resistance. Cardiac output was maintained by an increase in heart rate accompanied by a decrease in stroke volume (40). No direct measurements of fetal consequences of resistance exercise have been documented. However, Sorensen et al. (35) have demonstrated no change in umbilical artery blood flow with orthostatic stress, which resulted in greater changes in total peripheral resistance than unilateral knee extension isometric exercise at 15% of maximal voluntary contraction (MVC) sustained until fatigue (40).

Although theory suggests there are benefits to strength training during pregnancy, there has been only one research study to date that has evaluated strength training in pregnant women (16). Each subject (N = 452 exercisers) had an individual exercise prescription that included aerobic and strength training. The strength training was a highly supervised progressive resistance training program where load was increased when the subject could complete 12 repetitions. The muscle groups trained varied by subject, but generally included the whole body. More positive pregnancy outcomes such as lower cesarean section rate, higher Apgar scores, and shorter hospital stays were observed in the subjects who attended the most exercise sessions. There were no negative outcomes reported for any subjects. Exercising subjects subjectively reported an improved self-image, relieved tension, as well as fewer pregnancy-related discomforts. Those who stopped the program for more than two weeks reported more low back pain. This study suggests that the combination of strength and aerobic training provides benefits, with apparently very low risks in women with uncomplicated pregnancies. There is theoretical, but not empirical, evidence to suggest that women who are in late pregnancy should avoid movements that involve heavy loading at the ends of the range of motion. This is based on increased joint laxity due to the hormone relaxin, which is most pronounced in late pregnancy.

In 1985, the American College of Obstetricians and Gynecologists (ACOG) issued recommendations for exercise and pregnancy, although they did not differentiate between aerobic and resistance training. These recommendations were revised in 1994. The ACOG currently recommends an individual exercise prescription and emphasizes that their recommendations are not based on prospective, randomized clinical trials, but rather represent reasonable extrapolations from the existing literature. They note that there are no data for humans to indicate that pregnant women should limit exercise intensity due to potential adverse effects. The current recommendations (see table 8.2) are provided for pregnant women without any additional risk factors for adverse maternal or perinatal outcome (2).

TABLE 8.2 Pregnancy and Postpartum Recommendations of the ACOG (1994)

1. During pregnancy, women can continue to exercise and derive health benefits even from mild-to-moderate exercise routines. Regular exercise (at least three times per week) is preferable to intermittent activity.

2. Women should avoid exercise in the supine position after the first trimester. Such a position is associated with decreased cardiac output in most pregnant women; because the remaining cardiac output will be preferentially distributed away from splanchnic beds (including the uterus) during vigorous exercise, such regimens are best avoided during pregnancy. Prolonged periods of motionless standing should also be avoided.

3. Women should be aware of the decreased oxygen available for aerobic exercise during pregnancy. They should be encouraged to modify the intensity of their exercise according to maternal symptoms. Pregnant women should stop exercising when fatigued and not exercise to exhaustion. Weight-bearing exercises may under some circumstances be continued at intensities similar to those prior to pregnancy throughout pregnancy. Non-weight-bearing exercises such as cycling or swimming will minimize the risk of injury and facilitate the continuation of exercise during pregnancy.

4. Morphologic changes in pregnancy should serve as a relative contraindication to types of exercise in which loss of balance could be detrimental to maternal or fetal well-being, especially in the third trimester. Further, any type of exercise involving the potential for even mild abdominal trauma should be avoided.

(continued)

TABLE 8.2 *(continued)*

5. Pregnancy requires an additional 300 kcal/day in order to maintain metabolic homeostasis. Thus, women who exercise during pregnancy should be particularly careful to ensure an adequate diet.

6. Pregnant women who exercise in the first trimester should augment heat dissipation by ensuring adequate hydration, appropriate clothing, and optimal environmental surroundings during exercise.

7. Many of the physiological and morphologic changes of pregnancy persist 4-6 weeks postpartum. Thus, pre-pregnancy exercise routines should be resumed gradually based on a woman's physical capability.

From American College of Obstetricians and Gynecologists 1994 (2).

Summary

Although women are generally not as strong as men, their ability to increase strength is at least as great as their male counterparts. It is widely believed that the weight training prescription for most women should not differ from an age-matched male, except that the resistance is typically lower. There are very few cellular differences between male and female muscle, the most notable being a different hierarchy of fiber-type size. Resistance training is especially important as part of a comprehensive fitness program. Although most research studies have utilized aerobic training, there is increasing support for use of resistance training in the exercise prescription for various chronic diseases and medical conditions, which may include osteoporosis, diabetes, healthy aging, functional tasks, obesity, and weight loss as well as some conditions unique to women such as pregnancy and menopause.

References

1. Ades, P.A., D.L. Ballor, T. Ashikaga, J.L. Utton, and K.S. Nair. 1996. Weight training improves walking endurance in healthy elderly persons. *Annals of Internal Medicine* 124: 568-572.

2. American College of Obstetricians and Gynecologists. 1994. Exercise during pregnancy and the postpartum period. *International Journal of Gynecology and Obstetrics* 45: 65-70.

3. Berg, H., G. Berggren, and P. Tesch. 1994. Dynamic neck strength training effect on pain and function. *Archives of Physical Medicine and Rehabilitation* 75: 661-665.

4. Biolo, G., S.P. Maggi, B.D. Williams, K. Tipton, and R.R. Wolfe. 1995. Increased rates of muscle protein turnover and amino acid transport after resistance exercise in humans. *American Journal of Physiology (Endocrinology and Metabolism)* 268: E514-E520.

5. Bryner, R.W., I.H. Ullrich, J. Sauers, D. Donley, G. Hornsby, M. Kolar, and R. Yeater. 1999. Effects of resistance vs. aerobic training combined with an 800 calorie liquid diet on lean body mass and resting metabolic rate. *Journal of the American College of Nutrition* 18: 115-121.

6. Carraro, F., C.A. Stuart, W.H. Hartl, J. Rosenblatt, and R.R. Wolfe. 1990. Effect of exercise and recovery on muscle protein synthesis in human subjects. *American Journal of Physiology (Endocrinology and Metabolism)* 258: E821-E831.

7. Chandra, R.K. 1972. Immunocompetence in undernutrition. *Journal of Pediatrics* 81: 1194-1200.

8. Cumming, D., S.R. Wall, M.A. Galbraith, and A.N. Belcastro. 1987. Reproductive hormone responses to resistance exercise. *Medicine and Science in Sports and Exercise* 19: 234-238.

9. Cureton, K.J., M.A. Collins, D.W. Hill, and F.M. McElhannon. 1988. Muscle hypertrophy in men and women. *Medicine and Science in Sports and Exercise* 20: 338-344.

10. Donnelly, J.E., T. Sharp, J. Houmard, M.G. Carlson, J.O. Hill, J.E. Whatley, and R.G. Israel. 1993. Muscle hypertrophy with large-scale weight loss and resistance training. *Journal of Clinical Nutrition* 58: 561-565.

11. Evans, W.J. 1995. Effects of exercise on body composition and functional capacity of the elderly. *Journals of Gerontology. Series A, Biological Sciences and Medical Sciences* 50: 147-150.

12. Fahey, T.D., R. Rolph, P. Moungmee, J. Nagel, and S. Mortara. 1976. Serum testosterone, body composition and strength of young adults. *Medicine and Science in Sports and Exercise* 8: 31-34.

13. Fleck, S.J., and W.J. Kraemer. 1997. *Designing resistance training programs*. 2d ed. Champaign, IL: Human Kinetics.

14. Hakkinen, K. 1995. Neuromuscular fatigue and recovery in women at different ages during heavy resistance loading. *Electromyography and Clinical Neurophysiology* 35: 403-413.

15. Hale, R.W. 1985. *Women and exercise*. Paper presented at the American College of Obstretricians and Gynecologists, Washington, DC.

16. Hall, D.C., and D.A. Kaufmann. 1987. Effects of aerobic and strength conditioning on pregnancy outcomes. *American Journal of Obstetrics and Gynecology* 157: 1199-1203.

17. Henriksson, J. 1995. Influence of exercise on insulin sensitivity. *Journal of Cardiovascular Risk* 2: 303-309.

18. Kanaley, J.A., L.M. Fenicchia, C.S. Miller, K.S. Sagendorf, R. Carhart, R.S. Weinstock, J.L. Azevedo, and L.L. Ploutz-Snyder. 2000. Resistance training is effective in improving glucose concentrations in diabetic women. *Medicine and Science in Sports and Exercise* 32 (5): S291.

19. Kerr, D., A. Morton, I. Dick, and R. Prince. 1996. Exercise effects on bone mass in postmenopausal women are site-specific and load-dependent. *Journal of Bone and Mineral Research* 11: 218-225.

20. Knapik, J.J. 1997. The influence of physical fitness training on the manual material handling capability of women. *Applied Ergonomics* 28: 339-345.

21. Komi, P.V., J.T. Viitasalo, R. Rauramaa, and V. Vihko. 1978. Effect of isometric strength training on mechanical, electrical, and metabolic aspects of muscle function. *European Journal of Applied Physiology* 40: 45-55.

22. Kono, I., H. Kitao, M. Matsuda, S. Hagas, H. Fukushima, and H. Kashiwagi. 1988. Weight reduction in athletes may adversely affect the phagocytotic function of monocytes. *Physician and Sportsmedicine* 16: 56-65.

23. Kraemer, W., S. Gordon, S.J. Fleck, L.J. Marchitelli, R. Mello, J.E. Dziados, K. Friedl, E. Harman, C. Maresh, and A.C. Fry, 1991. Endogenous anabolic hormonal and growth factor responses to heavy resistance exercise in males and females. *International Journal of Sports Medicine* 12: 228-235.

24. Kraemer, W.J., S.J. Fleck, J.E. Dziados, E.A. Harman, L.J. Marchitelli, S.E. Gordon, R. Mello, P.N. Frykman, L.P. Koziris, and N.T. Triplett. 1993. Changes in hormonal concentrations after different heavy-resistance exercise protocols in women. *Journal of Applied Physiology* 75: 594-604.

25. Laubach, L.L. 1976. Comparative muscular strength of men and women: A review of the literature. *Aviation Space and Environmental Medicine* 47: 534-542.
26. Liu, H., P. Liu, and X. Qin. 1987. *Investigation of menstrual cycle in female weightlifters.* Beijing: Department of Exercise Physiology, National Institute of Sports Science.
27. Lotgering, F.K., A. van den Berg, P.C. Struijk, and H.C.S. Wallenberg. 1992. Arterial pressure response to maximal isometric exercise in pregnant women. *American Journal of Obstetrics and Gynecology* 66: 538-542.
28. Notelovitz, M., D. Martin, R. Tesar, F.Y. Khan, C. Probart, C. Fields, and L. McKenzie. 1991. Estrogen therapy and variable-resistance weight training increase bone mineral in surgically menopausal women. *Journal of Bone and Mineral Research* 6: 583-590.
29. Ploutz, L.L., D.L. Tatro, G.A. Dudley, and V.A. Convertino. 1993. Changes in plasma volume and baroreflex function following resistance exercise. *Clinical Physiology* 13: 429-438.
30. Ryan, A.S., R.E. Pratley, A.P. Goldberg, and D. Elahi. 1996. Resistive training increases insulin action in postmenopausal women. *Journals of Gerontology. Series A, Biological Sciences and Medical Sciences* 51: M199-M205.
31. Sanborn, D.F., B.J. Martin, and W.W. Wagner. 1982. Is athletic amenorrhea specific to runners? *American Journal of Obstetrics and Gynecology* 143: 859-861.
32. Scanga, C.B., T.J. Verde, A.M. Paolone, R.E. Andersen, and T.A. Wadden. 1998. Effects of weight loss and exercise training on natural killer cell activity in obese women. *Medicine and Science in Sports and Exercise* 30: 1666-1671.
33. Simoneau, J.A., G. Lortie, M.R. Boulay, and M. Marcotte. 1985. Human skeletal muscle fiber type alteration with high-intensity intermittent training. *European Journal of Applied Physiology* 54: 250-253.
34. Singh, M.A. 1998. Combined exercise and dietary intervention to optimize body composition in aging. *Annals of the New York Academy of Sciences* 20: 378-393.
35. Sorensen, T., S.K. Hendricks, T.R. Easterling, K.L. Carlson, and T.J. Benedetti. 1992. Effect of orthostatic stress on umbilical Dopler waveforms in normal and hypertensive pregnancy. *American Journal of Obstetrics and Gynecology* 167: 643-647.
36. Staron, R.S., R.S. Hikida, F.C. Hagerman, G.A. Dudley, and T. Murray. 1984. Human skeletal muscle fiber type adaptability to various workloads. *Journal of Histochemistry and Cytochemistry* 32: 146-152.
37. Staron, R.S., E.S. Malicky, M.J. Leonardi, J.E. Falkel, F.C. Hagerman, and G.A. Dudley. 1990. Muscle hypertrophy and fast fiber type conversions in heavy resistance-trained women. *European Journal of Applied Physiology* 60: 71-99.
38. Thomas, T.R., and M.B. Ridder. 1989. Resistance exercise program effects on abdominal function and physique. *Journal of Sports Medicine and Physical Fitness* 29: 45-48.
39. Tipton, K.D., A.A. Ferrando, B.D. Williams, and R.R. Wolfe. 1996. Muscle protein metabolism in female swimmers after a combination of resistance and endurance exercise. *Journal of Applied Physiology* 81: 2034-2038.
40. Van Hook, J.W., P. Gill, T.R. Easterling, B. Schmucker, K. Carlson, and T.J. Benedetti. 1993. The hemodynamic effects of isometric exercise during late normal pregnancy. *American Journal of Obstetrics and Gynecology* 169: 870-873.
41. Walberg, J.L., and C.S. Johnston. 1991. Menstrual function and eating behavior in female recreational weight lifters and competitive body builders. *Medicine and Science in Sports and Exercise* 23: 30-36.
42. Wang, N., R.S. Hikida, R.S. Staron, and J.A. Simoneau. 1993. Muscle fiber types of women after resistance training—quantitative ultrastructure and enzyme activity. *Pflugers Archives* 424: 494-502.
43. Weiss, L.W., K.J. Cureton, and F.N. Thompson. 1983. Comparison of serum testosterone and androstenedione responses to weight lifting in men and women. *European Journal of Applied Physiology and Occupational Physiology* 50: 413-419.

44. Wilmore, J.H. 1974. Alterations in strength, body composition, and anthropometric measurements consequent to a 10-week weight training program. *Medicine and Science in Sports and Exercise* 6: 133-138.

45. Wilmore, J.H., R.B. Parr, R.N. Girandola, P. Ward, P.A. Vodak, T.J. Barstow, T.V. Pipes, G.T. Romero, and P. Leslie. 1978. Physiological alterations consequent to circuit weight training. *Medicine and Science in Sports and Exercise* 10: 79-84.

9
CHAPTER

Resistance Exercise, Aging, and Weight Control

William J. Evans, PhD
University of Arkansas for Medical Sciences
and VA Medical Center

Advancing age is associated with a remarkable number of changes in body composition. Reductions in lean body mass have been well characterized and result primarily from losses in skeletal muscle mass (21, 58). This age-related loss in muscle mass has been termed *sarcopenia* (15). Loss in muscle mass accounts for the age-associated decreases in basal metabolic rate, muscle strength, and activity levels, which in turn are the causes of the decreased energy requirements of the elderly. In sedentary individuals, the main determinant of energy expenditure is fat-free mass, which declines by about 15% between the third and eighth decade of life. It also appears that declining caloric needs are not matched by an appropriate decline in caloric intake, ultimately resulting in an increased body-fat content with advancing age. Increased body fatness along with increased abdominal obesity are thought to be directly linked to the greatly increased incidence of type 2 diabetes among the elderly. This chapter describes the extent to which regularly performed exercise can affect protein and energy needs, with particular emphasis on adaptations by elderly people.

Sarcopenia

Sarcopenia, the age-associated loss of muscle mass (15), is a direct cause of the age-related decrease in muscle strength. Our laboratory (21) examined muscle strength and mass in 200 healthy 45-78-year-old men and women and concluded that muscle mass (not function) is the major determinant of the age- and sex-related differences in strength. This relationship is independent of muscle location (upper vs. lower extremities) and function (extension vs. flexion). Reduced muscle strength in the elderly is a major cause of their increased prevalence of disability. With advancing age and the very low activity levels seen in the very old, muscle strength and power are critical components of walking ability (3). The high prevalence of falls among the institutionalized elderly may be a consequence of their lower muscle strength.

This is the question that we have been attempting to address: To what extent are these changes inevitable consequences of aging? Data examining young and middle-aged endurance-trained men demonstrate that body-fat storage and maximal aerobic capacity are not related to age, but rather to the total number of hours these men exercised per week (42). Even among sedentary individuals, energy spent in daily activities explains more than 75% of the variability in body fatness among young and older men (49). These data and the results of other investigators indicate that levels of physical activity are important in determining energy expenditure and ultimately body-fat accumulation. However, the cross-sectional data of Klitgaard et al. indicated that older endurance athletes (runners and swimmers) display fat-free mass and muscle strength similar to that seen in sedentary age-matched controls (35, 36), an indication that endurance exercise alone may not prevent sarcopenia.

Aerobic Exercise

Maximal aerobic capacity ($\dot{V}O_2$max) declines with advancing age (9). This age-associated decrease in $\dot{V}O_2$max has been shown to be approximately 1% per year between the ages of 20 and 70. This decline is likely due to a number of factors, including decreased levels of physical activity, changing cardiac function (including decreased maximal cardiac output), and reduced muscle mass. Flegg and Lakatta determined that skeletal muscle mass accounted for most of the variability in $\dot{V}O_2$max in men and women above the age of 60 (20). Recently, Rosen et al. examined predictors of this age-associated decline in $\dot{V}O_2$max (50). They found $\dot{V}O_2$max declines at the same rate in athletic and sedentary men and that 35% of this decline is due to sarcopenia.

Aerobic exercise has long been an important recommendation for the prevention and treatment of many of the chronic diseases typically associated with old age. These include type 2 diabetes (and those with impaired glucose tolerance), hypertension, heart disease, and osteoporosis. Regularly performed aerobic exercise increases glucose tolerance and insulin action. The responses of initially sedentary young (age 20-30) and older (age 60-70) men and women to 3 months of aerobic conditioning (70% of maximal heart rate, 45 min/day, 3 days/week) were examined by Meredith et al (41). They found that the absolute gains in aerobic capacity were similar between the two age groups. However, the mechanism for adaptation to regular submaximal exercise appears to be different between old and young people. Muscle biopsies taken before and after training showed a more than twofold increase in oxidative capacity of the muscles of the older subjects, while that of the young subjects showed smaller improvements. In addition, skeletal muscle glycogen stores in the older subjects, significantly lower than those of the young men and women initially, increased significantly. The degree to which the elderly demonstrate increases in maximal cardiac output in response to endurance training is still largely unanswered. Seals et al. found no increases after one year of endurance training (54), while, more recently, Spina et al. observed that older men increased maximal cardiac output while healthy older women demonstrated no change in response to endurance exercise (56). If these gender-related differences in cardiovascular response are real, it may explain the lack of response in maximal cardiac output when older men and women are included in the same study population.

Exercise and Carbohydrate Metabolism

The two-hour (2 h) plasma glucose level during an oral glucose tolerance test (OGTT) increases by an average of 5.3 mg/dl per decade, and fasting plasma glucose increases by an average of 1 mg/dl per decade (14). The National Health and Nutrition Examination Survey II (NHANES II) study demonstrated a progressive increase of about 0.4 mmol per decade of life in mean plasma glucose value 2 h after a 75 g OGTT ($N =$ 1,678 men and 1,892 women) (26). Shimokata et al. examined glucose tolerance in community-dwelling men and women ranging in age from 17 to 92 (55). By assessing level of obesity, pattern of body-fat distribution, and activity and fitness levels, they attempted to examine the independent effect of age on glucose tolerance. They found no significant differences between the young and middle-aged groups; however, the older groups had significantly higher glucose and insulin values (following a glucose challenge) than young or middle-aged groups. They concluded, "The major finding of this study is that the decline in glucose tolerance from the early-adult to the middle-age years is entirely explained by secondary influences (fatness and fitness), whereas the decline from mid-life to old age still is also influenced by chronological age. This finding is unique. It is also unexplained" (55, p. 50). However, it must be pointed out that anthropometric determination of body fatness becomes increasingly less accurate with advancing age and does not reflect the intra-abdominal and intramuscular accumulation of fat that occurs with aging (5). The results of this study may be due more to an underestimation of true body-fat levels than to age per se. These age-associated changes in glucose tolerance can result in type 2 diabetes and the broad array of associated abnormalities. Stolk et al. recently noted that in a large population of elderly men and women (>55 years), serum glucose and fructosamine levels were seen to be higher in subjects with retinopathy compared with those without (57). Within the groups with retinopathy, serum glucose was significantly associated with the number of hemorrhages. These relationships were independent of body composition, abdominal obesity, or the presence of type 2 diabetes.

The relationship between aging, body composition, activity, and glucose tolerance was also examined in 270 female and 462 male factory workers aged 22 to 73 years, none of whom were retired (66). Plasma glucose levels, both fasting and after a glucose load, increased with age, but the correlation between age and total integrated glucose response following a glucose load was weak; in women, only 3% of the variance could be attributed to age. When activity levels and drug use were factored in, age accounted for only 1% of the variance in women and 6.25% in men.

The fact that aerobic exercise has significant effects on skeletal muscle may help explain its importance in the treatment of glucose intolerance and type 2 diabetes. Seals et al. found that a high-intensity training program produced greater improvements in the subjects' insulin response to an oral glucose load than lower-intensity aerobic exercise (53). However, their subjects began the study with normal glucose tolerance. Kirwan et al. found that 9 months of endurance training at 80% of the maximal heart rate (4 days/week) resulted in reduced glucose-stimulated insulin levels (34); however, no comparison was made to a lower-intensity exercise group. Hughes et al. demonstrated that regularly performed aerobic exercise without weight loss resulted in improved glucose tolerance, rate of insulin-stimulated glucose disposal, and increased skeletal muscle GLUT-4 (the glucose transporter protein in skeletal muscle) levels in older glucose intolerance subjects (31). In this investigation, a moderate-intensity aerobic exercise program was compared to a higher-intensity program (50% versus 75% of maximal heart rate reserve, 55 min/day, 4 days/week, for 12 weeks). No differences were seen between the moderate- and higher-intensity aerobic exercise on glucose tolerance, insulin sensitivity, or muscle GLUT-4 levels. Thus, a prescription of moderate aerobic exercise is recommended for older men or women with type 2 diabetes or at high risk for it to help ensure compliance with the program because people are less likely to comply with high-intensity activity.

Endurance training and dietary modifications are generally recommended as the primary treatment in the type 2 diabetic. Cross-sectional analysis of dietary intake supports the hypothesis that a low-carbohydrate/high-fat diet is associated with the onset of type 2 diabetes (40). This evidence, however, is not supported by prospective studies where dietary habits have not been related to the development of type 2 diabetes (17, 39). The effects of a high-carbohydrate diet on glucose tolerance have been equivocal (6, 23). Hughes et al. compared the effects of a high-carbohydrate (60% carbohydrate and 20% fat) / high-fiber (25 g dietary fiber/1000 kcal) diet with and without 3 months of high-intensity (75% max heart rate reserve, 50 min/day, 4 days/week) endurance exercise in older, glucose-intolerant men and women (30). Subjects were fed all of their food on a metabolic ward during the 3-month study and were not allowed to lose weight. These investigators observed no improvement in glucose tolerance or insulin-stimulated glucose uptake in either the diet or the diet plus exercise group. The exercise plus high-carbohydrate diet group demonstrated a significant and substantial increase in skeletal muscle glycogen content, and at the end of the training the muscle glycogen stores would be considered saturated. Since the primary site of glucose disposal is skeletal muscle glycogen stores, the extremely high muscle glycogen content associated with exercise and a high-carbohydrate diet likely limited the rate of glucose disposal. Thus, when combined with exercise and a weight-maintenance diet, a high-carbohydrate diet had a counter-regulatory effect. The value of a high-carbohydrate/high-fiber diet in the treatment of excess body fat is likely an important cause of the impaired glucose tolerance. Recently, Schaefer et al. demonstrated that older subjects consuming an ad libitum high-carbohydrate diet lost weight (52).

There appears to be no attenuation of the response of elderly men and women to regularly performed aerobic exercise compared to that seen in young subjects. Increased fitness levels are associated with reduced mortality and increased life expectancy. Helmrich et al. also showed that increased fitness levels prevent the occurrence of type 2 diabetes in individuals that are at the greatest risk for developing this disease (27). Thus, regularly performed aerobic exercise is an important way for older people to improve their glucose tolerance.

Strength Training

While endurance exercise has been the more traditional means of increasing cardiovascular fitness, strength or resistance training is currently recommended by the American College of Sports Medicine as an important component of an overall fitness program (1). This is particularly important in the elderly, where loss of muscle mass and weakness are prominent deficits.

Strength conditioning or progressive resistance training is generally defined as training in which the resistance that a muscle generates force against is progressively increased over time. Progressive resistance training involves few contractions against a heavy load. The metabolic and morphological adaptations resulting from resistance and endurance exercise are quite different. Muscle strength has been shown to increase in response to training between 60 and 100% of the one-repetition maximum (1-RM, the maximum amount of weight that can be lifted with one contraction). Strength conditioning will result in an increase in muscle size, and this increase in size is largely the result of increased contractile proteins. The mechanisms by which the mechanical events stimulate an increase in RNA synthesis and subsequent protein synthesis are not well understood. Lifting weight requires that a muscle shorten as it produces force. This is called a concentric contraction. Lowering the weight, on the other hand, forces the muscle to lengthen as it produces force. This is an eccentric muscle contraction. These lengthening muscle contractions have been shown to produce ultrastructural damage that may stimulate increased muscle protein turnover (16).

Our laboratory examined the effects of high-intensity resistance training of the knee extensors and flexors (80% of 1-RM, 3 days/week) in older men (age 60-72 years). The average increase in knee flexor and extensor strength were 227% and 107%, respectively. Computed tomography (CT) scans and muscle biopsies were used to determine muscle size. Total muscle area by CT analysis increased by 11.4%, while the muscle biopsies showed an increase of 33.5% in type I fiber area and 27.5% increase in type II fiber area. In addition, lower-body $\dot{V}O_2$max increased significantly while upper-body $\dot{V}O_2$max did not, indicating that increased muscle mass can increase maximal aerobic power. It appears that the age-related loss in muscle mass may be an important determinant in the reduced maximal aerobic capacity seen in elderly men and women (20). Improving muscle strength can enhance the capacity of many older men and women to perform many activities, such as climbing stairs, carrying packages, and even walking.

We have applied this same training program to a group of frail, institutionalized elderly men and women (mean age 90 ± 3 years, range 87-96) (18). After 8 weeks of training, the 10 subjects in this study increased muscle strength by almost 180% and muscle size by 11%. In a more recent study by Fiatarone et al., a similar intervention on frail nursing home residents demonstrated not only increases in muscle strength and size, but increased gait speed, stair-climbing power, and balance (19). In addition, spontaneous activity levels increased significantly, while the activity of a nonexercised control group was unchanged. In this study, the effects of a protein/calorie supplement (240 ml liquid supplying 360 kcal in the form of carbohydrate [60%], fat [23%], and soy-based protein [17%] designed to augment caloric intake by about 20% and provide one-third of the recommended daily allowance [RDA] of vitamins and minerals) combined with exercise was also examined. While no interaction was seen with muscle strength, functional capacity, or muscle size (no differences in improvements between the supplemented group and a nonsupplemented control group), the men and women that consumed the supplement and exercised gained weight compared to the three other groups examined (exercise/control, nonexercise supplemented, and nonexercise control). The nonexercising subjects who received the supplement reduced their habitual dietary energy intake so that total energy intake was unchanged. It should be pointed out that this was a very old, very frail population with diagnoses of multiple chronic diseases. The increase in overall levels of physical activity have been a common observation in our studies (19, 22, 44). Since muscle weakness is a primary deficit in many older individuals, increased strength may stimulate more aerobic activities like walking and cycling.

Strength training may increase balance by strengthening the muscle involved in walking. Indeed, ankle weakness has been demonstrated to be associated with increased risk of falling in nursing home patients (60). However, balance training, which may demonstrate very little improvement in muscle strength, size, or cardiovascular changes, has also been demonstrated to decrease the risk of falls in older people (63). Tai Chi, a form of dynamic balance training that requires no new technology or equipment, has been demonstrated to reduce the risk of falling in older people by almost 50% (62). As a component of the National Institute on Aging FICSIT trials (Frailty and Injuries: Cooperative Studies of Intervention Techniques), individuals aged 70+ were randomized to Tai Chi (TC), individualized balance training (BT), and exercise control education (ED) groups for 15 weeks (38). In a follow-up assessment 4 months postintervention, 130 subjects responded to exit interview questions asking about perceived benefits of participation. Both TC and BT subjects reported increased confidence in balance and movement, but only TC subjects reported that their daily activities and their overall life had been affected; many of these subjects had changed their normal physical activity to incorporate ongoing TC practice. The data suggest that when mental as well as physical control is perceived to be enhanced, with a generalized sense of improvement in overall well-being, older persons' motivation to continue exercising also increases. Province et al.

examined the overall effect of many different exercise interventions in the FICSIT trials on reducing falls (47). While these separate interventions alone were not powerful enough to allow conclusions to be made about their effects on the incidence of falls in an elderly population, investigators did conclude that "all training domains, taken together under the heading of 'general exercise,' showed an effect on falls." This probably demonstrates the 'rising tide raises all boats' principle, in which training that targets one domain may improve performance somewhat in other domains as a consequence. If this is so, then the differences seen on fall risk due to the exact nature of the training may not be as critical compared with the differences in not training at all. Recently, the use of a community-based exercise program for frail older people was examined (29). Participants were predominantly sedentary women over age 70 with multiple chronic conditions. The program was conducted with peer leaders to facilitate its continuation after the research demonstration phase. In addition to having positive health outcomes related to functional mobility, blood pressure maintenance, and overall well-being, this intervention was successful in sustaining active participation in regular physical activity through the use of peer leaders selected by the program participants.

Exercise and Weight Loss

In addition to its effect on increasing muscle mass and function, resistance training can also have an important effect on energy balance of elderly men and women (11). Men and women participating in a resistance training program of the upper- and lower-body muscles required approximately 15% more calories to maintain body weight after 12 weeks of training compared to their pretraining energy requirements. This increase in energy needs resulted from an increased resting metabolic rate, the small energy cost of the exercise, and what was presumed to be an increase in activity levels. While endurance training has been demonstrated to be an important adjunct to weight loss programs in young men and women by increasing their daily energy expenditure, its utility in treating obesity in the elderly may not be great. This is because many sedentary older men and women do not spend many calories when they perform endurance exercise, due to their low fitness levels. Thirty to forty minutes of exercise may increase energy expenditure by only 100 to 200 kcals, with very little residual effect on calorie expenditure. Aerobic exercise training will not preserve lean body mass to any great extent during weight loss. Because resistance training can preserve or even increase muscle mass during weight loss, this type of exercise for those older men and women who must lose weight may be of genuine benefit.

We have recently observed clear gender-related responses to resistance exercise training in older individuals (32). Moderately overweight men ($n = 18$) and women ($n = 17$) (aged 54-71 years, body mass index [BMI] 26-36 kg · m^{-2}) participated in a 12-week progressive resistance training program (3 days/week, 80% of 1-RM). Seventeen of the men completed 23 exercise sessions (100% compliance) and one man completed 22 sessions (95.7%). Each of the women completed all of the sessions. No special diet or dietary restrictions were imposed on these subjects, and they were all free-living during the time of the experiment. As a result of the training, a significant time-by-sex interaction was observed. The men had an increase in fat-free mass (FFM) and a decrease in percent body fat (%BF) and fat mass (FM), while the women demonstrated no change in FFM, %BF, or FM (see figure 9.1). These data indicate clear gender-related differences in response to resistance exercise training and indicate that responses of men and women should be examined separately. We also examined the effects of resistance exercise on muscle strength and power in elderly versus young men and women (33). While no age-related differences were seen in strength gain, a

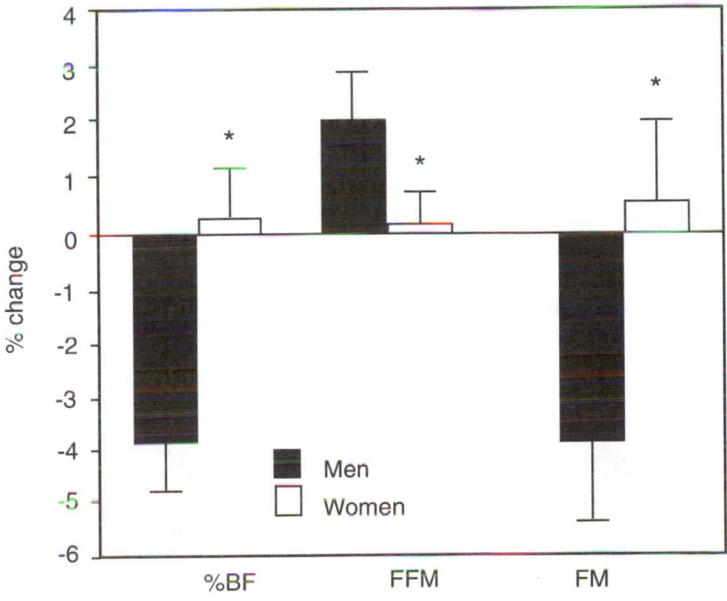

Figure 9.1 Comparison of relative change in body composition after 12 weeks of high-intensity progressive resistance exercise training. These data demonstrate a greater gain in FFM and reduction in FM in men versus women performing similar exercise training. * Significant time-by-sex interaction, $p < 0.05$.

Adapted from Joseph et al. 1999 (32).

gender-related difference was seen, with old and young men gaining more absolute and relative strength than women in response to the same exercise training regimen.

Aerobic exercise is generally prescribed as an important adjunct to a weight loss program. Aerobic exercise combined with weight loss has been demonstrated to increase insulin action to a greater extent than weight loss through diet restriction alone. In the study by Bogardus et al., diet therapy alone improved glucose tolerance, mainly by reducing basal endogenous glucose production and improving hepatic sensitivity to insulin (4). Aerobic exercise training, on the other hand, increased carbohydrate storage rates, and therefore "diet therapy plus physical training produced a more significant approach toward normal" (4, p. 318). However, aerobic exercise (as opposed to resistance training) combined with a hypocaloric diet has been demonstrated to result in a greater reduction in resting metabolic rate (RMR) than diet alone (46). Heymsfield et al. found aerobic exercise combined with caloric restriction did not preserve FFM and did not further accelerate weight loss when compared with diet alone (28). This lack of an effect of aerobic exercise may have been due to a greater decrease in RMR in the exercising group. In perhaps the most comprehensive study of its kind, Goran and Poehlman examined components of energy metabolism in older men and women engaged in regular endurance training (25). They found that endurance training did not increase total daily energy expenditure, due to a compensatory decline in physical activity during the remainder of the day. In other words, when elderly subjects participated in a regular walking program, they rested more, so activities outside of walking decreased, and thus 24 h calorie expenditure was unchanged. However, older individuals who had been participating in endurance exercise for most of their lives have been shown to have a greater RMR and total daily energy expenditure than did age-matched sedentary controls (61). Bryner et al. compared the effects of aerobic exercise (AE; walking, biking 1 h/day, 4 days/week) + very low-calorie diet (VLCD; 800 kcal/d) versus resistance exercise (RE) + VLCD (7). They found that maximum oxygen consumption increased significantly ($p < 0.05$) but equally in both groups. Body weight decreased significantly more ($p < 0.01$) in the AE group than in those participating in RE. The AE group lost a significant ($p < 0.05$) amount of fat-free mass (FFM; 51 to 47 kg), while no change was observed in the RE group. In addition, the RE group demonstrated an increase ($p < 0.05$) in RMR O_2 ml $\cdot$ kg^{-1} $\cdot$ min^{-1} (2.6 to 3.1). The 24 h RMR decreased ($p < 0.05$) in the AE group. The authors concluded that the addition of an intensive, high-volume resistance training program resulted in preservation of lean body weight (LBW) and RMR during weight loss with a VLCD.

Ballor et al. compared the effects of resistance training to those of diet restriction alone in obese women (2). They found that resistance exercise training results in increased strength and gains in muscle size as well as a preservation of FFM during weight loss. These data are similar to the results of Pavlou et al., who used both aerobic and resistance training as an adjunct to a weight loss program in obese men (45). Kraemer et al. found no significant difference between regular aerobic exercise versus resistance exercise training (when combined with a hypocaloric diet) on visceral fat content, preservation of muscle size, and oral glucose (37). In this study, the exercise groups demonstrated a significantly greater loss of visceral fat and preservation of muscle size than with diet alone. Similarly, Rice et al. found no difference between diet with aerobic exercise and diet with resistance exercise on visceral fat and oral glucose tolerance, and both groups demonstrated greater effects than with diet alone (48). In both studies (37, 48), improved glucose tolerance was significantly related to reductions in visceral fat content.

Protein Needs and Aging

Previous estimates of dietary protein needs of the elderly using nitrogen (N) balance have ranged from 0.59 to $0.8\,g \cdot kg^{-1} \cdot d^{-1}$ (24, 59, 65). However, the low value was reported by Zanni et al., who preceded their 10-day dietary protein feeding with a 17-day protein-free diet, which was likely to improve nitrogen retention during the 10-day balance period (65). Recently, we (10) reassessed the N-balance studies mentioned above using the currently accepted 1985 World Health Organization (WHO) N-balance formula (64). These newly recalculated data were combined with N-balance data collected on 12 healthy older men and women (age range 56-80 years, 8 men and 4 women) consuming the current RDA for protein or double this amount ($0.8\,g \cdot kg^{-1} \cdot d^{-1}$ and $1.6\,g \cdot kg^{-1} \cdot d^{-1}$, respectively) in our laboratory. Our subjects consumed the diet for 11 consecutive days, and N-balance ($mg\,N \cdot kg^{-1} \cdot d^{-1}$) was measured during days 6 to 11. The estimated mean protein requirements from the three retrospectively assessed studies and the current study can be combined by weighted averaging to produce an overall protein requirement estimate of $0.91 \pm 0.043\,g \cdot kg^{-1} \cdot d^{-1}$. The combined estimate excluding the data from our 12 subjects is 0.894 ± 0.048 g protein $\cdot kg^{-1} \cdot d^{-1}$.

The current RDA in the United States of $0.8\,g \cdot kg^{-1} \cdot d^{-1}$ is based on data collected, for the most part, on young subjects. The RDA includes an upward adjustment based on the coefficient of variability (CV) of the average requirement established in these studies ($0.6\,g \cdot kg^{-1} \cdot d^{-1}$). Based on the CV previously established for N-balance studies, an adequate dietary protein level for 97.5% of the elderly population would be provided by an intake of 25% (twice the standard deviation [SD]) above the mean protein requirement. Our data suggests that the safe protein intake for elderly adults is 1.25 g · kg^{-1} · d^{-1}. On the basis of the current and recalculated short-term N-balance results, a safe recommended protein intake for older men and women should be set at 1.0-1.25 g of high-quality protein · kg^{-1} · d^{-1}. Sahyoun reported that approximately 50% of 946 healthy free-living men and women above the age of 60 living in the Boston, Massachusetts, area consumed less than this amount of protein, and 25% of the elderly men and women in this survey consumed <0.86 g and <0.81 g protein · kg^{-1} · d^{-1}, respectively (51). As noted in a study by Bunker et al., a large percentage of homebound elderly people consuming their habitual dietary protein intake (0.67 g mixed protein · kg^{-1} · d^{-1}) have been shown to be in negative N-balance (8).

We examined the effects of marginal dietary protein intake in 12 sedentary healthy women, aged 66-79 (13). They were admitted into a 9-week metabolic study and consumed a meat-free diet containing 0.45 or 0.93 g protein · kg^{-1} · d^{-1}. The nonprotein energy in the diet was provided by carbohydrates (65%) and fat (35%). Six-day N-balance periods were measured during study days 16-21 (week 3) and days 56-61 (week 9). In addition to the N-balance, body composition (total body potassium, body density [underwater weighing], and dual-energy X-ray absorptiometry), whole-body leucine kinetics ([1 – ^{13}C] leucine infusion), muscle fiber area, immune function (delayed hypersensitivity), urinary creatinine and 3-methylhistidine, muscle strength, and plasma IGF-1 (insulin-like growth factor) were measured while the women consumed 1.2 g protein · kg^{-1} · d^{-1} at baseline and after adaptation to the two different dietary protein levels (week 9). This study demonstrated that long-term adaptation to 0.45 g protein · kg^{-1} · d^{-1} resulted in an accommodation, which led to reductions in ^{40}K (active cell mass), skeletal muscle mass, muscle strength, and immune function. Leucine oxidation rates were a more sensitive index of the adequacy of protein intake than synthesis, flux, or metabolic rate. N-balance was negative in the low-protein group. The greatest losses in body nitrogen occurred during the first balance period; however, the women on the low-protein intake remained in negative N-balance throughout the trial. The change in IGF-1 levels was significantly associated with the change in N-balance, body cell mass, muscle fiber size, and skeletal muscle and immune function. Inadequate dietary protein intake may be an important cause of sarcopenia. These data demonstrate that the compensatory response to long-term decreases in dietary protein intake is a loss in lean body mass.

We recently examined the adequacy of the current RDA for protein for healthy elderly men and women by examining the effects of long-term consumption (15 weeks) of a eucaloric diet providing 0.8 g protein · kg^{-1} · d^{-1} (12). Subjects demonstrated a significant and continued reduction in urinary nitrogen losses throughout the period of the study, indicating a significant accommodation to the diet. CT scans of the thigh muscle showed that the subjects who consumed the RDA for protein and did not exercise lost a significant amount of skeletal muscle, confirming our hypothesis that the RDA for protein is inadequate for older individuals. The reduction in muscle area observed by CT and the change in urinary nitrogen excretion were significantly related. Muscle biopsies taken from the medial vastus lateralis confirm the CT scan data by demonstrating a significant reduction in the muscle fiber area of type II muscle cells in the sedentary group of subjects. This study demonstrates that healthy elderly people may have a greater need for dietary protein than previous estimates, and the current RDA may not meet these needs.

High-intensity resistance training appears to have profoundly anabolic effects in the elderly. Data from our laboratory demonstrate a 10-15% decrease in N-excretion at the initiation of training that persists for 12 weeks. That is, progressive resistance training improved N-balance; thus older subjects performing resistance training have a lower mean protein requirement than do sedentary subjects. These results are somewhat at variance with our previous research (43) demonstrating that regularly performed aerobic exercise causes an increase in the mean protein requirement of middle-aged and young endurance athletes. This difference likely results from increased oxidation of amino acids during aerobic exercise that may not be present during resistance training.

We recently examined the effects of resistance training on N-balance in subjects with mild to moderate chronic renal failure (CRF; unpublished observation). Five women (62 ± 10 years old, BMI = 30.3 ± 4 kg/m^2, creatinine clearance = 56 ± 22 ml/min) were studied before and after a 4-week resistance training protocol (2 upper-body and 3 lower-body exercises, 3 sets of 8 repetitions, at 80% of 1-RM, 3 days/week) (unpublished observation). All of the women consumed a diet providing 0.6 g $\cdot$ kg$^{-1} \cdot$ d^{-1} protein for 3 weeks before and during the training period. Body weight was maintained at ± 0.5 kg of baseline weight. At week 3 of baseline and week 4 of resistance training, 24 h urine collections and food homogenates were collected during 4 consecutive days and analyzed for total nitrogen by the Kjeldahl method. With resistance training, strength increased $11 \pm 6\%$ for the upper body ($p < 0.05$) and $17 \pm 6\%$ ($p < 0.01$) for the lower body. Glomerular filtration rate estimated by insulin clearance (57 ± 26 ml/min), renal plasma flow estimated by p-aminohyppurate clearance (277 ± 146 ml/min), and %BF ($42.3 \pm 6.2\%$) and FFM estimated by underwater weighing (44.8 ± 4.2 kg) did not change during the intervention. Urinary nitrogen excretion decreased $10.7 \pm 7.9\%$ (0.56 ± 0.4 g N/day, $p < 0.05$), and estimated N-balance increased from -0.34 ± 0.58 to 0.08 ± 0.41 g N/day ($p < 0.05$). These results demonstrate that resistance training in CRF patients is safe, increases nitrogen retention, and reduces renal handling of nitrogen. Strength training may, therefore, be an important clinical tool in the treatment of CRF, especially to prevent muscle wasting.

Muscle Strength Training in the Elderly

In conclusion, there is no other group in our society that can benefit more from regularly performed exercise than the elderly. While both aerobic and strength conditioning are highly recommended, only strength training can stop or reverse sarcopenia. Increased muscle strength and mass in the elderly can be the first step toward a lifetime of increased physical activity and a realistic strategy for maintaining functional status and independence.

References

1. American College of Sports Medicine. 1998. The recommended quantity and quality of exercise for developing and maintaining cardiorespiratory and muscular fitness, and flexibility in healthy adults. *Medicine and Science in Sports and Exercise* 30: 975-991.
2. Ballor, D.L., V.L. Katch, M.D. Becque, and C.R. Marks. 1988. Resistance weight training during caloric restriction enhances lean body weight maintenance. *American Journal of Clinical Nutrition* 47: 19-25.
3. Bassey, E.J., M.A. Fiatarone, E.F. O'Neill, M. Kelly, L.A. Lipsitz, and W.J. Evans. 1992. Leg extensor power and functional performance in very old men and women. *Clinical Science* 82: 321-327.
4. Bogardus, C., E. Ravussin, D.C. Robbins, R.R. Wolfe, E.S. Horton, and E.A.H. Sims. 1984. Effects of physical training and diet therapy on carbohydrate metabolism in patients with glucose intolerance and non-insulin-dependent diabetes mellitus. *Diabetes* 33: 311-318.
5. Borkan, G.A., D.E. Hultz, and A.F. Gerzoff. 1983. Age changes in body composition revealed by computed tomography. *Journal of Gerontology* 38: 673-677.
6. Borkman, M., L.V. Campbell, D.J. Chisholm, and L.H. Storlien. 1991. Comparison of the effects on insulin sensitivity of high carbohydrate and high fat diets in normal subjects. *Journal of Clinical Endocrinology* 72: 432-437.
7. Bryner, R.W., I.H. Ullrich, J. Sauers, D. Donley, G. Hornsby, M. Kolar, and R. Yeater. 1999. Effects of resistance vs. aerobic training combined with an 800 calorie liquid diet on lean body mass and resting metabolic rate. *Journal of the American College of Nutrition* 18: 115-121.
8. Bunker, V., M. Lawson, M. Stansfield, and B. Clayton. 1987. Nitrogen balance studies in apparently healthy elderly people and those who are housebound. *British Journal of Nutrition* 57: 211-221.
9. Buskirk, E.R., and J.L. Hodgson. 1987. Age and aerobic power: The rate of change in men and women. *Federation Proceedings* 46: 1824-1829.
10. Campbell, W.W., M.C. Crim, G.E. Dallal, V.R. Young, and W.J. Evans. 1994. Increased protein requirements in the elderly: New data and retrospective reassessments. *American Journal of Clinical Nutrition* 60: 167-175.
11. Campbell, W.W., M.C. Crim, V.R. Young, and W.J. Evans. 1994. Increased energy requirements and body composition changes with resistance training in older adults. *American Journal of Clinical Nutrition* 60: 167-175.

12. Campbell, W.W., T.A. Trappe, R.R. Wolfe, and W.J. Evans. In review. Older people who consume the Recommended Dietary Allowance for protein accommodate with decreased skeletal muscle.

13. Castaneda, C., G.G. Dolnikowski, G.E. Dallal, W.J. Evans, and M.C. Crim. 1995. Protein turnover and energy metabolism of elderly women fed a low-protein diet. *American Journal of Clinical Nutrition* 62: 40-48.

14. Davidson, M.B. 1979. The effect of aging on carbohydrate metabolism. A review of the English literature and a practical approach to the diagnosis of diabetes mellitus in the elderly. *Metabolism* 28: 688-705.

15. Evans, W. 1995. What is sarcopenia? *Journal of Gerontology* 50A (special issue): 5-8.

16. Evans, W.J., and J.G. Cannon. 1991. The metabolic effects of exercise-induced muscle damage. In *Exercise and sport sciences reviews,* edited by J.O. Holloszy, 99-126. Baltimore: Williams & Wilkins.

17. Feskens, E.J.M., and D. Kromhout. 1989. Cardiovascular risk factors and the 25-year incidence of diabetes mellitus in middle-aged men. *American Journal of Epidemiology* 130: 1101-1108.

18. Fiatarone, M.A., E.C. Marks, N.D. Ryan, C.N. Meredith, L.A. Lipsitz, and W.J. Evans. 1990. High-intensity strength training in nonagenarians. Effects on skeletal muscle. *Journal of the American Medical Association* 263: 3029-3034.

19. Fiatarone, M.A., E.F. O'Neill, N.D. Ryan, K.M. Clements, G.R. Solares, M.E. Nelson, S.B. Roberts, J.J. Kehayias, L.A. Lipsitz, and W.J. Evans. 1994. Exercise training and nutritional supplementation for physical frailty in very elderly people. *New England Journal of Medicine* 330: 1769-1775.

20. Flegg, J.L., and E.G. Lakatta. 1988. Role of muscle loss in the age-associated reduction in VO_2max. *Journal of Applied Physiology* 65: 1147-1151.

21. Frontera, W.R., V.A. Hughes, and W.J. Evans. 1991. A cross-sectional study of upper and lower extremity muscle strength in 45-78-year-old men and women. *Journal of Applied Physiology* 71: 644-650.

22. Frontera, W.R., C.N. Meredith, K.P. O'Reilly, and W.J. Evans. 1990. Strength training and determinants of VO_2max in older men. *Journal of Applied Physiology* 68: 329-333.

23. Garg, A., S.M. Grundy, and R.H. Unger. 1992. Comparison of effects of high and low carbohydrate diets on plasma lipoprotein and insulin sensitivity in patients with mild NIDDM. *Diabetes* 41: 1278-1285.

24. Gersovitz, M., H. Munro, N. Scrimshaw, and V. Young. 1982. Human protein requirements: Assessment of the adequacy of the current recommended dietary allowance for dietary protein in elderly men and women. *American Journal of Clinical Nutrition* 35: 6-14.

25. Goran, M.I., and E.T. Poehlman. 1992. Endurance training does not enhance total energy expenditure in healthy elderly persons. *American Journal of Physiology* 263: E950-E957.

26. Hadden, W.C., and M.I. Harris. 1987. *Prevalence of diagnosed diabetes, undiagnosed diabetes, and impaired glucose tolerance in adults 20-74 years of age: United States, 1976-1980.* DHHS PHS Publication No. 87-1687. Washington, DC: U.S. Government Printing Office.

27. Helmrich, S.P., D.R. Ragland, R.W. Leung, and R.S. Paffenbarger Jr. 1991. Physical activity and reduced occurrence of non-insulin-dependent diabetes mellitus. *New England Journal of Medicine* 325: 147-152.

28. Heymsfield, S.B., K. Casper, J. Hearn, and D. Guy. 1989. Rate of weight loss during underfeeding: Relation to level of physical activity. *Metabolism* 38: 215-223.

29. Hickey, T., P.A. Sharpe, F.M. Wolf, L.S. Robins, M.B. Wagner, and W. Harik. 1996. Exercise participation in a frail elderly population. *Journal of Health Care for the Poor and Underserved* 7: 219-231.

30. Hughes, V.A., M.A. Fiatarone, R.A. Fielding, C.M. Ferrara, D. Elahi, and W.J. Evans. 1995. Long-term effects of a high carbohydrate diet and exercise on insulin action in older subjects with impaired glucose tolerance. *American Journal of Clinical Nutrition* 62: 426-433.

31. Hughes, V.A., M.A. Fiatarone, R.A. Fielding, B.B. Kahn, C.M. Ferrara, P. Shepherd, E.C. Fisher, R.R. Wolfe, D. Elahi, and W.J. Evans. 1993. Exercise increases muscle GLUT 4 levels and insulin action in subjects with impaired glucose tolerance. *American Journal of Physiology* 264: E855-E862.

32. Joseph, L.J.O., S.L. Davey, W.J. Evans, and W.W. Campbell. 1999. Differential effect of resistance training on body composition and lipoprotein-lipid profile in older men and women. *Metabolism* 48: 1474-1480.

33. Jozsi, A.C., W.W. Campbell, L. Joseph, S.L. Davey, and W.J. Evans. 1999. Changes in power with resistance training in older and younger men and women. *Journal of Gerontology* 54A (11): M591-M596.

34. Kirwan, J.P., W.M. Kohrt, D.M. Wojta, R.E. Bourey, and J.O. Holloszy. 1993. Endurance exercise training reduces glucose-stimulated insulin levels in 60- to 70-year-old men and women. *Journal of Gerontology* 48: M84-M90.

35. Klitgaard, H., M. Mantoni, S. Schiaffino, S. Ausoni, L. Gorza, C. Laurent-Winter, P. Schnohr, and B. Saltin. 1990. Function, morphology and protein expression of ageing skeletal muscle: A cross-sectional study of elderly men with different training backgrounds. *Acta Physiologica Scandinavica* 140: 41-54.

36. Klitgaard, H., M. Zhou, S. Schiaffino, R. Betto, G. Salviati, and B. Saltin. 1990. Ageing alters the myosin heavy chain composition of single fibres from human skeletal muscle. *Acta Physiologica Scandinavica* 140: 55-62.

37. Kraemer, W.J., J.S. Volek, K.L. Clark, S.E. Gordon, S.M. Puhl, L.P. Koziris, J.M. McBride, N.T. Triplett-McBride, M. Putukian, R.U. Newton, K. Hakkinen, J.A. Bush, and W.J. Sebastianelli. 1999. Influence of exercise training on physiological and performance changes with weight loss in men. *Medicine and Science in Sports and Exercise* 31: 1320-1329.

38. Kutner, N.G., H. Barnhart, S.L. Wolf, E. McNeely, and T. Xu. 1997. Self-report benefits of Tai Chi practice by older adults. *Journals of Gerontology. Series B, Psychological Sciences and Social Sciences* 52: P242-P246.

39. Lundgren, J., C. Bengtsson, G. Blohme, B. Isaksson, L. Lapidus, R.A. Lenner, A. Jaaek, and E. Winther. 1989. Dietary habits and incidence of noninsulin-dependent diabetes mellitus in a population study of women in Gothenburg, Sweden. *American Journal of Clinical Nutrition* 52: 708-712.

40. Marshall, J.A., R.F. Hamman, and J. Baxter. 1991. High-fat, low-carbohydrate diet and the etiology of non-insulin-dependent diabetes mellitus: The San Luis Valley Diabetes Study. *American Journal of Epidemiology* 134: 590-603.

41. Meredith, C.N., W.R. Frontera, E.C. Fisher, V.A. Hughes, J.C. Herland, J. Edwards, and W.J. Evans. 1989. Peripheral effects of endurance training in young and old subjects. *Journal of Applied Physiology* 66: 2844-2849.

42. Meredith, C.N., M.J. Zackin, W.R. Frontera, and W.J. Evans. 1987. Body composition and aerobic capacity in young and middle-aged endurance-trained men. *Medicine and Science in Sports and Exercise* 19: 557-563.

43. Meredith, C.N., M.J. Zackin, W.R. Frontera, and W.J. Evans. 1989. Dietary protein requirements and body protein metabolism in endurance-trained men. *Journal of Applied Physiology* 66: 2850-2856.

44. Nelson, M.E., M.A. Fiatarone, C.M. Morganti, I. Trice, R.A. Greenberg, and W.J. Evans. 1994. Effects of high-intensity strength training on multiple risk factors for osteoporotic fractures. *Journal of the American Medical Association* 272: 1909-1914.

45. Pavlou, K.N., W.P. Steffee, R.H. Lerman, and B.A. Burrows. 1985. Effects of dieting and exercise on lean body mass, oxygen uptake, and strength. *Medicine and Science in Sports and Exercise* 17: 466-471.

46. Phinney, S.D., B.M. LaGrange, M. O'Connell, and E. Danforth Jr. 1988. Effects of aerobic exercise on energy expenditure and nitrogen balance during very low calorie dieting. *Metabolism* 37: 758-765.

47. Province, M.A., E.C. Hadley, M.C. Hornbrook, L.A. Lipsitz, J.P. Miller, C.D. Mulrow, M.G. Ory, R.W. Sattin, M.E. Tinetti, and S.L. Wolf. 1995. The effects of exercise on falls in elderly patients: A preplanned meta-analysis of the FICSIT trials. *Journal of the American Medical Association* 273: 1341-1347.

48. Rice, B., I. Janssen, R. Hudson, and R. Ross. 1999. Effects of aerobic or resistance exercise and/or diet on glucose tolerance and plasma insulin levels in obese men. *Diabetes Care* 22: 684-691.

49. Roberts, S.B., V.R. Young, P. Fuss, M.B. Heyman, M.A. Fiatarone, G.E. Dallal, J. Cortiella, and W.J. Evans. 1992. What are the dietary energy needs of adults? *International Journal of Obesity* 16: 969-976.

50. Rosen, M.J., J.D. Sorkin, A.P. Goldberg, J.M. Hagberg, and L.I. Katzel. 1998. Predictors of age-associated decline in maximal aerobic capacity: A comparison of four statistical models. *Journal of Applied Physiology* 84: 2163-2170.

51. Sahyoun, N. Nutrient intake by the NSS elderly population. 1992. In *Nutrition in the elderly: The Boston Nutritional Status Survey*, edited by S.C. Hartz, R.M. Russell, and I.H. Rosenberg, 31-44. London: Smith-Gordon.

52. Schaefer, E.J., A.H. Lichtenstein, S. Lamon-Fava, J.R. McNamara, M.M. Schaefer, H. Rasmussen, and J.O. Ordovas. 1995. Body weight and low-density lipoprotein cholesterol changes after consumption of a low-fat ad libitum diet. *Journal of the American Medical Association* 274: 1450-1455.

53. Seals, D.R., J.M. Hagberg, B.F. Hurley, A.A. Ehsani, and J.O. Holloszy. 1984. Effects of endurance training on glucose tolerance and plasma lipid levels in older men and women. *Journal of the American Medical Association* 252: 645-649.

54. Seals, D.R., J.M. Hagberg, B.F. Hurley, A.A. Ehsani, and J.O. Holloszy. 1984. Endurance training in older men and women: Cardiovascular responses to exercise. *Journal of Applied Physiology: Respiratory, Environmental and Exercise Physiology* 57: 1024-1029.

55. Shimokata, H., D.C. Muller, J.L. Fleg, J. Sorkin, A.W. Ziemba, and R. Andes. 1991. Age as independent determinant of glucose tolerance. *Diabetes* 40: 44-51.

56. Spina, R.J., T. Ogawa, W.M. Kohrt, W.H. Martin III, J.O. Holloszy, and A.A. Ehsani. 1993. Differences in cardiovascular adaptation to endurance exercise training between older men and women. *Journal of Applied Physiology* 75: 849-855.

57. Stolk, R.P., J.R. Vingerling, P.T.V.M. de Jong, I. Dielemans, A. Hofman, W.J. Lamberts, H.A.P. Pols, and D.E. Grobbee. 1995. Retinopathy, glucose and insulin in an elderly population: The Rotterdam study. *Diabetes* 44: 11-15.

58. Tzankoff, S.P., and A.H. Norris. 1978. Longitudinal changes in basal metabolic rate in man. *Journal of Applied Physiology* 33: 536-539.

59. Uauy, R., N. Scrimshaw, and V. Young. 1978. Human protein requirements: Nitrogen balance response to graded levels of egg protein in elderly men and women. *American Journal of Clinical Nutrition* 31: 779-785.

60. Whipple, R.H., L.I. Wolfson, and P.M. Amerman. 1987. The relationship of knee and ankle weakness to falls in nursing home residents. *Journal of the American Geriatrics Society* 35: 13-20.

61. Withers, R.T., D.A. Smith, R.C. Tucker, M. Brinkman, and D.G. Clark. 1998. Energy metabolism in sedentary and active 49- to 70-year-old women. *Journal of Applied Physiology* 84: 1333-1340.

62. Wolf, S.L., H.X. Barnhart, N.G. Kutner, E. McNeely, C. Coogler, and T. Xu. 1996. Reducing frailty and falls in older persons: An investigation of Tai Chi and computerized balance training. Atlanta FICSIT Group. Frailty and Injuries: Cooperative Studies of Intervention Techniques [see comments]. *Journal of the American Geriatrics Society* 44: 489-497.

63. Wolfson, L., R. Whipple, J. Judge, P. Amerman, C. Derby, and M. King. 1993. Training balance and strength in the elderly to improve function. *Journal of the American Geriatrics Society* 41: 341-343.

64. World Health Organization. 1985. Energy and protein requirements. *WHO Technical Report Series* 724.
65. Zanni, E., D. Calloway, and A. Zezulka. 1979. Protein requirements of elderly men. *Journal of Nutrition* 109: 513-524.
66. Zavaroni, I., E. Dall'Aglio, F. Bruschi, E. Bonora, O. Alpi, A. Pezzarossa, and U. Butturini. 1986. Effect of age and environmental factors on glucose tolerance and insulin secretion in a worker population. *Journal of the American Geriatrics Society* 34: 271-275.

10
CHAPTER

Resistance Training and Musculoskeletal Injury

Lorelee L. Stock, MD
Ralph K. Requa, MSPH
James G. Garrick, MD
Saint Francis Memorial Hospital

Introduction

The increasing use of resistance training over the last four decades has played an important role in improving athletic performance in high-level competitive sports. Although the International Weightlifting Federation was founded in 1905 (27), it took some time for the utility of resistance training for improving performance in many other sports to be recognized. Indeed, in the United States in the 1940s, athletes devoted only about 10% of their total training time to the development of power and strength (14).

Currently, resistance training has become more than merely part of the training for specific sports. It has become a popular physical fitness activity in itself. Whether weight machines or free weights are used, resistance training has become a common component of recreational exercise for many active people.

As competitive athletes and their coaches discovered many years ago, resistance training can enhance sports performance and may prevent musculoskeletal injuries. Prior to the popularity of resistance training for sports like football and wrestling in the 1960s and 1970s, many team sport coaches, especially in basketball and baseball, believed that weightlifting made an athlete "tight" and could compromise the fine muscle control needed to perform optimally. Efforts have been and are still being made to disseminate scientific information to educate coaches and athletes about the benefits of an intelligent resistance training program, but the success stories of well-known coaches using resistance training have probably had greater influence on its acceptance. In addition to increasing performance from adding strength and endurance, resistance training is believed to enhance and increase the strength of connective tissue sheaths within the muscle, joint cartilage, tendons, and ligaments. The mechanical strain and loading of weights also contribute to increasing bone mineral content. Although resistance training is becoming more common among children, adolescents, and to some degree the elderly, the benefits in these populations are not as well documented.

Most of the documented information on weightlifting injuries arises from those injuries sustained while training for or participating in an Olympic-style weightlifting or powerlifting competition. This type of training involves performing a maximal lift one or two times. In contrast, a majority of the resistance training programs for enhancing sport performance are aimed at improving conditioning and often are designed to enhance strength to do specific tasks involving complex motor movements (e.g., a jump in figure skating, repetitive movements such as throwing a football or hitting a tennis ball for several matches in a row). Resistance training as a recreational activity may have elements of a sports-specific training program for, say, a tennis player, but frequently is aimed at building or maintaining general strength and conditioning; for many people, improving physical appearance is also an important goal (9).

In today's fitness environment, resistance training is generally a solitary endeavor, which does not include a team roster, coach or athletic trainer, preparticipation physical, or signing a waiver consent form. No medical records are kept, injuries are not documented, and there is no way of knowing the total time of participation to calculate injury rates. Few cohort studies exist, and for the most part information is documented from case reports. The case reports that are documented tend to involve the serious injuries, leaving the minor injuries largely undocumented.

We will first discuss the most common acute and overuse (chronic) injuries, briefly discuss treatment protocols, and then provide recommendations to help prevent weightlifting injuries.

Injury Types

We will discuss the injuries reported in resistance training in four categories: recreational resistance training, Olympic-style lifting, powerlifting, and bodybuilding.

Recreational Resistance Training

Recreational resistance training is generally not competitive and usually not considered a sport in itself nor practiced as a primary activity. Instead it may be a part of a general fitness program or used to improve performance in another activity. Clearly, some of the interest in it has arisen from the desire to appear physically fit and healthy. For a variety of reasons, there has been a growing participation in recreational weightlifting over the past two decades. The literature discussing injuries in recreational resistance training is sparse.

One study followed 986 recreational athletes from 15 fitness clubs in the San Francisco Bay Area for a 3-month period (30). Injury definitions were the same across sports, allowing meaningful comparisons between activities. Subjects worked out at least 4 days a week in more than one major activity, or, if aerobic dancers, at least 3 days a week. Rates of time-loss injury for free weights and weight machines were essentially similar, between 4-5 injuries per 1000 hours of participation (the participants averaged slightly less than 300 hours per year of fitness activities). Upper-extremity injuries predominated, accounting for about two-thirds of the injuries. The shoulder was most often injured (29.6%), followed by the upper arm (13.6%), knee (12.3%), and back (11.1%). Gradual onset injuries were the rule; only two acute injuries were reported. Women reported similar or slightly lower injury rates compared with men for most resistance training activity (free weights and weight machines). The injury rates for resistance training were lower than for competitive team sports but higher than for noncompetitive, noncontact activities like hiking, walking, and exercise bicycling.

The most prevalent injuries in recreational weightlifters documented in other sources are muscle strains and ligament sprains, which account for 40% of all reported injuries (32). Contusions and abrasions account for 20%. The highest percentage of fractures in resistance training occur in recreational lifters (33).

Olympic-Style Lifting

Weightlifting was part of the first modern Olympic Games in 1896. Two events were included: the snatch and the clean-and-jerk. Today, these two events are referred to as Olympic-style weightlifting.

The most prevalent injuries in Olympic-style lifting are ligament sprains, which account for 30-45% of the total. Muscle strains are the next most prevalent injury, constituting approximately 30%. There is a lower percentage of fractures, perhaps attributable to good technique and skeletal muscular development (13).

Powerlifting

Distinct from Olympic-style weightlifting, which is a highly technical sport where weight is lifted over one's head, powerlifting involves brute strength. Powerlifting consists of three lifts: the squat, bench press, and deadlift.

Muscle strains make up about 60% of the total injuries in adolescent male powerlifters, 11% in women, and 6% in males (9). Arthritis and degenerative joint changes are more common, as were chronic and overuse injuries, among a group of adult athletes (9).

Bodybuilding

Bodybuilding refers to weightlifting for the purpose of developing skeletal muscle mass and definition. It is characterized by high-volume resistance training accompanied by strict dietary regimens to minimize body fat.

In female lifters the most common diagnosis is tendinitis, accounting for one-third of the problems. Male lifters have reported chronic overuse injuries such as degenerative joint disease, arthritis, and tendinitis (9). However, there are no comparative data for women.

Risk Factors Associated with Resistance Training Injuries

There is very little published information on risk factors for resistance training injuries. However, steroid abuse (ergogenic aids), skeletal immaturity, improper technique, and equipment itself have been implicated as contributing factors, along with genetic predisposition for injury, lack of supervision, exercise intensity, and training sessions (21).

Steroids

Steroid usage has been associated with many acute musculoskeletal injuries as well as medical conditions. The physiologic changes in muscle, tendon, and ligaments that may make them more susceptible to failure and rupture are usually associated with the performance of heavy demands. Complete spontaneous ligament ruptures potentially related to steroid use have been reported only with the ACL (anterior cruciate ligament) (8). The medical side effects include testicular atrophy, liver function abnormalities and hepatomas, myocardial ischemia, gynecomastia, hypertension, strokes, aggressive behavior, baldness, acne, and death (6).

Skeletal Immaturity

Growth plate injuries have been reported with weightlifting. Therefore, the American Academy of Pediatrics has issued guidelines for resistance training in children. These guidelines recommend a qualified trainer and medical clearance before a child begins weightlifting and advise that an adolescent should have reached the Tanner 5 stage (well-developed secondary sex characteristics) before performing strenuous weightlifting (15).

Improper Technique

Lifting with poor mechanics, or too quickly, may place sudden loads on a vulnerable orthopedic system. All athletes or individuals that are starting a resistance training program should go through a formal instruction session on utilization of free weights or weight machines. They should then be monitored periodically until they become more experienced at lifting programs.

Lift technique is often compromised by even world-class weightlifters. If an athlete loses concentration, becomes fatigued, or rushed with his or her lifting routine, injuries may occur. The use of too many repetitions, excessive weight, and ballistic exercise routines predispose an athlete to injuries. Frequently, conditioning programs are not balanced and appropriate for the individual (1).

Equipment Risks

There are a few risk factors associated with different pieces of equipment. In the free-weight bench press, the most common complication is dropping the weight on extremities or on the chest or neck, thought to occur when there is no lifting partner to act as a spotter. Other problems have to do with appropriate upkeep and maintenance of equipment in workout gyms. It is not uncommon for a cable to break, a chain to stick, or a weight stack to fall.

Types of Musculoskeletal Injuries With Resistance Training

Injuries can be categorized as acute and overuse (gradual onset) injuries. Chronic injuries are often confused with overuse injuries. Acute injuries often result from weight room accidents, improper warm-up techniques, or being overzealous. A chronic injury is best defined as an acute injury that doesn't get better within a reasonable period of time. This is different from an overuse injury, which has a gradual onset, though it too may become chronic.

Acute Injuries

The most commonly reported acute injuries are sprains and strains. A sprain is defined as the stretching or tearing of ligaments and may result in permanent laxity and thus a decrease in joint stability. A strain refers to stretching or tearing of a muscle or tendon and may result from active contraction against (too much) resistance or passive stretching.

Ligament Sprains

Ligaments function to stabilize joints. Sprains may be divided into different degrees of severity: beginning with pain without ligament laxity, increasing to slight laxity with pain, and progressing to gross instability often without much pain, which translates to a complete ligament tear. Medial and lateral collateral ligament sprains of the knee occur during squats, lunges, and leg press or with improper lower-extremity placement. Knee sprains associated with rotational movements and stress have been associated with meniscus or cartilage tears. These types of injuries can occur with squatting and dead lifts (3).

Muscle Strains and Ruptures

Acute muscle strains are painful and present with limited range of motion, loss of strength, and tenderness. These are graded as I, no muscle weakness; II, muscle weakness; and III, rupture and weakness of the muscle-tendon unit. The tendons that most frequently rupture include the hamstring, biceps, patellar, pectoralis major, and triceps. The treatment for a young athlete with an avulsion tear is usually surgical repair.

One of the most common strains involves the paraspinous musculature. If this injury is treated appropriately at time of acute onset, the injury will generally resolve through treatment and activity modifications.

Pelvic Avulsion

Excessive tension placed on a tendon insertion into bone can cause an avulsion fracture. The most common are avulsion of the anterior superior iliac spine (ASIS), the ischial apophysis, and hamstrings origin. Most apophyseal avulsions occur in skeletally immature athletes (31). Examples include the following:

1. ASIS: The mechanism of injury is usually forceful hip extension with the knee flexed and lumbar hyperextension (e.g., dead lifts). Avulsion fracture of ASIS occurs in adolescents involved in competitive sports or vigorous exercise in which the sartorius and tensor fascia lata

muscles are contracted strongly and suddenly against a hyperextended trunk (31).

2. Ischial apophysis: Avulsions occur with sprinting, running, and jumping activities or dead lifts, hamstring curls, or squats, when the hamstring muscle avulses the ischial tuberosity from the pelvis. These injuries may also be associated with trauma or a blow to the back of the leg, or with squatting heavy loads of weight (25).

Biceps Tendon Rupture
A biceps tendon rupture usually occurs when an individual is lifting a heavy object. In the past these injuries were frequently work related. Currently, most such reported injuries occur with weightlifting activities, most commonly biceps curls (26).

Acute Fractures
There are few reported fractures caused by weightlifting. Most are upper-extremity fractures. Two fractures were reported in adolescents performing clean-and-jerk lifts. They lost control of the overhead weight and sustained bilateral radius and ulna fractures. A scaphoid fracture was sustained in a 17-year-old boy who developed wrist pain while attempting a 430 lb (195 kg) bench press (29). A 22-year-old competitive weightlifter presented with complaints of anterior shoulder pain. This was thought to be caused by repeated muscle torque on the humerus from the pectoralis major muscle, apparently resulting in a fatigue fracture (10). A transchondral fracture of the dome of the talus was reported to have occurred during the performance of a "power squat" (20).

Overuse Injuries

Chronic injuries often result from overuse injuries, particularly if the injury is ignored. In weightlifting, the body is required to put heavy stress on the ligaments, tendons, and musculature. Tendinitis is probably the most common overuse injury seen in resistance training (3.5-12%) (28). Often overuse injuries occur because of incorrect exercise technique or excessive repetition of movements performed against resistance.

Rotator Cuff Injury
Rotator cuff injuries are often the result of muscle imbalances, weakness, and repetitive loading activities. The rotator cuff stabilizes the humerus so the larger muscles can lift heavier weights. The rotator cuff strain is often the result of the weight attempted posing too much stress for the small cuff muscles used to stabilize the joint. Resistance training activities associated with these injuries include the military press, rowing, bench press, and pectoralis machines.

Therefore, it is important to access the strength of all the musculature in the shoulder (especially the posterior shoulder and external rotators). Rehabilitation of these weak muscles is often the key to resolving pain. Secondly, the range of motion in the shoulder needs to be tested and corrected. Often the external and internal rotator muscles become tight and limit the range.

Anterior Shoulder Instability

An athlete with anterior shoulder instability will report looseness, transient numbness, and apprehension about the shoulder "going out of joint." This feeling often occurs with the arm abducted and externally rotated. The relocation test (pushing the humeral head posteriorly) will relieve the symptoms of apprehension. The bench press produces hyperextension of the shoulder musculature and can cause repetitive shoulder capsule trauma and may also disrupt the AC (acromioclavicular) joint. An often problematic exercise is the reverse behind-the-neck military pull-down. This exercise often causes shoulder capsule loading and inferior glenohumeral ligament sprain.

A study done on occult instability in weightlifters found that by strengthening the shoulder abductor and external rotators and toning the periscapular stabilizers, 50% of those patients with anterior instability and pain become pain free. The other 50% required surgical correction (18).

Neuropathies

Nerve injuries, often the result of constriction from muscle hypertrophy, present with pain or parasthesias as well as muscle weakness. Repetitive traction on the nerve can also produce similar symptoms. These injuries occur over months of repetitive stress or increase in muscle size. The most commonly reported injuries of this type, to be discussed in the following paragraphs, include suprascapular and musculocutaneous neuropathy, long thoracic nerve injury, thoracic outlet syndrome, lateral plantar nerve entrapment, and ulnar nerve neuritis.

Suprascapular Neuropathy

Compression of the suprascapular nerve within the suprascapular notch produces shoulder pain, muscle weakness, and atrophy. Often this diagnosis is missed. The etiology for this disorder includes impingement of the suprascapular nerve, brachial plexus injuries, direct trauma to the scapular region, dislocation of the shoulder, or fracture of the scapula. This disorder presents with insidious onset of pain after the individual has performed abductor strengthening exercises or used dumbbells to perform shoulder abductions. These symptoms present as infraspinatus and supraspinatus muscle weakness and atrophy. (If only the supraspinatus muscle shows atrophy, the diagnosis is most likely supraspinatus tear.) An EMG study will show reduced motor unit recruitment for the involved muscles. An MRI of the shoulder may be helpful in identifying other causes such as a neuroma or cyst in the suprascapular notch.

Long Thoracic Nerve Injury

Long thoracic nerve injury results in scapular winging and weakness of the serratus anterior muscle. There is no specific reproducible injury mechanism, but the injury may be a result of pressure of the machine pads resting against that nerve. In this injury, scapular winging is more prominent at the inferior border of the scapula compared with accessory nerve palsies, which cause superior medial scapular winging.

This disorder is best diagnosed with EMG studies and treated with rest, ice, and removal of the pressure against the nerve. Spontaneously these usually resolve within 3 to 24 months (27).

Musculocutaneous Neuropathy

Musculocutaneous neuropathy may be brought on by repetitive biceps curls. The pain and weakness are thought to be caused by impingement of the musculocutaneous nerve from the coracobrachialis muscle hypertrophy. An EMG differentiates this disorder from C-5 or C-6 cervical radiculopathy, brachial plexopathy, or biceps rupture.

The treatment is activity restriction and is nonoperative. This strength returns about 3 months after rest (2).

Thoracic Outlet Syndrome

Thoracic outlet syndrome is thought to occur in weightlifters through hypertrophy of the scalene muscles, which impinge the subclavian vessels and the brachial plexus in the scalene or costoclavicular triangles. Pectoralis minor hypertrophy may also impinge these nerves, especially with hyperabduction and external rotation of the shoulder (e.g., bench press, dumbbell free weights, and neck-strengthening machines involving lateral sidebending, flexion, and rotation), or result in shoulder girdle protraction that places the bracheal plexus under tension.

The symptoms include insidious upper-limb pain of ulnar nerve distribution, with ulnar hand parasthesias and thenar weakness. There is no definitive test for this disorder. A patient is taken through provocative maneuvers to reproduce pain. The examiner should rule out arterial compression by examining the supraclavicular or infraclavicular fossa for a mass or bruit. Treatment focuses on muscle strength balance between the anterior and posterior thorax, stretching of the pectoral muscles, and the anterior shoulder. The patient should avoid positions that reproduce the pain and should strengthen the posterior scapular stabilizers (rhomboids and trapezium).

Lateral Plantar Nerve Entrapment

Lateral plantar nerve entrapment was described in a weightlifter that complained of burning pain below the medial malleolus radiating to the plantar surface of the foot (11). The pain was worse with powerlifting because the intrinsic muscles of the foot become activated in an attempt to prevent pronation of the subtalar joint and collapse of the longitudinal arch of the foot. The intrinsic muscle activity and tension on the lateral arch of the foot produce lateral plantar nerve compression. An EMG revealed segmental neuropathy of the lateral plantar nerve. The patient was found to have flattening of the medial longitudinal arch with weightlifting. The patient was treated with rigid foot orthosis and became pain free. The EMG study was repeated after treatment and no longer showed segmental neuropathy of the lateral plantar nerve.

Ulnar Nerve Neuritis

Ulnar nerve neuritis has been well described and is thought to be secondary to traction, friction, or compression at the elbow. The presenting symptoms include insidious onset of parasthenia over the ulnar aspect of the hand and progressive grip weakness. The problem is often accompanied by atrophy of the hypothenar eminence and adductor pollicis muscle (a positive Wartenburg's sign). This is usually best treated surgically by an anterior transposition, medial epicondylectomy, or decompression by division of the fascial band that connects the two heads of the flexor carpi ulnaris muscle (5).

Bony Disorders

A variety of bony disorders have been reported in weightlifters. The most common are stress fractures, osteoarthritis, osteolysis, and back disorders such as spondylolysis and spondylolisthesis.

Stress Fractures

Stress fractures of the humerus, sternum, and lumbar ring apophysis have all been associated with resistance training. The presenting symptoms include progressive focal or point tenderness and exacerbation of local pain with deep pressure, or increased pain with loading the bone. A bone scan is the "gold standard" and may turn out positive before changes are visible on standard X ray.

Osteoarthritis

Many competitive weightlifters have patellofemoral osteoarthritis. Researchers have documented the fact that this disorder is found more in lifters than in runners or soccer players (16). This is thought to be due in part to suboptimal technique. Squats are done with heavy loads, with the thighs descending below 90°, placing stress on the articular cartilage of the patella and on the thinnest part of the femoral articular cartilage. The most successful treatment strategies address patellar alignment and include vastus medialis strengthening and placing the knee "over the foot" when undertaking squat-type lifts. X-ray findings of narrowing of the compartment allow diagnosis. Treatment includes closed-chain kinetic strengthening exercises and an orthotic wedge to unload the involved compartment.

Atraumatic Osteolysis of the Distal Clavicle

Atraumatic osteolysis of the distal clavicle was described in a group of weight trainers. The patients complained of insidious aching pain of the AC region that was prompted by overhead activities, horizontal adduction, and resistance training. The mechanism of osteolysis is thought to be caused by protraction of the shoulder, which loads the AC joint during bench press-type activities. X rays show subchondral osteolysis. A study done by Cahill reported that 46 men without trauma had osteolysis of the distal clavicle (4). Initial treatment includes avoidance of the painful lifts, and scapular retraction exercises. Thirty-seven out of 40 athletes that had surgery with excision of the distal clavicle returned to weightlifting without pain (4).

Back Disorders

The use of weightlifting equipment was initially thought to cause back pain or herniated disk problems. An epidemiological study done by Mundt et al. showed that there is a very small risk of herniated disk in lifting weights when proper technique is used (24). In fact, lifting weights is a means of strengthening the back and decreasing the stress on the back.

Spondylolysis is a defect (stress fracture) or congenital defect in the pars interarticularis that probably arises from repeated back extensions in the presence of a predisposing bony weakness. While often observed in oblique radiographs of the lumbar spine, a radioisotope bone scan is usually positive far in advance of the radiographic changes. The treatment includes pain-free activities for 6-8 weeks. Thoracolumbosacral bracing may enhance comfort. Flexion activities are stressed and extension activities are avoided (17). Flexion exercises (abdominal strengthening) may help to lessen the often-present lumbar lordosis.

Spondylolisthesis

Spondylolisthesis is the anterior subluxation of one vertebral body relative to the one below. This injury is seen in weightlifters who do squats and clean-and-jerk lifts. About one-half of the disorders are asymptomatic. If the slippage is less than 30% and asymptomatic, it is left alone. If it is more than 30% and symptomatic, it is followed with serial X rays and avoidance of extension activities. This is best studied by a lateral radiographic view of the spine (17). Surgical stabilization is done if the subluxation continues to be problematic.

Prevention of Injuries

Scientific research indicates that resistance training can play an important role in injury prevention. The physiological mechanisms that aid in injury prevention include increased strength of tendons, ligaments, joint cartilage, connective tissue, and tendon-to-bone and ligament-to-bone junction.

Without epidemiological information concerning injuries associated with weightlifting or training, strategies for injury prevention are based more on common sense than science. Losing control of free weights or abruptly increasing either the number of repetitions or amount of weight are frequently cited causes of problems. Joint pain, swelling, or loss of motion are often indications of impending injuries and should not be ignored.

Recommendations

General recommendations to prevent musculoskeletal injury include the following:

- Warming up
- Good technique
- Assess imbalances/preexisting conditions and deal with them
- Use of weight belt when lifting heavy loads
- Alternate upper-extremity and lower-extremity workout days
- Proper shoe wear while lifting
- Equipment orientation
- Adequate sleep and diet
- If injured acutely, seek medical attention before the condition causes compensation injuries (19)

Conclusion

Future research is needed to better define the incidence and types of injuries acquired in various kinds of strength training both for high-level competitive sport and in the recreational setting. A few studies have been done that look at injuries in resistance training, but most of our information is anecdotal. Case reports of injuries from resistance training are useful in identifying potential hazards but do not provide definitive values for risk or permit comparisons to be made. Studies of younger and older participants are particularly needed.

There are injury issues related to the type of weights used. Free weights generally take more time to set up and require awareness of good technique and body mechanics; some exercises require a spotter. Free weights, unlike weight machines, are not contained and can present hazards to both the exerciser and others nearby if control is not maintained. Injuries have been reported, some quite serious, from loss of control of free weights. Free weights have an advantage in that they allow one to move in three planes and simulate performing sport-specific movements. Weight machines, on the other hand, generally do not require a spotter, are already set up and ready to use, and are more forgiving of poor technique and body mechanics. Good supervision is particularly important with free weights, but weight machines can also be used improperly, subjecting their users to potential injury. Supervision may be even more important for groups who are at potentially higher risk, such as adolescents and the elderly.

The American College of Sports Medicine recommended in 1990 that moderate resistance training be included in fitness programs as an integral component (1). Resistance training has shown beneficial effects in fitness programs by improving muscle strength, neuromuscular pathways, and cardiovascular endurance, and decreasing the percent body fat (18). The multiple benefits—physical and mental—include strengthening of musculature and bones (5, 12, 23) and decreased symptoms of depressions and arthritis (22). The elderly even benefit by counteracting muscle weakness and physical frailty, which improves quality of life by maintaining strength to carry out daily living activities and achieving more independence in daily living (7).

References

1. American College of Sports Medicine. 1990. The recommended quantity and quality of exercise for developing and maintaining cardiorespiratory and muscular fitness in healthy adults. *Medicine and Science in Sports and Exercise* 22 (2): 265-274.
2. Braddom, R.L., and C. Wolfe. 1978. Musculocutaneous nerve injury after heavy exercise. *Archives of Physical Medicine and Rehabilitation* 59 (6): 290-293.
3. Brady, T.A., B.R. Cahill, and L.M. Bodnar. 1982. Weight training-related injuries in the high school athlete. *American Journal of Sports Medicine* 10 (1): 1-5.
4. Cahill, B.R. 1982. Osteolysis of the distal part of the clavicle in male athletes. *Journal of Bone and Joint Surgery (American Volume)* 64 (7): 1053-1058.
5. Dangles, C.J., and Z.J. Bilos. 1980. Ulnar nerve neuritis in a world champion weightlifter. *American Journal of Sports Medicine* 8 (6): 443-445.
6. Dickerman, R.D., F. Schaller, I. Prather, and W.J. McConathy. 1995. Sudden cardiac death in a 20-year-old bodybuilder using anabolic steroids. *Cardiology* 86 (2): 172-173.
7. Fiatarone, M.A., E.F. O'Neill, N.D. Ryan, et al. 1994. Exercise training and nutritional supplementation for physical frailty in very elderly people [see comments]. *New England Journal of Medicine* 330 (25): 1769-1775.

8. Freeman, B.J., and G.D. Rooker. 1995. Spontaneous rupture of the anterior cruciate ligament after anabolic steroids. *British Journal of Sports Medicine* 29 (4): 274-275.

9. Goertzen, M., K. Schöppe, G. Lange, and K.P. Schulitz. 1989. Verletzungen und Uberlastungsschäden beim Bodybuilding und Powerlifting [Injuries and damage caused by excess stress in body building and power lifting]. *Sportverletzung Sportschaden* 3 (1): 32-36.

10. Horwitz, B.R., and V. DiStefano. 1995. Stress fracture of the humerus in a weight lifter. *Orthopedics* (Thorofare, NJ) 18 (2): 185-187.

11. Johnson, E.R., K. Kirby, and J.S. Lieberman. 1992. Lateral plantar nerve entrapment: Foot pain in a power lifter. *American Journal of Sports Medicine* 20 (5): 619-620.

12. Karlsson, M.K., O. Johnell, and K.J. Obrant. 1993. Bone mineral density in weight lifters. *Calcified Tissue International* 52 (3): 212-215.

13. König M., and K. Biener. 1990. Sportartspezifische Verletzungen im Gewichtheben [Sport-specific injuries in weightlifting]. *Schweizerische Zeitschrift fur Sportmedizin* 38 (1): 25-30.

14. Kraemer, W.J., N.D. Duncan, and J.S. Volek. 1998. Resistance training and elite athletes: Adaptations and program considerations. *Journal of Orthopaedic and Sports Physical Therapy* 28 (2): 110-119.

15. Kraemer, W.J., S.E. Gordon, S.J. Fleck, et al. 1991. Endogenous anabolic hormonal and growth factor responses to heavy resistance exercise in males and females. *International Journal of Sports Medicine* 12 (2): 228-235.

16. Kujala, U.M., J. Kettunen, H. Paananen, et al. 1995. Knee osteoarthritis in former runners, soccer players, weight lifters, and shooters. *Arthritis and Rheumatism* 38 (4): 539-546.

17. Kulund, D.N., J.B. Dewey, C.E. Brubaker, and J.R. Roberts. 1978. Olympic weight-lifting injuries. *Physician and Sportsmedicine* 6 (11): 111-119.

18. Lombardi, V. 1989. *Beginning weight training: The safe and effective way.* Dubuque, IA: Brown.

19. Lombardi, V. 1996. Resistance training. In *Epidemiology of sports injuries*, edited by D. Caine, C.G. Caine, and K.J. Lindner. Champaign, IL: Human Kinetics.

20. Mannis, C.I. 1983. Transchondral fracture of the dome of the talus sustained during weight training. *American Journal of Sports Medicine* 11 (5): 354-356.

21. Mazur, L.J., R.J. Yetman, and W.L. Risser. 1993. Weight-training injuries. Common injuries and preventative methods. *Sports Medicine* 16 (1): 57-63.

22. McCubbin, J.A. 1990. Resistance exercise training for persons with arthritis. *Rheumatic Diseases Clinics of North America* 16 (4): 931-943.

23. Menkes, A., S. Mazel, R.A. Redmond, et al. 1993. Strength training increases regional bone mineral density and bone remodeling in middle-aged and older men. *Journal of Applied Physiology* 74 (5): 2478-2484.

24. Mundt, D.J., J.L. Kelsey, A.L. Golden, et al. 1993. An epidemiologic study of sports and weight lifting as possible risk factors for herniated lumbar and cervical discs. The Northeast Collaborative Group on Low Back Pain. *American Journal of Sports Medicine* 21 (6): 854-860.

25. Orava, S., and M. Kujala. 1995. Rupture of the ischial origin of the hamstring muscles. *American Journal of Sports Medicine* 21 (6): 702-705.

26. Rantanen, J., and S. Orava. 1999. Rupture of the distal biceps tendon. A report of 19 patients treated with anatomic reinsertion, and a meta-analysis of 147 cases found in the literature. *American Journal of Sports Medicine* 27 (2): 128-132.

27. Reeves, R.K., E.R. Laskowiski, and J. Smith. 1998. Weight training injuries: Part 1: Diagnosing and managing acute conditions. *Physician and Sportsmedicine* 26 (2): 67-83.

28. Reeves, R.K., E.R. Laskowiski, and J. Smith. 1998. Weight training injuries: Part 2: Diagnosing and managing chronic conditions. *Physician and Sportsmedicine* 26 (3): 54-96.

29. Reider, B., J. Yurokofsky, and D. Mass. 1993. Scaphoid wrist fracture in a weight lifter: Case report. *American Journal of Sports Medicine* 21 (2): 329-331.

30. Requa, R.K., L.N. DeAvilla, and J.G. Garrick. 1993. Injuries in recreational adult fitness activities. *American Journal of Sports Medicine* 21 (3): 461-467.

31. Thanikachalam, M., J.G. Petros, and S. O'Donnell. 1995. Avulsion fracture of the anterior superior iliac spine presenting as acute-onset meralgia paresthetica. *Annals of Emergency Medicine* 26 (4): 515-517.

32. U.S. Consumer Product Safety Commission National Injury Information Clearing-house, 1993. *Estimates and injury detail reports: National electronic injury surveillance system: Weight lifting* (code 3264 and 3265). Washington, DC: USCPSC.

33. U.S. Consumer Product Safety Commission National Injury Information Clearing-house, 1990. *Explanation sheet for NEISS estimates report.* Washington, DC: USCPSC.

11

CHAPTER

Elderly Patients and Frailty

Maria A. Fiatarone Singh, MD
University of Sydney and Tufts University

Exercise and the Health of the Older Population

Policy makers and health care professionals have gradually become aware of the centrality of appropriate exercise habits to major public health outcomes. For example, in the current draft of Healthy People 2010, the goal suggested in the realm of physical activity is to "improve the health, fitness, and quality of life of all Americans through the adoption and maintenance of regular, daily physical activity" (119). It has been known for decades that physical activity prevents heart disease, but more recent data suggest that, on average, physically active people outlive those who are inactive (9, 63) and that regular physical activity helps to maintain the functional independence of older adults and enhance the quality of life for people of all ages.

Unfortunately, disparities in levels of physical activity exist among population groups and exaggerate the negative health consequences of a sedentary lifestyle. According to the 1996 *Physical Activity and Health: A Report of the Surgeon General* (120), demographic groups at highest risk for inactivity are the elderly, women, minorities, those with low income or low educational background, and those with disabilities or chronic health conditions. So, for example, 43% of adults aged 65 and older were sedentary (no regular physical activity) in 1985, and 29% in 1991, in figures from this report. Notably, these are the same demographic groups that both bear a large burden of the diseases amenable to prevention and treatment with exercise, and yet often have the least access and opportunity for health promotion efforts related to physical activity. This lack of education, access, and promotion by the health care community is most pronounced in the specific exercise modality this volume is concerned with, that of progressive resistance training.

Previous objectives for the nation have primarily focused on physical activities designed to improve cardiorespiratory fitness and prolong life. However, it is now recognized that everyone also could benefit from physical activities designed to ensure functional independence throughout life. The specific physical fitness components that provide continued physical function as individuals age include muscle strength, muscle endurance, balance, and flexibility. Resistance training has been shown to enhance fitness in each of these four domains, thus providing a unique opportunity to practice economy of prescription with a large potential for health-related benefit. Conversely, cardiovascular training, balance training, and flexibility training do not typically by themselves enhance muscle mass and strength and cannot be substituted for resistance training if this is a primary goal of the activity. The problems of mobility impairment, falls, arthritis, osteoporotic fractures, and frailty and functional decline are clearly related to muscle strength and mass (41, 122), and thus strengthening activities, while important for all age groups, are particularly important for older adults. Age-related loss of strength, muscle mass, and bone density, which are most dramatic in women, may be attenuated by strengthening exercises (71, 84), and regained even long afterward with appropriate resistance training (98).

Women, because of their longer life expectancy, make up an increasingly larger proportion of the elderly with advancing age, outnumbering men by 2-3:1 over the age of 85. They are at higher risk for sarcopenia, muscle weakness, functional decline, and injurious falls than are age-matched men, due to a variety of physiological, pathological, and psychosocial factors. The potential utility of exercise as a preventive and rehabilitative tool to combat these problems is therefore particularly attractive in this demographic subgroup. Unfortunately, national survey data indicate that women in general report lower than average adult participation levels for strength training (11% vs. 16%). Additionally, despite the evidence on safety and efficacy in even frail elders (35, 36, 80), the prevalence rate for resistance exercise is even lower among the old (6% at ages 65-74) or the very old

(4% above age 75). Data on those over the age of 85 (predominantly women) are currently lacking, but are likely to be less than 1% currently. Thus, health promotion efforts directed specifically at this high-risk population are vitally needed if the benefits of resistance training noted in this and other chapters of this volume are to be realized.

The needs of an older, chronically ill, or disabled population in relation to physical activity are more complicated than the straightforward elements of the basic exercise prescription for younger adults (2). Thus, an understanding of the relationship of exercise to aging and disease, and the specificity of training adaptations that occur, is critical to the care of the older patient, and is the focus of this chapter.

Integrating Disciplines

In this overview, we will consider the interaction of habitual physical activity and chronic disease expression in the older patient, with an aim to identify the intersection of these fields as they relate to optimization of aging processes as well as both prevention and treatment of common diseases and syndromes relevant to aging. The rationale for integrating a prescription for resistance training into geriatric health care is based on four essential concepts that will be reviewed in detail in the sections that follow. First, there is a great similarity between the physiologic changes attributable to musculoskeletal and other kinds of disuse and those typically observed in aging populations, leading to the speculation that the way we age may in fact be greatly modulated by attention to activity levels (13). Second, chronic diseases increase with age, and resistive exercise (as well as cardiovascular exercise) has now been shown to be a potential adjunctive treatment for many of the causes of morbidity and mortality in Western societies, a potential currently vastly underutilized. Third, traditional medical interventions don't typically address disuse syndromes accompanying chronic disease, which may be responsible for much of an older patient's associated disability. Resistive exercise is particularly good at targeting syndromes of disuse of the neuromuscular, but also the cardiovascular system. Finally, many pathophysiological aberrations that are central to a disease or secondary to its treatment are specifically addressed only by exercise, which therefore deserves a place in the mainstream of medical care, not just as an optional adjunct.

Relationship of Resistance Training to Physiological Aging

Many of the physiological changes associated with aging can be attributed to a sedentary lifestyle. Participation in regular physical activity can attenuate and often reverse unfavorable physiological aging.

Retarding the Aging Process

Some of the most visible changes we recognize as aging, such as changes in hair color and volume, development of presbyopia, altered skin texture and elasticity, reductions in height, and even changes in speed of cognitive processing, will have little direct impact on the ability to exercise or remain functionally independent in advanced years, whereas others (e.g., loss of strength and muscle mass) may have a far greater impact. In most physiologic systems, the normal aging processes do not result in significant impairment or dysfunction in the absence of pathology and under resting conditions. However, in response to a stress, the age-related reduction in physiologic reserves causes a loss of homeostatic balance. This process has been termed *homeostenosis*, or a lessened capacity for fine-tuning of the system. On the one hand, these changes limit the maximal performance or work capacity in a given domain. This may be seen in tests of maximal muscle strength, muscle power, muscle endurance, aerobic capacity, static or dynamic balance, or flexibility, for example. Although such changes will be immediately noticeable and disastrous for an elite athlete (49), they may accrue insidiously in nonathletic populations over many years without much effect on daily life. This is because most sedentary individuals rarely call on themselves to exert maximal effort in physical domains. Thus, subtle changes in physical activity patterns over the adult lifespan allow most people not engaged in athletic pursuits to lose a very large proportion of their physical work capacity before they even notice that something is wrong or find that they have crossed a threshold of disability (122). Women are particularly susceptible here, because their initial reserve of muscle mass is so much lower than that of men because of gender differences in anabolic hormonal milieu (28, 34, 43). They will therefore cross this threshold where losses of musculoskeletal capacity impact on functional status at least 10 years before men do, in most cases (48).

The second consequence of age-related changes in physiologic capacity is the increased perception of effort associated with submaximal work. For example, between youth and middle age, an untrained man or woman may find that walking briskly results in increased blood pressure, heart rate, respiratory rate, and an earlier sense of overall and leg muscle fatigue than previously (127). Again, this changing physical capacity has the unfortunate negative side effect of increasing the tendency to avoid activity contributed to by changing job requirements or retirement, societal roles and expectations, and other psychosocial influences (47). Thus a vicious cycle is set up: "usual" aging leading to decreasing exercise capacity, resulting in an elevated perception of effort, subsequently causing avoidance of activity, and finally feeding back to exacerbation of the age-related declines themselves secondary to disuse. The major decrements in exercise capacity observed in normal aging are summarized in table 11.1 and will be reviewed briefly in the following paragraphs.

Cardiovascular endurance capacity, or aerobic capacity, depends primarily on cardiac output (stroke volume × heart rate), oxygen-carrying capacity of the blood, capillary density, extraction of oxygen by the working muscles, and oxidative capacity of the muscle fibers, including oxidative enzyme content, mitochondrial volume density, proportion of type I (slow-twitch) fibers, and storage of glycogen for fuel. There are two major reasons for the reduced maximal aerobic capacity with aging: the diminished maximal heart rate in response to exercise, which appears to be limited by an age-related decreased sensitivity of the myocardium to beta-adrenergic stimulation (52, 64), and the loss of muscle mass itself, which is thought to explain at least 40% of the decline in maximal aerobic capacity with aging (40).

Musculoskeletal function (strength, power, muscle endurance) is dictated largely by the size of the muscle mass that is contracting and to a somewhat lesser extent in normal aging by changes in surrounding connective tissue in the joint (cartilage, tendons, and ligaments) and neural recruitment, conduction velocities, and fatigue patterns. Sedentary individuals lose large amounts of muscle mass over the course of adult life (20-50%), and this loss plays a major role in the similarly large losses in muscle strength observed in both cross-sectional and longitudinal studies (3, 43, 62). However, unlike many other changes that impact on exercise capacity, muscle mass cannot be maintained into old age even with habitual aerobic activities in either typical individuals (94) or master athletes (95). Only loading of muscle via resistive exercise has been shown to avert losses of muscle mass (and also strength) in older individuals (59). In his study, Klitgaard found that elderly men who swam or ran had similar measures of muscle size and strength as their sedentary peers, whereas the muscle of older men who had been weightlifting for 12-17 years was almost indistinguishable, and even

TABLE 11.1   Age-Related Changes in Physiology That Impair Exercise Capacity

Decreased anaerobic threshold

Decreased joint range of motion (flexibility)

Decreased maximal aerobic capacity (0.5-1.0% per year)

Decreased muscle force, endurance, and power (1-2% per year)

Impaired coordination and speed of movement

Impaired static and dynamic balance

Increased cardiovascular response, perception of effort, and lactate response to submaximal aerobic work superior in some aspects, to healthy men 40 to 50 years younger than them.

Similarity of Disuse and Aging

One of the major goals of gerontological research over the past several decades has been to separate the true physiologic changes of aging from changes due to disease or environmental factors, including disuse or underuse of body systems. Numerous studies point out the superior physical condition of those who exercise regularly compared with their more sedentary peers, even in the tenth decade of life (12, 102). On the other hand, research indicates that years of physiologic aging of diverse organ systems and metabolic functions can be mimicked by short periods of enforced inactivity such as bed rest, casting, denervation, or loss of gravitational forces. These two types of studies have led to a theory of disuse and aging that suggests that aging as we now know it in modern society is, in many ways, an exercise deficiency syndrome (13), implying that we may have far more control over the rate and extent of the aging process than we previously thought.

Conversely, many studies suggest that chronic adaptation to physical activity can markedly attenuate decrements in exercise capacity that would otherwise occur with aging. Although peak workload achievable (e.g., peak torque) is almost always lower in aged individuals, the musculoskeletal adaptations to chronic resistive exercise, as detailed in chapter 3, will enable the trained individual to sustain higher submaximal workloads for a longer period of time with less overall and musculo-skeletal fatigue. Thus, adaptations in muscle endurance seen after resistance training can overcome much of the day-to-day functional limitations that might otherwise be imposed by the physiological changes of aging and disuse (90). Even in the absence of any aerobic training at all, measures of cardiorespiratory endurance will improve significantly as well after resistance training, due to the contribution of muscle mass and metabolism to aerobic capacity noted above (1).

Appropriate progressive resistance training programs lasting 3-12 months have been shown to increase muscle strength by an average of 40-150%, depending on the subject's characteristics and intensity of the program, and to increase total body muscle mass by several kilograms (22, 24, 36, 72, 100, 108). Thus, even if some of the neural control of muscle and absolute number of motor units remaining is not affected by exercise, the adaptation to muscle loading, even in very old age, causes neural, metabolic, and structural changes in muscle that can completely compensate for the strength losses, and to some extent the atrophy, of aging.

Some of the most important physiological adaptations at both the muscle fiber and whole-body level that have been documented after high-intensity progressive resistance training in the older adult are outlined in table 11.2. It should be noted that studies demonstrating such adaptations have all used exercise prescriptions of moderate- to high-intensity progressive resistance training (see chapters 2 and 7), and that little adaptation occurs with low-intensity training in the elderly. These adaptations are seen in both healthy (84) and frail subjects (36, 38), and thus the presence of chronic disease or disability itself does not appear to be a barrier to successful adaptation in this realm.

Prevention: Minimizing Risk Factors for Chronic Disease

Another way to integrate resistive and other forms of exercise into health care is to view them in light of their potential to reduce risk factors for chronic diseases. Most epidemiological data on disease prevention and exercise relate to cardiovascular activities, as muscle strengthening activities are rarely seen in populations at high enough rates to analyze

TABLE 11.2   Physiological Adaptations to Resistance Training in the Older Adult

Activation of satellite cells

Appearance of insulin-like growth factor 1 (IGF-1) in muscle fibers

Decreased total and visceral adipose tissue mass

Decreased aerobic exercise-induced ischemia

Improved static and dynamic balance

Improved tolerance to orthostatic stressors

Increased maximal aerobic capacity

Increased bone density

Increased glycogen storage, GLUT-4 receptors in muscle

Increased insulin sensitivity

Increased joint range of motion

Increased muscle fiber area, total muscle mass

Increased muscle force, endurance, and power

Increased myofibrillar protein synthesis rate; increased protein turnover

Increased nitrogen retention from diet

Increased oxidative enzyme capacity

Increased total energy expenditure (resting, activity, muscle mass, protein turnover, increased thermic effect of feeding)

Increased gastrointestinal transit time

Myofibrillar damage

and are not appropriately captured in most older survey instruments (8, 89). The major causes of morbidity and mortality (heart disease, stroke, diabetes, cancer, arthritis, functional dependency, hip fracture) in the older population are all more prevalent in individuals who are sedentary than in their more active peers (91). Theoretically, there is reason to suspect (based on the adaptations noted in table 11.2) that habitual resistive exercise would provide protection from osteoporosis, diabetes, other diseases linked to visceral adiposity, and functional dependency and frailty itself, but such epidemiological evidence is still largely lacking.

One of the most promising uses of progressive resistance training in preventive medicine lies in its ability to modify typical age-associated changes in body composition. In this conceptual model, one can categorize chronic diseases and geriatric syndromes that are potentially modifiable by exercise if an underlying derangement in body composition is addressed. For example, a stabilization or increase in bone mass is achievable by resistive exercise and may be useful for both prevention and treatment of osteoporosis and related fractures and disability (see chapter 20). Decreases in adipose tissue accumulation are achievable by both resistive training (as noted in chapter 9) and aerobic training, usually in conjunction with an energy-restricted diet. This may be both preventive and therapeutic for many of the most common chronic diseases of old age, and preventive in the cases of cardiovascular disease, diabetes, hypertension, arthritis, cancer, stroke, and vascular impotence. There is evidence of reduction in intra-abdominal fat stores with resistance training in two studies of healthy, normal weight elders (117, 118); such reduction would be metabolically advantageous if achievable in those with visceral obesity and associated syndromes characterized by insulin resistance, such as type 2 diabetes mellitus. Reduced adiposity is also important for the prevention and treatment of osteoarthritis, mobility impairments, and sleep-disordered breathing.

A substantial increase in muscle mass is achievable only with progressive resistance training or generalized weight gain (33), and could have a role in preventing diabetes, functional dependency, falls, and fractures. Currently, increased muscle mass is thought to be important primarily for the treatment of the numerous chronic diseases and disabilities (34) that are accompanied by disuse and sarcopenia. It is notable that the treatment of disease-related sarcopenia with exercise is an area not addressed at all by the pharmacological management of conditions such as congestive heart failure and Parkinson's disease, and therefore it is likely that such adjunctive treatment will impact significantly on related morbidity in these patients. For some diseases, like type 2 diabetes mellitus or osteoarthritis, there are advantages to both minimizing fat tissue as well as maximizing muscle tissue, since these compartments have opposite, independent effects on disease expression and disease-related disability in the elderly (26).

There are numerous studies of normal healthy older adults that indicate that high-intensity resistance training is associated with increases in lean body mass or muscle area, usually with minimal alteration of total body weight (22, 24, 67, 72). However, the observed adaptive response of skeletal muscle to resistance training in these studies is quite variable, likely influenced by the intensity and duration of the intervention, subject characteristics, and the precision of the measurement technique itself (22, 30, 83).

Unfortunately, most studies to date have included only healthy individuals (17, 21, 24, 44, 61, 65, 100) and little clinical information other than age to allow insight into the wide range of muscle tissue responsiveness to weightlifting regimens. It is clear from these studies and our own (36, 98) including frail elders that advancing age impairs the hypertrophic response to resistance training, for reasons not yet identified. The existing literature suggests that both exercise-related variables and individual characteristics contribute to the wide range of lean tissue responsiveness to resistance training. It is possible to see changes in whole-body lean tissue with progressive resistance training even in the face of hypocaloric dieting in healthy middle-aged and older women (4, 5). However, we have found that in chronically diseased elderly, even eucaloric energy intake appears insufficient for optimal muscle growth, and energy supplementation was necessary to induce significant hypertrophy with weightlifting exercise (38). Further research is required to separate out the effects of advanced age, nutritional deficiencies, hormonal status, disease attributes, and extreme sedentariness in clinical populations that may impair their ability to augment lean tissue with this mode of exercise as compared with healthy peers.

There is now much literature to suggest that exercise is useful in combating the typical age-associated increases in fat mass and decreases in lean mass (muscle and bone) that are seen in older adults. Exercise is adjunctive to energy restriction in the treatment of generalized and central obesity and will therefore contribute to the management of this risk factor for many chronic diseases. Resistance training, in the presence of adequate energy intake, will augment muscle mass and bone density and is therefore theoretically of central importance in preventing functional impairment and osteoporotic fractures in older men and women, although there are yet no data from randomized controlled trials on its efficacy for prevention of falls or osteoporotic fracture.

Finally, since resistive exercise increases energy expenditure and therefore requirements in a variety of ways, it may also counteract the risk for macro- and micronutrient deficiencies, which may be seen in older adults who consume a very small volume of food because of their reduced energy requirements and/or anorexia from chronic disease. We have seen that multinutrient supplementation fails to augment total dietary intake in frail elders unless accompanied by resistance training, for example (36), and that older adults consuming a multinutrient supplement during resistance training exhibit more hypertrophy than those receiving exercise alone (38). Thus, understanding such interactions of diet and exercise is critical to a successful approach to the sarcopenia of undernutrition and disuse in the elderly, and further long-term studies are needed in this field to refine recommendations for practice.

Treatment: Adjunctive and Primary Treatment of Chronic Disease in the Elderly

Resistive exercise has a potential direct role in a variety of diseases because of its ability to treat the pathophysiology of the disease itself. Examples of this use of exercise with different diseases are given in table 11.3; many are covered in detail in other chapters of this volume. In some cases, resistive exercise may provide quantitatively similar benefits to standard pharmacotherapy (e.g., for major depressions; 107); in others, it may act through an entirely different complementary pathway. In treating diabetes, for example, where insulin can replace the missing endogenous hormone, resistive exercise increases sensitivity to insulin and the ability to transport glucose into cells and store it as glycogen, without altering insulin secretion (54, 103). Thus, the two treatments are complementary to each other, and it is possible that exercise can delay the need for insulin injections or can lower the dosages required. In congestive heart failure, medical therapies improve fluid balance and cardiac contractility, prevent myocardial ischemia and arrhythmias, and decrease afterload, while exercise improves exercise tolerance by targeting the peripheral abnormalities (decreased capillary density, decreased mitochondrial density and oxidative enzyme capacity, and myopathy of type I skeletal muscles). So again, these two different forms of treatment in combination may offer a far superior approach to disease management than either one alone. In depression, resistive exercise appears to have about the same potency as pharmacological management, in that about 70 percent of clinically depressed older people will respond in a meaningful way to both treatments (11, 107), providing a significant therapeutic alternative.

Thus, deciding when to use exercise in a given individual may depend on the constellation of other diseases present, and therefore the risks and benefits relevant to each mode of treatment, as well as the personal preferences of the patient. The chronic treatment of hypertension and

TABLE 11.3   Diseases for Which Progressive Resistance Training in Older Adults Can Provide Adjunctive Treatment

Chronic obstructive pulmonary disease (COPD)

Congestive heart failure (CHF)

Coronary artery disease (CAD)

Depression

Diabetes mellitus

Hypertension

Inflammatory arthritis

Neuromuscular disease

Obesity

Osteoarthritis

Osteoporosis

Parkinson's disease, other degenerative neurological diseases

Stroke

coronary artery disease is clearly a case for adjunctive management with standard medical treatments and exercise, and resistance training is now becoming recognized as safe and effective in this population, in addition to the better-known benefits of cardiovascular forms of exercise (6, 7, 73).

Treating Disuse Accompanying Chronic Disease

For a great many diseases, gradual reduction in activity levels is a nearly universal accompaniment to the chronic illness. This may be due to pain, as in arthritis or osteoporosis, or exercise intolerance, as in peripheral vascular disease, chronic lung disease, stroke, or congestive heart failure. In this situation, there is inevitable atrophy and disuse of many physiologic systems, which will exacerbate age-related changes in these domains and thus markedly accelerate functional decline. Standard medical treatments unfortunately do not address these syndromes of disuse, which result in cardiovascular deconditioning, muscle atrophy and weakness, postural hypotension due to loss of baroreceptor sensitivity, venous stasis, insulin insensitivity and/or glucose intolerance, and immune dysfunction, among other things. However, resistive as well as aerobic exercise retains the capacity to prevent or treat much of the disuse in these systems, just as they do in the healthy aged individual. For some conditions, such as loss of baroreceptor sensitivity or venous stasis, the specific efficacy of progressive resistance training is based on physiological responses of normal individuals to laboratory stressors (66), and therapeutic efficacy remains to be demonstrated in clinical situations. Overall, using resistance exercise to treat the disuse accompanying chronic diseases may be one of the most powerful and underutilized therapies in the health care of older individuals.

The benefits of treating disuse are often most dramatic in individuals in whom medical treatment is already optimized and cannot be pushed further, or when the pathophysiology of the disease itself is not amenable to change. For example, in congestive heart failure, once fluid status has been stabilized, exercise tolerance may still be very limited due to peripheral skeletal muscle atrophy and inability to effectively extract oxygen and utilize it for aerobic work from years of disuse, poor nutrition, and the myopathy of the disease itself (25, 50). However, such peripheral abnormalities can be directly and effectively targeted and treated with progressive resistance training, which has been shown to significantly improve exercise tolerance in such patients even after optimization of pharmacological management (98, 99). Therefore, not using exercise as an adjunct to medical therapy is clearly an incomplete approach to treatment, in this as in many other conditions. Disuse is also common in arthritis and joint replacement, stroke, Parkinson's disease, gait and balance disorders, chronic pain syndromes, osteoporotic or other fractures, prolonged or recurrent hospitalizations, catabolic illness, or periods of bed or chair rest. These should always provoke exploration of adjunctive resistive exercise treatment both acutely and chronically. In most cases, if disuse has been prolonged or severe, it is prudent to begin with muscle reconditioning prior to initiating cardiovascular activities, because walking and similar pursuits may not be possible to be done safely until sufficient strength and balance have been regained through retraining of the musculoskeletal system.

Combating the Side Effects of Dietary or Pharmacological Management of Disease in Older Adults

In addition to its usefulness in optimal aging and the prevention and treatment of disease, exercise may be considered as a specific intervention to offset adverse side effects of standard medical therapies, as summarized in table 11.4. Multiple medications may be implicated in anorexia and decreased nutritional intake in the older patient, with resultant weight loss and depletion of lean tissue. Progressive resistance training has been shown to allow augmentation of energy intake in frail elders through a nutritional supplement, whereas sedentary peers had no increase in total energy intake when given the same supplement (36). Chronic corticosteroid therapy causes large losses of muscle and bone

TABLE 11.4 Counteracting Disease Treatment Side Effects With Exercise

Disease treatment	Adverse consequence	Effective exercise modalities
Anorexia secondary to drug therapy (digoxin, serotonin re-uptake inhibitors, theophylline, multiple drug regimens)	Weight loss, sarcopenia	Progressive resistance exercise*
Corticosteroid treatment for chronic pulmonary disease, rheumatologic disease, organ transplantation	Myopathy	Progressive resistance exercise
	Osteopenia, osteoporotic fracture	Progressive resistance exercise or endurance exercise
Hypocaloric dieting for obesity	Loss of lean body mass (muscle and bone)	Progressive resistance exercise
Low-protein diet for chronic renal failure or liver failure	Weight loss, sarcopenia	Progressive resistance exercise
Postural hypotension secondary to drug therapy (diuretics, anti-hypertensives, Parkinsonian drugs, antidepressants)	Postural symptoms, falls, fractures	Progressive resistance exercise or endurance exercise*
Slowed gastrointestinal motility secondary to anticholinergics, narcotics, calcium channel blockers, iron therapy	Constipation, fecal impaction, reduced food intake	Progressive resistance exercise or endurance exercise*
Thyroid replacement for hypo-thyroidism	Osteopenia	Progressive resistance exercise and endurance exercise*
Treatment with beta-blockers or alphamethyl dopa for hypertension or heart disease	Depression	Progressive resistance exercise or endurance exercise*

*Clinical trial evidence not yet available; recommendation based on laboratory data or known physiological adaptations in healthy individuals.

mass, as well as a proximal myopathy, which is reversible with progressive resistance training, even in heart transplant recipients (14, 15). This finding has very significant implications for patients with rheumatoid arthritis, chronic lung disease, other organ transplantation, and other illnesses where long periods of immunosuppressive therapy are indicated. Restriction of energy intake in obesity (4, 5) and protein intake in chronic renal failure (23) both result in losses of muscle mass and strength, which can be completely offset in the elderly by the concurrent prescription of progressive resistance training. This work has important implications for the clinical management of chronic renal failure and liver disease, in that the necessary protein restriction can be accomplished without the negative consequences on health and functioning that would otherwise occur. In other older patients, protein intake may be low, not due to Iatrogenic prescriptions, but simply to small volumes of food consumed, avoidance of certain food groups for financial reasons or preferences, and so on. In these situations as well, the tendency to waste skeletal muscle to preserve visceral protein stores for metabolism and immune function may be offset by the addition of the anabolic influence of progressive resistance training. This improved nitrogen retention with weightlifting exercise has not been demonstrated to occur with aerobic exercise in older adults. Therefore, if this is one of the goals of the exercise prescription, it is important to advise the correct modality of exercise needed to achieve such goals.

For some conditions (slowed gastrointestinal transit time, depression, osteopenia related to drug therapy), aerobic training may provide similar benefits to resistance training, and the choice of which modality to use may be made in the context of other clinical features and individual preferences. In general, it is advisable to think about the adjunctive use of exercise for these and other common side effects of standard treatment before beginning a second medication to treat the side effects of the first. The benefits of this approach include not only the avoidance of polypharmacy and unwanted medication interactions, but also cost savings and improved fitness levels and other health benefits attributable to exercise itself.

Treatment of Disease Clusters

Another way to consolidate treatment is to use exercise in older patients who present with clusters of diseases that are all responsive in some way to appropriate levels of physical activity. For example, it would not be uncommon for an older woman with central and generalized obesity to present at age 65 with osteoarthritis, type 2 diabetes, hypertension, coronary artery disease, peripheral vascular disease, varicose veins, hyperlipidemia, mobility impairment, insomnia, and depression. Even if only one drug were given for each of these conditions (often it is two or more), a list of eight to ten different medications may be quickly generated. Although exercise is unlikely to eliminate the need for all medications, it certainly has the potential to replace some and reduce dosages of others. At the same time, it will provide conditioning effects and other benefits previously unrealized with drug therapy alone. Therefore, a thorough review of all diagnoses and medications is warranted in all older patients, to see where substitutions and alterations can be made to reduce the burden of treatment and suffering and increase quality of life and functioning. It is critical to reevaluate what has been prescribed every 2-3 months, to see whether clinical disease control and risk factors are improved with this change in management and to assess current needs.

Use of Exercise in Frailty and Functional Decline

It was once thought that vigorous physical activity was not appropriate for older adults. Risk of orthopedic injury and heart attack were the primary concerns. Recent research, however, has demonstrated that previously sedentary men and women can benefit from a properly prescribed exercise program well into their 90s.

Rationale and Benefits

In the past, exercise, and especially progressive resistance training, has been generally considered inappropriate for frail or very aged individuals, due to both low expectations of benefit as well as exaggerated fears of exercise-related injury. The past decade has seen an accumulation of data that dispels myths of futility, and additionally provides reassurance of the safety of exercise in the oldest old (34). The benefits are wide ranging, including physiologic, metabolic, psychological, and functional adaptations to resistance training that can substantially contribute to quality of life in older adults with disabilities. Goals of exercise appropriate to younger adults (46), such as prevention of cardiovascular disease, cancer, or diabetes, or increases in longevity itself (60), are replaced in the oldest old (over the age of 85) with a new set of goals that include minimizing biological changes of aging (33), reversing disuse syndromes (12), contributing to the control of chronic diseases (29, 84, 87), maximizing psychological health (106, 107), mobility, and function (36, 80, 88), and assisting with rehabilitation from acute and chronic illnesses. For many of the geriatric syndromes common to this vulnerable population, in fact, a targeted exercise prescription offers benefits that cannot be achieved with any other therapeutic modality. It is important to understand the diverse pathophysiology of frailty in order to utilize exercise appropriately in this setting.

The Etiology of Frailty

Biological aging, high burdens of chronic disease, malnutrition, psychosocial vulnerability, and extreme sedentariness are the primary contributors to a common pathway that results in the syndrome of physical frailty. Frailty is not specific to the elderly, but is increasingly prevalent with aging, particularly after the age of 80 (48). Anorexia and undernutrition are commonly seen in frail, sedentary elders. Exercise has been of interest as a way to boost energy requirements, and thus appetite and voluntary food intake, in such individuals, thus reducing the risk of malnutrition as a contributor to frailty (79). In institutionalized older men and women, resistance training has been shown to prevent the decrease in habitual food intake seen with administration of a liquid multinutrient supplement (36). This may have important clinical implications, since the assumption is that such liquid supplements augment total caloric intake, as opposed to simply substituting one form of calories for another. It is not currently known if aerobic training would provide the same benefit in frail elders. Further studies are required to define the long-term benefit of treating undernourished individuals with a combination of resistance training exercise and nutritional supplements in comparison to supplementation alone. The psychosocial factors related to frailty include depressive symptoms, low self-efficacy, low self-esteem, isolation, loneliness, age discrimination and negative societal expectations, and inadequate social support networks (57). These may exert as powerful an influence as physiological decline in some individuals. Resistance training and other forms of exercise in healthy, depressed, and clinical populations of older adults have been shown to significantly improve depressive symptoms, morale, self-efficacy, and social integrations (7, 31, 107, 113). Such efforts serve to enhance adherence and adaptation to the new exercise behavior, as well as directly improving functional status and quality of life (32).

Resistance Training for the Frail Elderly

The principles of specificity that apply to younger adults are of equal relevance in the frail elderly. Increases in muscle mass and strength are seen following high-intensity progressive resistance training (i.e., approximately 80% of the one-repetition maximum [1-RM]) (36), whereas lower-intensity regimens (body weight, elastic bands or tubing, resistance to a therapist, or light weights) result in little if any significant gains in strength (81). Muscle weakness and atrophy are probably the most functionally relevant and reversible parameters related to exercise in this population, so attempts to reverse these deficits and minimize the clinical consequences (functional decline, immobility, poor balance, falls, low energy requirements and intake) should focus on scientifically proven strategies rather than nonspecific "movement" programs for the aged. The literature on exercise training in the frail elderly in nursing homes, between the ages of 80 and 100, includes no reports to date of serious cardiovascular incidents, sudden death, myocardial infarction, or exacerbation of metabolic control of hypertension (10, 35, 36, 42, 55, 56, 75, 77, 80, 81, 82, 93, 97, 104, 105, 110). Resistive exercise-related events that have been described include exacerbation of a pre-existing hernia (35), and underlying arthritis or other joint abnormalities requiring modification of the exercises prescribed (36). No adverse events related to resistance training in small groups with free weights have been reported in a large randomized controlled trial of nursing home residents exercising over a 12-month period (80). Therefore, sedentariness appears a far more dangerous condition than physical activity in the very old, based on the available evidence.

As summarized in table 11.5, resistance training in frail elders results in a range of clinical adaptations that are relevant to the targeted disability, which is almost always a multifactorial phenomenon. Associated with gains in strength after resistance training in the frail elderly are improvements in gait velocity, balance, ability to rise from a chair, stair-climbing power, aerobic capacity, performance-based tests of functional independence, self-reported disability, morale, depressive symptoms, and energy intake (35, 36, 80, 85, 97, 98, 104). Balance enhancement is clearly possible after resistance training in the frail elderly and may be one of the most robust adaptations to exercise in this cohort (35, 84, 99). We are currently testing the efficacy of one year of standing resistance training exercises with reduced hand and visual support as a means of enhancing balance and ultimately preventing falls (37). In healthier elderly subjects, resistance training has also been shown to increase bone density, resting metabolic rate, insulin sensitivity, and gastrointestinal transit time, to decrease pain and disability from arthritis, to reduce body fat and central adiposity, and to improve sleep quality; but it remains to be demonstrated that these adaptations in fact occur in the very frail as well.

Many common geriatric syndromes contributing to frailty are improved after increased levels of appropriate physical activity. Improving these syndromes is one of the most effective ways to use exercise, but to be effective it must be done in a rational way, applied in the correct modality, dose, and, in some cases, time of day. For example, if someone complains of weakness, it will not benefit them very much to advise

TABLE 11.5 Clinical Improvements Associated With Progressive Resistance Training in the Elderly

Aerobic capacity (maximal workload and submaximal tolerance)	
Balance	Muscle mass
Depression	Muscle strength and endurance
Fall risk	Nutritional intake
Flexibility	Overall physical activity level
Gait speed and stability	Perceived quality of life
Mobility tasks	Self-efficacy
Morale	

taking a walk or engaging in some other low-intensity cardiovascular form of exercise. In some cases, the modality of exercise does not seem to be critical, whereas the time of day does, as in the case of insomnia (for which exercise is optimally prescribed 4-8 h before desired bedtime). The relative potencies of different modalities of exercise on various risk factors for functional impairment are outlined in table 11.6.

The major physiologic deficits that are relevant and treatable by exercise training include muscle weakness, low muscle mass, low bone density, cardiovascular deconditioning, depression, and poor balance and gait. The most evidence for early functional and mobility benefit exists with programs that include resistance training and balance training; and higher-intensity training is more beneficial and just as safe as lower-intensity training. Therefore, most exercise programs for the frail elderly should include progressive resistance training of the major muscle groups of the upper and lower extremities and trunk if possible.

TABLE 11.6   Risk Factors for Frailty Addressed by Various Exercise Modalities

Risk factor	Aerobic training	Resistance training	Balance training	Flexibility training
Aerobic deconditioning	Yes	Yes	No	No
Chronic disease prevention	Yes	?	?	No
Chronic disease treatment	Yes	Yes	Yes	Yes
Dementia	No	No	No	No
Depression	Yes	Yes	No	No
Impaired range of motion	No	Yes	No	Yes
Low muscle power	No	Yes*	No	No
Low self-efficacy	Yes	Yes	?	?
Muscle weakness	No	Yes	No	No
Obesity	Yes	Yes	No	No
Poor balance	No	Yes	Yes	?
Sarcopenia	No	Yes	No	No
Sedentariness	Yes	Yes	?	?
Slow gait velocity	No	Yes	Yes	?
Social isolation	?	?	?	?
Undernutrition	Yes	Yes	No	No
Visual impairment	No	No	No	No

? = Theoretically of benefit, but no direct evidence available.
* = If high-velocity, high-force training modality is used (power training).

Balance training should also be incorporated, either as part of the resistance training (e.g., progressive decrease in hand support and visual cues during standing resistive exercises with free weights) or as a separate modality if time and functional status permit. Improving muscle strength, joint stability, and balance, as described above, may significantly improve the tolerance to weight-bearing activity such as walking and thereby allow adoption of a prescription for cardiovascular exercises as well.

General guidelines for the use of exercise to treat common geriatric syndromes, based on currently available evidence, are given in table 11.7. In some cases, the capacity of the individual, rather than the intended goals of exercise, forms the basis for the choice of modality. For example, clinical depression and insomnia are equally benefited by aerobic and resistive exercise in the elderly (11, 58, 106, 107). In someone with severe osteoarthritis of the knee, gait and balance disorder, amputation, low threshold for ischemic symptoms, or desaturation secondary to obstructive pulmonary disease, resistance training may be the only

TABLE 11.7   Choice of Exercise for Common Geriatric Syndromes

Syndrome—Therapeutic exercise recommendation

Anorexia—Resistance training

Constipation—Endurance or resistance exercise

Depression, anxiety, low self-efficacy, low morale, loneliness, low self-esteem— Individual or group exercises including endurance or resistive exercises at moderate to high intensity

Fatigue—Endurance training in the morning hours (increase duration and intensity as tolerated); muscle endurance training

Functional dependency—Stair climbing for endurance; resistance training of upper and lower extremities; power training; balance training

Incontinence (stress)—Pelvic muscle strengthening (Kegel exercises); mobility improvement with endurance, balance, and resistance training as needed

Insomnia—Endurance or resistance exercise in early to mid afternoon

Low back pain, spinal stenosis—Resistance training to strengthen the back extensor muscles, rectus abdominus, and hip and knee extensor muscle groups

Recurrent falls, gait and balance disorders—Lower-extremity resistance training for hip, knee, and ankle, including lateral movements; balance training, Tai Chi, yoga, ballet; training in use of ambulatory devices and functional mobility (e.g., stairs, obstacles) as needed

Weakness and sarcopenia—Moderate- to high-intensity resistance training for all major muscle groups feasible choice, despite the theoretical benefits of aerobic training as well. In some cases, symptoms may improve enough to allow the addition or substitution of cardiovascular exercise; in others, a more permanent inability to walk or bear weight may be present. Such flexibility in prescription, based on a thoughtful integration of therapeutic efficacy, individual limitations, and personal preferences, is much more likely to engender long-term adoption and adherence in such older persons than rigid protocols.

Neuropsychological Effects of Resistance Training in the Elderly

The benefits of physical activity in older adults extend beyond morphological changes and improvements in functional (physical work) capacity. Participation in an appropriate level of exercise also enhances psychological well-being by reducing symptoms of depression, improving sleep quality, and preventing cognitive impairment.

Depression and Depressive Symptoms

A large literature supports the antidepressant effect of exercise (86). The rationale for the use of exercise as an antidepressant is based on its favorable risk/benefit ratio compared with current pharmacological therapies and the cost associated with various forms of group and psychotherapy in selected populations. While improvements continue to be made in side effect profiles of drugs used to treat depression, data on effectiveness and side effect profiles of these drugs in the elderly are limited, with as yet no convincing evidence of a reduction in falls risk compared with older agents.

The majority of studies have used aerobic exercise as the intervention, since early work suggested that an aerobic training effect was required to elicit depression reduction. Two subsequent studies in young subjects comparing aerobic to nonaerobic training have shown equivalent antidepressant effects (27, 70). For subjects over the age of 60, two aerobic (11, 76) and one resistance training (107) randomized controlled trials have been conducted and published regarding depressed elders over the age of 60. Low- to moderate-intensity walking was not better than attention control (76) (about 30% reduction in depressive symptoms), but both high-intensity progressive resistance training (107) and moderate-to high-intensity jogging (11) have now been shown to be equipotent to pharmacological management (60-70% effective in relief of depression). Low-intensity progressive resistance training is not more effective than referral to a general practitioner (approximately 30% improvement) (112). Thus, adequate intensity of training appears to be necessary for both physiological adaptation and psychological improvement in this cohort. There is no adequate study of unsupervised exercise as an initial treatment in clinically depressed elders; although we have seen that antidepressant effect is maintained and increased further when resistance training changes from a supervised to an unsupervised setting after 10 weeks (107). Further studies on long-term relapse rates and changes in functional status using this approach are needed, particularly in older adults who are frail or institutionalized, as well as depressed.

Insomnia

Although sleep problems are not generally life threatening, we do spend one-third of our lives in sleep, and this time may profoundly influence quality of life in the elderly, among whom sleep complaints are frequent. Insomnia has been associated with increased risk of accidents, falls, nursing home placement, and an increased mortality (121), and so is relevant to the treatment of frail elders. Two randomized controlled trials in older adults with moderate sleep impairment have been published. In a clinically depressed group, it was demonstrated that weightlifting exercise significantly improved sleep quality over 10 weeks compared with an attention control group (106). In a study using aerobic exercise, King targeted a group free of clinically diagnosable sleep disorders or a medical or psychiatric condition responsible for sleep complaints. Global sleep quality, total sleep time, and sleep onset latency were significantly improved by 16 weeks of aerobic exercise (58) compared with wait-listed controls. Therefore, exercise has the advantage of having an effect on sleep disturbance in elders with and without depression. A direct comparison of the two modalities of exercise would be required to determine which is most effective, has higher compliance and feasibility, or lower rates of injury in older adults. No evidence is currently available regarding the efficacy of either form of exercise for insomnia in institutionalized elders. Such evidence would be very useful, since this population has a very high prevalence of sleep disturbance and is at high risk for sedative-induced side effects and injuries, including hip fracture (101).

Data on exercise frequency, volume, and intensity required for improvement in insomnia can be based only on the two published randomized trials in sleep-disturbed elders. These were four 30-40 min sessions a week at 60-75% of heart rate reserve (moderate intensity) for aerobic exercise (58), and three 45-60 min sessions per week, at 3 sets of 8 repetitions using a load of 80% of the 1-RM (high intensity) for resistance training (106). Exercise is optimal for insomnia when performed between 4-8 h before desired sleep time. Less than 4 h and greater than 8 h leads to an attenuation of its effect and possibly a worsening of sleep. Less exposure to light is postulated as one reason why the elderly may not sleep as well as the young. In young normals there appears to be a sleep benefit to outdoor exercise compared with indoor exercise, but whether this is related to increased light exposure is unknown. In the two positive trials in symptomatic elderly, exercise classes were performed indoors with undefined light exposure, suggesting that increased light exposure was not the primary mechanism of the exercise-induced improvement in sleep. Thus, when planning programs for institutionalized or homebound elderly, or in residential settings, one should not have to depend on the availability of outdoor or sun-exposed exercise venues for success.

Cognitive Impairment

Cognitive decline is a major factor in the development of functional dependency in old age (19). There is no hard scientific evidence that resistance training or any form of exercise can prevent or treat dementia directly. Small changes in attention span, alertness, mood, communication skills, activity levels, and reaction time tests have been noted in some trials of aerobic exercise in adults with dementia or long-standing mental illness (42, 68, 77, 110), but a definitive role for any exercise regimen in the improvement of global cognitive function or memory has not been demonstrated.

However, this does not mean that exercise is to be avoided in patients with dementia. On the one hand, assuming that attention span and behavior do not preclude even supervised exercise, physiological improvements may be as robust in demented individuals as in the cognitively intact (36). In addition, functional decline in those with dementia may be significantly slowed with attention to the other, more reversible contributors to frailty (see table 11.6). The exercise prescription needs to be modified in terms of delivery (setting, supervision, length of sessions, time of day) to accommodate cognitive impairment, but the other elements of training (frequency, intensity, volume) in general do not. One-on-one training in the home or institutional setting may be carried out by family members, volunteers, caregivers, or other staff, and may substitute for more sedentary forms of interaction ("baby-sitting," watching TV, playing board games, etc.) without extending the cost, length, or frequency of encounters. Administrative consent and creative restructuring of job descriptions, volunteer training programs, and family education packages for Alzheimer's disease and related disorders are necessary to implement such programs successfully.

Disorders of Gait and Balance

Falls are an extremely heterogeneous problem in the older adult, with many extrinsic and intrinsic contributing factors (45, 51, 69, 109, 114, 123-

125). Psychological risk factors include depression and low self-efficacy. Central nervous system pathology may include changes in reaction time, dementia, cerebellar dysfunction, subcortical changes, stroke, and neurodegenerative diseases. The peripheral nervous system may be etiologic in the form of visual impairment, vestibular dysfunction, loss of proprioception, vibration or light touch sensation, and even decreased hearing. Musculoskeletal abnormalities that have been associated with falling include sarcopenia, muscle weakness and low endurance, loss of coordination, poor range of motion across joints, degenerative changes of bone and soft tissues around weight-bearing joints, osteoporotic deformities, and pediatric problems. Cardiovascular factors that have been implicated in abnormal gait include peripheral vascular disease, edema, postural hypotension, conduction system disturbances, and congestive heart failure. Environmental features include polypharmacy and particular categories of medications, hazardous obstacles, lack of supportive structures, poor lighting, use of suboptimal corrective lenses and footwear, inclement weather, and slippery surfaces. Given this plethora of interacting risk factors, it is unlikely that a single intervention will ever be shown to be effective in a broad population of fallers. The best approach would appear to be thorough assessment to identify potentially remediable factors in the individual and the environment, and subsequent robust, targeted intervention in these areas (114, 115).

Resistance training has a strong potential role in the prevention of falls and injurious falls because of its known effects on depression, self-efficacy, muscle mass, muscle strength, balance, postural reflexes, and bone density, as reviewed already. Although no trials have been conducted using high-intensity progressive resistance training as an isolated intervention to prevent falls as a primary outcome, low- to moderate-intensity strengthening exercises have been shown to reduce falls in combination with balance training (20, 96) as has moderate- to high-intensity resistance training in combination with aerobic training (18) in the elderly. No studies have yet demonstrated reduction in hip fracture or other injuries secondary to resistance training or any form of exercise. Much remains to be learned about the targeting of appropriate individuals; dose-response relationships; optimal muscle groups to train; the efficacy of combined nutritional, psychological, and exercise interventions; and the long-term benefits of this approach to falls reduction. However, based on the available data, it seems sensible to

1. screen for deficits in muscle strength, muscle power, and balance in fallers;
2. offer a combined program of balance training and progressive resistance training, including hip and knee extensors, hip abductors, and dorsiflexors among exercises;

3. attempt to substitute exercise for hazardous drugs (e.g., sedatives, antidepressants) when treating depression or insomnia in at-risk elders; and
4. treat other remediable factors (visual impairment, environment, postural hypotension) concurrently, as possible.

Parkinson's Disease and Other Neurodegenerative Conditions

Even when relatively good control of tremor and bradykinesia are provided by pharmacotherapy, functional status and quality of life may continue to deteriorate in individuals with Parkinson's disease. This may be ascribable in part to a host of disease sequelae, including loss of muscle mass (sarcopenia), low muscle power, autonomic neuropathy resulting in postural hypotension, poor balance, impaired gait and elevated risk of falling, depression, cognitive decline, nutritional inadequacies secondary to swallowing difficulty, increased work of breathing and constipation, and low physical activity levels. Unfortunately, standard medical care of these patients does not optimally address this constellation of problems, which result in significant disability and reduced health-related quality of life.

Progressive resistance training (weightlifting) exercise offers a potential means to intervene in this cascade of events in Parkinson's disease and thus augment quality of life in this population substantially. In studies of non-Parkinson populations by our laboratory and others, resistance training has been shown to increase muscle mass (36, 84), muscle strength (35, 39, 78), flexibility (112), and balance (36, 84), improve gait velocity (36), reduce risk factors for falls (84), increase overall activity levels (36, 84), improve nutritional intake (36), increase tolerance to hypotensive stressors (66), increase gastrointestinal transit time (53), and treat depression (107).

All of these outcomes are of great relevance to patients with Parkinson's disease, who have deficits in these areas compared with age-matched normals. For example, in patients with Parkinson's disease, muscle strength and range of motion at the knee and ankle have been shown to be critical for the maintenance of equilibrium (116). Therefore, the high risk for falls and impaired mobility in these patients potentially may be ameliorated by an intervention that could simultaneously increase strength, range of motion, balance, and postural stability. Patients with Parkinson's disease tend to have muscle wasting because of their high energy expenditure secondary to muscle tremor and difficulty maintaining food intake secondary to swallowing difficulty and constipation. Thus, an intervention that could boost appetite and improve gastrointestinal transit time should theoretically combat the catabolic effects of this illness on skeletal muscle, which compound the neurologically mediated impairment. In another realm, the prevalence of depression is a major factor in Parkinson's disease, responsible for much disability and reduced quality of life. The potent effect of resistance training for the treatment of clinical depression does not carry with it the negative side effects of many antidepressant medications (postural hypotension, weight loss, gastrointestinal disturbance, elevated fall risk) that often make these medications intolerable in this population (2, 74).

Thus there is a substantial literature supporting the rationale for the application of resistance training to Parkinson's disease. Previous studies on physiological capacity in Parkinson's disease indicate that aerobic capacity is often not significantly reduced compared with controls (111), whereas muscle strength and speed of movement are. Therefore, an exercise intervention that seeks to address the specific physiological derangement in this condition, as well as the associated metabolic and other abnormalities noted above, would seemingly need to include an anabolic mode of exercise. Power training (training for both high-force and high-velocity movements) is ideally suited to these requirements. We have shown that in frail elders, muscle power is the single most important physiological determinant of functional independence (41) and thus a desirable target when functional status is a clinical outcome. However, to date, published exercise interventions in Parkinson's disease have included only aerobic training or flexibility exercises (126), or trunk muscle strengthening in addition to aerobic exercise (16), and thus definitive data on efficacy are lacking.

Potential benefits of true progressive resistance training or power training of relevance in older adults with Parkinson's disease would include

- increased muscle strength,
- increased muscle mass,
- increased gait stability,
- improved balance,
- increased flexibility,
- increased habitual activity level,
- improved nutritional intake,
- increased gastrointestinal transit time,
- increased resistance to postural stress,
- decreased depressive symptoms,
- improved functional status, and
- improved health-related quality of life.

Randomized controlled trials of progressive resistance training are currently lacking in Parkinson's disease, and only a small number of controlled exercise studies (four) have been reported in the literature in this condition (92). Such data are urgently needed to assess the true relevance of resistance training to this and other neurodegenerative conditions of aging.

Issues of Adoption and Adherence in the Older Adult

Most frail elders live in environments and among caregivers in which and for whom exercise is still an unfamiliar and perhaps frightening concept. So there is a great need to change the physical surroundings, recreational programming options, and staff training to allow the above recommendations to be instituted in private homes, senior apartment complexes, life-care communities, and nursing homes. By eliminating unnecessary barriers to optimal mobility and fitness among the oldest old, substantial health benefits may be realized via both prevention of new disabilities as well as rehabilitation from chronic conditions. Barriers may also exist on a personal level. The most common of these in the older adult are perceived lack of time, exaggerated fear of injury, misconceptions about the role of exercise in chronic disease, reduced expectation of benefit, negative attitudes toward aging, the caregiving role of the spouse, and lack of transportation. Once education on these topics is provided, many older adults *would* exercise if it were not for the substantial societal and institutional barriers that exist, such as lack of financial reimbursement, limited access to appropriate facilities and qualified trainers, regulations prohibiting certain activities (such as stair climbing in nursing homes), and negative societal stereotypes. We have shown that providing access to a resistance training program in nursing homes that is sanctioned by the administration and carried out by the clinical staff can result in optimal adherence (>10 sessions per month) in about one-third of residents of typical facilities over a 12-month period (80). Staffing shortages that do not allow individualized training and inclusion of nonambulatory residents are the greatest roadblock in such programs.

Most importantly, an educational process that integrates exercise therapy and geriatric medicine into a holistic vision of health care for the older patient is still missing from the core training of many health care practitioners at this time. This omission poses a significant barrier for the aged-care institutions and health care systems that the elderly must rely on. Changing this will require extensive education of health care practitioners so that they recognize the importance of physical activity for

- prevention of age-related declines,
- primary risk factor prevention,
- treatment of established disease,
- treatment of accompanying disuse syndromes,
- treatment of medication/diet prescription side effects,

- benefits outside of the target disease, treatment of disease clusters and geriatric syndromes, and
- optimization of quality of life and functional independence.

The optimal health and functioning of the older adult is obviously a multifactorial process, dependent on genetic substrate, environmental design, social or political forces, psychological factors, support networks, and lifestyle choices, among other things. Recognizing the benefits of progressive resistance training in this cohort becomes increasingly important as we seek to identify modifiable elements that will prevent or delay the onset of many chronic diseases and disabilities.

References

1. Ades, P.A., D.L. Ballor, T. Ashikaga, J.L. Utton, and K.S. Nair. 1996. Weight training improves walking endurance in healthy elderly persons. *Annals of Internal Medicine* 124: 568-572.
2. American College of Sports Medicine. 1995. *ACSM's guidelines for exercise testing and prescription*. Philadelphia: Williams & Wilkins.
3. Asmussen, E., and K. Heeboll-Nielsen. 1961. Isometric muscle strength of adult men and women. In *Community testing observation*, edited by E. Asmussen, A. Fredsted, and E. Ryge, 1-43. Institute for the Danish National Association for Infantile Paralysis.
4. Ballor, D.L., J.R. Harvey-Berino, P.A. Ades, J. Cryan, and J. Calles-Escandon. 1996. Contrasting effects of resistance and aerobic training on body composition and metabolism after diet-induced weight loss. *Metabolism: Clinical and Experimental* 45: 179-183.
5. Ballor, D.L., V.L. Katch, M.D. Becque, and C.R. Marks. 1988. Resistance weight training during caloric restriction enhances lean body weight maintenance. *American Journal of Clinical Nutrition* 47: 19-25.
6. Beniamini, Y., J. Rubenstein, A. Faigenbaum, A. Lichtenstein, and M. Crim. 1999. High-intensity strength training of patients enrolled in an outpatient cardiac rehabilitation program. *Journal of Cardiopulmonary Rehabilitation* 19: 8-17.
7. Beniamini, Y., J.J. Rubenstein, L.D. Zaichkowsky, and M.C. Crim. 1997. Effects of high-intensity strength training on quality-of-life parameters in cardiac rehabilitation patients. *American Journal of Cardiology* 80: 841-846.
8. Blair, S.N., J.B. Kampert, H.W. Kohl, C.E. Barlow, C.A. Macera, R.S. Paffenbarger, and L.W. Gibbons. 1996. Influences of cardiovascular fitness and other precursors on cardiovascular disease and all-cause mortality in men and women. *Journal of the American Medical Association* 276: 205-210.
9. Blair, S.N., H. Kohl, C. Barlow, R.S. Paffenbarger, L. Gibbons, and C. Macera. 1995. Changes in physical fitness and all-cause mortality: A prospective study of healthy and unhealthy men. *Journal of the American Medical Association* 273: 1093-1098.
10. Blankfort-Doyle, W., H. Waxman, and K. Coughey. 1989. An exercise program for nursing home residents. In *Aging and motor behavior*, edited by A.C. Ostrow, 201-206. Indianapolis: Benchmark Press.
11. Blumenthal, J., M. Babyak, K. Moore, E. Craighead, S. Herman, P. Khatri, R. Waugh, M. Napolitano, L. Forman, M. Appelbaum, M. Doraiswamy, and R. Krishnan. 1999. Effects of exercise training on older patients with major depression. *Archives of Internal Medicine* 159: 2349-2356.
12. Bortz, W.M. 1982. Disuse and aging. *Journal of the American Medical Association* 248: 1203-1208.
13. Bortz, W.M. 1989. Redefining human aging. *Journal of the American Geriatrics Society* 37: 1092-1096.

14. Braith, R., R. Mills, M. Welsch, J. Keller, and M. Pollock. 1996. Resistance exercise training restores bone mineral density in heart transplant recipients. *Journal of the American College of Cardiology* 28: 1471-1477.
15. Braith, R., M. Welsch, R. Mills, J. Keller, and M. Pollock. 1998. Resistance exercise prevents glucocorticoid-induced myopathy in heart transplant recipients. *Medicine and Science in Sports and Exercise* 30 (4): 483-489.
16. Bridgewater, K., and M. Sharpe. 1997. Trunk muscle training and early Parkinson's disease. *Physiotherapy Theory and Practice* 13: 139-153.
17. Brown, A., N. McCartney, and D. Sale. 1990. Positive adaptations to weight-lifting training in the elderly. *Journal of Applied Physiology* 69: 1725-1733.
18. Buchner, D.M., M.E. Cress, B.J. de Lateur, P.C. Esselman, A.J. Margherita, R. Price, and E.H. Wagner. 1997. The effect of strength and endurance training on gait, balance, fall risk, and health services use in community-living older adults. *Journal of the American Geriatrics Society* 52A: M218-M224.
19. Buchner, D.M., and E.H. Wagner. 1992. Preventing frail health. *Clinics in Geriatric Medicine* 8: 1-17.
20. Campbell, A., M. Robertson, M. Gardner, R. Norton, M. Tilyard, and D. Buchner. 1997. Randomised controlled trial of a general practice programme of home based exercise to prevent falls in elderly women. *British Medical Journal* 315: 1065-1069.
21. Campbell, W.W., M.C. Crim, V.R. Young, and W.J. Evans. 1994. Increased energy requirements and changes in body composition with resistance training in older adults. *American Journal of Clinical Nutrition* 60: 167-175.
22. Cartee, G.D. 1994. Aging skeletal muscle: Response to exercise. *Exercise and Sport Sciences Reviews* 22: 91-120.
23. Castaneda, C., P. Gordon, K. Uhlin, J. Kehayias, A. Levey, J. Dwyer, R. Roubenoff, and M. Fiatarone Singh. 1999. Resistance training prevents muscle wasting in renal disease. *Federation of American Societies for Experimental Biology Journal* 13: A877.
24. Charette, S., L. McEvoy, G. Pyka, C. Snow-Harter, D. Guido, R. Wiswell, and R. Marcus. 1991. Muscle hypertrophy response to resistance training in older women. *Journal of Applied Physiology* 70: 1912-1916.
25. Coats, A.J., A.L. Clark, M. Peipoli, M. Volterrani, and P.A. Poole-Wilson. 1994. Symptoms and quality of life in heart failure: The muscle hypothesis. *British Heart Journal* 72: S36-S39.
26. Despres, J.-P. 1998. Body fat distribution, exercise and nutrition: Implications for prevention of atherogenic dyslipidemia, coronary heart disease, and non-insulin dependent diabetes mellitus. In *Perspectives in exercise science and sports medicine: Exercise, nutrition, and weight control*, edited by D. Lamb and R. Murray, 107-150. Carmel, IN: Cooper.
27. Doyne, E.J., D.J. Ossip-Klein, E.D. Bowman, K.M. Osborn, I.B. McDougall-Wilson, and R.A. Neimeyer. 1987. Running versus weight lifting in the treatment of depression. *Journal of Consulting and Clinical Psychology* 55: 748-754.
28. Evans, W., and W. Campbell. 1993. Sarcopenia and age-related changes in body composition and functional capacity. *Journal of Nutrition* 123: 465-468.
29. Evans, W., V. Hughes, C. Ferrara, R. Fielding, M. Fiatarone, E. Fisher, and D. Elahi. 1991. Effects of training intensity on glucose homeostasis in glucose intolerant adults. *Medicine and Science in Sports and Exercise* 23: S152.
30. Evans, W.J. 1996. Reversing sarcopenia: How weight training can build strength and vitality. *Geriatrics* 51: 46-47, 51-53; quiz 54.
31. Ewart, C. 1989. Psychological effects of resistive weight training: Implications for cardiac patients. *Medicine and Science in Sports and Exercise* 21: 683-688.
32. Ewart, C., K. Stewart, R. Gillian, and M. Keleman. 1986. Self-efficacy mediates strength gains during circuit weight training in men with coronary artery disease. *Medicine and Science in Sports and Exercise* 18: 531-540.
33. Fiatarone, M., and W. Evans. 1993. The etiology and reversibility of muscle dysfunction in the elderly. *Journal of Gerontology* 48: 77-83.

34. Fiatarone, M.A., and W.J. Evans. 1990. Exercise in the oldest old. *Topics in Geriatric Rehabilitation* 5: 63-77.

35. Fiatarone, M.A., E.C. Marks, N.D. Ryan, C.N. Meredith, L.A. Lipsitz, and W.J. Evans. 1990. High-intensity strength training in nonagenarians: Effects on skeletal muscle. *Journal of the American Medical Association* 263: 3029-3034.

36. Fiatarone, M.A., E.F. O'Neill, N.D. Ryan, K.M. Clements, G.R. Solares, M.E. Nelson, S.R. Roberts, J.K. Kehayias, L.A. Lipsitz, and W.J. Evans. 1994. Exercise training and nutritional supplementation for physical frailty in very elderly people. *New England Journal of Medicine* 330: 1769-1775.

37. Fiatarone Singh, M. In press. Soft tissue responses to exercise in the elderly. In *Sports medicine for specific client groups*, edited by N. Maffuli, K. Chan, R. MacDonald, R. Malino, and A. Parker. Edinburgh, UK: Churchill Livingstone.

38. Fiatarone Singh, M., W. Ding, T. Manfredi, G. Solares, E. O'Neill, K. Clements, N. Ryan, J. Kehayias, R. Fielding, and W. Evans. 1999. Insulin-like growth factor I in skeletal muscle after weight-lifting exercise in frail elders. *American Journal of Physiology (Endocrinology and Metabolism)* 277: E136-E143.

39. Fiatarone Singh, M., C. Pu, M. Johnson, D. Forman, J. Hausdorff, R. Roubenoff, and R. Fielding. In press. The effects of progressive resistance training on skeletal muscle and exercise performance in older women with heart failure. *Australian and New Zealand Journal of Medicine*.

40. Fleg, J., and E. Lakatta. 1988. Role of muscle loss in age-associated reduction in VO_2max. *Journal of Applied Physiology* 65: 1147-1151.

41. Foldvari, M., M. Clark, L. Laviolette, M. Bernstein, C. Castaneda, C. Pu, J. Hausdorff, R. Fielding, and M. Fiatarone Singh. 2000. Association of muscle power with functional status in community-dwelling elderly women. *Journals of Gerontology. Series A, Biological Sciences and Medical Sciences* 55 (4): M192-M199.

42. Friedman, R., and R. Tappen. 1991. Effect of planned walking on commuication in Alzheimer's disease. *Journal of the American Geriatrics Society* 39: 650-654.

43. Frontera, W., V. Hughes, K. Lutz, and W. Evans. 1991. A cross-sectional study of muscle strength and mass in 45- to 78-yr-old men and women. *Journal of Applied Physiology* 71: 644-650.

44. Frontera, W.R., C.N. Meredith, K.P. O'Reilly, H.G. Knuttgen, and W.J. Evans. 1988. Strength conditioning in older men: Skeletal muscle hypertrophy and improved function. *Journal of Applied Physiology* 64: 1038-1044.

45. Gehlsen, G.M., and M.H. Whaley. 1990. Falls in the elderly: Part II. Balance, strength, and flexibility. *Archives of Physical Medicine and Rehabilitation* 71: 739-741.

46. Goldberg, T., and S. Chavin. 1997. Preventive medicine and screening for older adults. *Journal of the American Geriatrics Society* 45: 344-354.

47. Grembowski, D., D. Patrick, P. Diehr, M. Durham, S. Beresford, E. Kay, and J. Hecht. 1993. Self-efficacy and health behavior among older adults. *Journal of Health and Social Behavior* 34: 89-104.

48. Guralnik, J., A. LaCroix, R.D. Abbott, L.F. Berkman, S. Satterfield, D.A. Evans, and R.B. Wallace. 1993. Maintaining mobility in late life. I. Demographic characteristics and chronic conditions. *American Journal of Epidemiology* 137: 845-857.

49. Hagerman, F., R. Fielding, M. Fiatarone, J. Gault, D. Kirkendall, K. Ragg, and W. Evans. 1996. A 20-year longitudinal study of Olympic oarsmen. *Medicine and Science in Sports and Exercise* 28: 1150-1156.

50. Harrington, D., S. Anker, T. Chua, K. Webb-Peploe, P. Ponikowski, P. Poole-Wilson, and A. Coats. 1997. Skeletal muscle function and its relation to exercise tolerance in chronic heart failure. *Journal of American College of Cardiology* 30: 1758-1764.

51. Hausdorff, J., M. Cudkowicz, R. Firtion, J. Wei, and A. Goldberger. 1998. Gait variability and basal ganglia disorders: Stride-to-stride variations of gait cycle timing in Parkinson's disease and Huntington's disease. *Movement Disorders* 13: 428-437.

52. Heath, G., J. Hagberg, A. Ehsani, and J. Holloszy. 1981. A physiological comparison of young and older endurance athletes. *Journal of Applied Physiology* 51: 634-640.

53. Hurley, B.F. 1995. Age, gender, and muscular strength. *Journal of Gerontology* 50A: 41-44.

54. Ishii, T., T. Yamakita, T. Sato, S. Tanaka, and S. Fuji. 1998. Resistance training improves insulin sensitivity in NIDDM subjects without altering maximal oxygen uptake. *Diabetes Care* 21: 1353-1355.

55. Jirovec, M. 1991. The impact of daily exercise on the mobility, balance, and urine control of cognitively impaired nursing home residents. *International Journal of Nursing Studies* 28: 145-151.

56. Karl, C.A. 1982. The effects of an exercise program on self-care activities for the institutionalized elderly. *Journal of Gerontological Nursing* 8 (5): 282-285.

57. Katz, S., A.B. Ford, R.A. Moskowitz, B.A. Jackson, and M.W. Jaffe. 1963. The index of ADL: A standard measure of biological and psychosocial function. *Journal of the American Medical Association* 185: 914-919.

58. King, A.C., R. Oman, G.S. Brassington, D. Bliwise, and W. Haskell. 1997. Moderate-intensity exercise and self-rated quality of sleep in older adults. *Journal of the American Medical Association* 277: 32-37.

59. Klitgaard, H., M. Mantoni, S. Schiaffino, S. Ausoni, L. Gorza, C. Laurent-Winter, P. Schnohr, and B. Saltin. 1990. Function, morphology and protein expression of aging skeletal muscle: A cross-sectional study of elderly men with different training backgrounds. *Acta Physiologica Scandinavica* 140: 41-54.

60. LaCroix, A., S. Leveille, and J. Hecht. 1996. Does walking decrease the risk of cardiovascular disease, hospitalizations and death in older adults? *Journal of the American Geriatrics Society* 44 (2): 113-120.

61. Larsson, L. 1982. Physical training effects on muscle morphology in sedentary males at different ages. *Medicine and Science in Sports and Exercise* 14: 203-206.

62. Larsson, L.G., G. Grimby, and J. Karlsson. 1979. Muscle strength and speed of movement in relation to age and muscle morphology. *Journal of Applied Physiology* 46: 451-456.

63. Lee, I., C. Hsieh, and R. Paffenbarger. 1995. Exercise intensity and longevity in men: The Harvard alumni health study. *Journal of the American Medical Association* 273: 1179-1184.

64. Lehmann, M., P. Schmid, and J. Keul. 1984. Age- and exercise-related sympathetic activity in untrained volunteers, trained athletes and patients with impaired left-ventricular contractility. *European Heart Journal* 5: 1-7.

65. Lexell, J., D. Downham, Y. Larsson, E. Bruhn, and B. Morsing. 1995. Heavy-resistance training in older Scandinavian men and women: Short- and long-term effects on arm and leg muscles. *Scandinavian Journal of Medicine and Science in Sports* 5: 329-341.

66. Lightfoot, T., D. Torok, T. Journell, M. Turner, and R. Clayton. 1994. Resistance training increases lower body negative pressure tolerance. *Medicine and Science in Sports and Exercise* 26: 1005-1011.

67. Lillegard, W.A., and J.D. Terrio. 1994. Appropriate strength training. *Medical Clinics of North America* 78: 457-477.

68. Lindemuth, G., and B. Moose. 1990. Improving cognitive abilities of elderly Alzheimer's disease patients with intense exercise therapy. *American Journal of Alzheimer's Care and Related Disorders Research* 5: 31-33.

69. Lord, S.R., and J.A. Ward. 1994. Age-associated differences in sensor-motor function and balance in community dwelling women. *Age and Ageing* 23: 452-460.

70. Martinsen, E.W., A. Hoffart, and O. Solberg. 1989. Comparing aerobic and nonaerobic forms of exercise in the treatment of clinical depression: A randomized trial. *Comprehensive Psychiatry* 30: 324-331.

71. Mazzeo, R., P. Cavanaugh, W. Evans, M. Fiatarone, J. Hagberg, E. McAuley, and J. Startzell. 1998. Exercise and physical activity for older adults. *Medicine and Science in Sports and Exercise* 30: 992-1008.

72. McCartney, N., A. Hicks, J. Martin, and C. Webber. 1995. Long-term resistance training in the elderly: Effects on dynamic strength, exercise capacity, muscle, and bone. *Journal of Gerontology* 50A: B97-B104.

73. McCartney, N., R. McKelvie, D. Haslam, and N. Jones. 1991. Usefulness of weightlifting training in improving strength and maximal power output in coronary artery disease. *American Journal of Cardiology* 67: 939-945.

74. McDonagh, T.A., S.B. Davison, J. Norrie, C.E. Morrison, J.J. McMurray, H. Tunstall-Pedoe, and H.J. Dargie. 1994. The effect of psychological depression on functional capacity. *Circulation* 90: I-162.

75. McMurdo M.E., and L.M. Rennie. 1994. Improvements in quadriceps strength with regular seated exercise in the institutionalized elderly. *Archives of Physical Medicine and Rehabilitation* 75: 600-603.

76. McNeil, J.K., E.M. LeBlanc, and M. Joyner. 1991. The effect of exercise on depressive symptoms in the moderately depressed elderly. *Psychology and Aging* 6: 467-488.

77. Molloy, D., L. Delaquerriere-Richardson, and R. Crilly. 1988. The effects of a three-month exercise programme on neuropsychological function in elderly institutionalized women: A randomized controlled trial. *Age and Ageing* 17: 303-310.

78. Morganti, C.M., M.E. Nelson, M.A. Fiatarone, G.E. Dallal, C.D. Economos, B.M. Crasford, and W.J. Evans. 1995. Strength improvements with 1 yr of progressive resistance training in older women. *Medicine and Science in Sports and Exercise* 27: 906-912.

79. Morley, J. 1996. Anorexia in older persons: Epidemiology and optimal treatment. *Drugs and Aging* 8: 134-155.

80. Morris, J., M. Fiatarone, D. Kiely, P. Belleville-Taylor, K. Murphy, S. Littlehale, W. Ooi, E. O'Neill, and N. Doyle. 1999. Nursing rehabilitation and exercise strategies in the nursing home. *Journal of Gerontology* 54A: M494-M500.

81. Mulrow, C., M. Gerety, D. Kanten, J. Cornell, L. Chiodo, C. Aguilar, M. O'Neil, J. Rosenberg, and R. Solis. 1994. A randomized trial of physical rehabilitation for very frail nursing home residents. *Journal of the American Medical Association* 271: 519-524.

82. Naso, F., E. Carrier, and C.K. Blankfort-Doyle. 1990. Endurance training in the elderly nursing home patient. *Archives of Physical Medicine and Rehabilitation* 71: 241-243.

83. Nelson, M., M. Fiatarone, J. Layne, I. Trice, C. Economos, R. Fielding, R. Ma, R. Pierson, and W. Evans. 1996. Analysis of body-composition techniques and models for detecting change in soft tissue with strength training. *American Journal of Clinical Nutrition* 63: 678-686.

84. Nelson, M., M. Fiatarone, C. Morganti, I. Trice, R. Greenberg, and W. Evans. 1994. Effects of high-intensity strength training on multiple risk factors for osteoporotic fractures. *Journal of the American Medical Association* 272: 1909-1914.

85. Nelson, M., J. Layne, A. Nuernberger, M. Allen, J. Judge, D. Kaliton, and M. Fiatarone. 1997. Home-based exercise training in the frail elderly: Effects on physical performance. *Medicine and Science in Sports and Exercise* 29: S110.

86. North, T., P. McCullagh, and Z. Tran. 1990. The effect of exercise on depression. *Exercise and Sport Sciences Reviews* 18: 379-415.

87. Oddis, C. 1996. New perspectives on osteoarthritis. *American Journal of Medicine* 100 (2A): 10S-15S.

88. Ory, M.G., K.B. Schechtman, J.P. Miller, E.C. Hudley, M.A. Fiatarone, M.A. Province, C.L. Arfken, D. Morgan, S. Weiss, M. Kaplan, and the FICSIT Group. 1993. Frailty and injuries in later life: The FICSIT trials. *Journal of the American Geriatrics Society* 41: 283-296.

89. Paffenbarger, R., R. Hyde, A. Wing, and C.-C. Hsieh. 1986. Physical activity and longevity of college alumni. *New England Journal of Medicine* 315: 399-401.

90. Panton, L.B., G.J. Guillen, L. Williams, J.E. Graves, C. Vivas, M. Cediel, M.L. Pollock, L. Garzarella, J. Krumerman, H. Derendorf, et al. 1995. The lack of effect of aerobic exercise training on propranolol pharmacokinetics in young and elderly adults. *Journal of Clinical Pharmacology* 35: 885-894.

91. Pate, R.R., M. Pratt, S.N. Blair, W.L. Haskell, C.A. Macera, C. Bouchard, D. Buchner, C.J. Caspersen, W. Ettinger, G.W. Heath, A.C. King, A. Kriska, A.S. Leon, B.H. Marcus, J. Morris, R.S. Paffenbarger Jr, K. Patrick, M.L. Pollock, J.M. Rippe, J. Sallis, and J.H. Wilmore. 1995. Physical activity and public health: A recommendation from the Centers for Disease Control and Prevention and the American College of Sports Medicine. *Journal of the American Medical Association* 273: 402-407.

92. Pelissier, J., and D. Perennou. 2000. Exercise progam and rehabilitation of motor disorders in Parkinson's disease. *Revue Neurologique* 156 (supp 3): 190-200.

93. Perkins, K., S. Rapp, C. Carlson, and C. Wallace. 1986. Behavioral interventions to increase exercise. *Gerontologist* 26: 479-481.

94. Pollock, M., H. Miller, R. Janeway, A. Linnerud, B. Robertson, and R. Valentino. 1971. Effects of walking on body composition and cardiovascular function of middle-aged men. *Journal of Applied Physiology* 30: 126-130.

95. Pollock, M.L., C. Foster, D. Knapp, J.L. Rod, and D.H. Schmidt. 1987. Effect of age and training on aerobic capacity and body composition of master athletes. *Journal of Applied Physiology* 62: 725-731.

96. Province, M.A., E.C. Hadley, M.C. Hombrook, L.A. Lipsitz, P. Miller, C.D. Mulrow, M.G. Ory, R.W. Sattin, M.E. Tinetti, and S.L. Wolf. 1995. The effects of exercise on falls in elderly patients: A preplanned meta-analysis of the FICSIT trials. *Journal of the American Medical Association* 273: 1341-1347.

97. Pu, C., M. Johnson, D. Forman, J. Hausdorff, R. Roubenoff, R.A. Fielding, and M. Fiatarone Singh. In press. The effects of high-intensity strength training on skeletal muscle and exercise performance in older women with heart failure: A randomized controlled trial. *Journal of Applied Physiology*.

98. Pu, C., M. Johnson, D. Forman, L. Piazza, and M. Fiatarone. 1997. High-intensity progressive resistance training in older women with chronic heart failure. *Medicine and Science in Sports and Exercise* 29: S148.

99. Pu, C., M. Johnson, D. Forman, L. Piazza, and M. Fiatarone. 1997. Performance-based functional changes after strength training in elderly women with heart failure. *Journal of the American Geriatrics Society* 45: S3.

100. Pyka, G., D.R. Taaffe, and R. Marcus. 1994. Effect of a sustained program of resistance training on the acute growth hormone response to resistance exercise in older adults. *Hormone and Metabolic Research* 26: 330-333.

101. Ray, W.A., M.R. Griffen, W. Scheffner, N.K. Baugh, and L.J. Melton. 1987. Psychotropic drug use and the risk of hip fracture. *New England Journal of Medicine* 316: 313-319.

102. Rickli, R., and J. Jones. 1999. Development and validation of a functional fitness test for community-residing older adults. *Journal of Aging and Physical Activity* 7: 129-161.

103. Ryan, A., R. Pratley, A. Goldberg, and D. Elahi. 1996. Resistive training increases insulin action in postmenopausal women. *Journal of Gerontology. Series A, Biological Sciences and Medical Sciences* 51A: M199-M205.

104. Sauvage, L.R., Jr., B.M. Myklebust, J. Crow-Pan, S. Novak, P. Millington, M.D. Hoffman, A.J. Hartz, and D. Rudman. 1992. A clinical trial of strengthening and aerobic exercise to improve gait and balance in elderly male nursing home residents. *American Journal of Physical Medicine and Rehabilitation* 71: 333-342.

105. Schnelle, J., P. MacRae, J. Ouslander, S. Simmons, and M. Nitta. 1995. Functional incidental training, mobility performance, and incontinence care with nursing home residents. *Journal of the American Geriatrics Society* 43: 1356-1362.

106. Singh, N.A., K.M. Clements, and M.A. Fiatarone. 1997. A randomised controlled trial of the effect of exercise on sleep. *Sleep* 20: 95-101.

107. Singh, N.A., K.M. Clements, and M.A. Fiatarone. 1997. A randomized controlled trial of progressive resistance training in depressed elders. *Journal of Gerontology* 52A: M27-35.

108. Skelton, D.A., A. Young, C.A. Greig, and K.E. Malbut. 1995. Effects of resistance training on strength, power, and selected functional abilities of women aged 75 and older. *Journal*

of the American Geriatrics Society 43: 1081-1087.

109. Smidt, G. 1990. Aging and gait. In *Gait in rehabilitation,* edited by G. Smidt, 185-198. New York: Churchill Livingstone.

110. Stamford, B.A., W. Hambacker, and A. Fallica. 1974. Effects of daily physical exercise on the psychiatric state of institutionalized geriatric mental patients. *Research Quarterly* 45 (1): 34-41.

111. Stanley, R., E. Protas, and J. Jankovic. 1999. Exercise performance in those having Parkinson's disease and healthy normals. *Medicine and Science in Sports and Exercise* 31: 761-766.

112. Stavrinos, T., Y. Skarbek, G. Galambos, M. Fiatarone Singh, and N. Singh. 2000. The effects of low intensity versus high intensity progressive resistance weight training on shoulder function in the elderly: A randomized controlled trial. *Australian and New Zealand Journal of Medicine* 30 (2): 305.

113. Stewart, A.L., A.C. King, and W.L. Haskell. 1993. Endurance exercise and health-related quality of life in 50-65-year-old adults. *Gerontologist* 33: 782-789.

114. Tinetti, M., D. Baker, and G. McAvay. 1994. A multifactorial intervention to reduce the risk of falling among elderly people living in the community. *New England Journal of Medicine* 331: 821-827.

115. Tinetti, M.E., M. Speechley, and S.F. Ginter. 1988. Risk factors for falls among elderly persons living in the community. *New England Journal of Medicine* 319: 1701-1707.

116. Toole, T., S. Park, M. Hirsch, D. Lehman, and C. Maitland. 1996. The multicomponent nature of equilibrium in persons with parkinsonism: A regression approach. *Journal of Neural Transmission* 103: 561-580.

117. Treuth, M., G. Hunter, T. Szabo, R. Weinsier, M. Goran, and L. Berland. 1995. Reduction in intra-abdominal adipose tissue after strength training in older women. *Journal of Applied Physiology* 78: 1425-1431.

118. Treuth, M., A. Ryan, R. Pratley, M. Rubin, J. Miller, B. Nicklas, J. Sorkin, S. Harman, A. Goldberg, and B. Hurley. 1994. Effects of strength training on total and regional body composition in older men. *Journal of Applied Physiology* 77: 614-620.

119. U.S. Department of Health and Human Services. 1999. Healthy People 2010. Draft for public comment.

120. U.S. Department of Health and Human Services. 1996. *Physical activity and health: A report of the surgeon general.* Atlanta: U.S. Department of Health and Human Services, Centers for Disease Control and Prevention, National Center for Chronic Disease Prevention and Health Promotion.

121. Vellas, B., and J.E. Morley. 1994. Sleep disorders and insomnia in the elderly. *Clinical Geriatrics* 2: 50-51.

122. Wagnar, E.H., A.Z. Lacroix, D.M. Buchner, and E.B. Larson. 1992. Effects of physical activity on health status in older adults. *Annual Review of Public Health* 13: 451-468.

123. Wickham, C., C. Cooper, B.M. Margetts, and D.J.P. Barker. 1989. Muscle strength, activity, housing, and the risk of falls in elderly people. *Age and Ageing* 18: 47-51.

124. Wolfson, L., J. Judge, R. Whipple, and M. King. 1995. Strength is a major factor in balance, gait, and the occurrence of falls. *Journal of Gerontology* 50A: 64-67.

125. Woolley, S.M., S.J. Czaja, and C.G. Drury. 1997. An assessment of falls in elderly men and women. *Journal of Gerontology* 52A: M80-M87.

126. Wright, J. 1999. Nonpharmacological management strategies. *Medical Clinics in North America* 83: 499-508.

127. Zauner, C.W., M. Notelovitz, C.D. Fields, K.M. Clair, W.J. Clair, and R.B. Vogel. 1984. Cardiorespiratory efficiency at submaximal work in young and middle-aged women. *American Journal of Obstetrics and Gynecology* 150: 712-715.

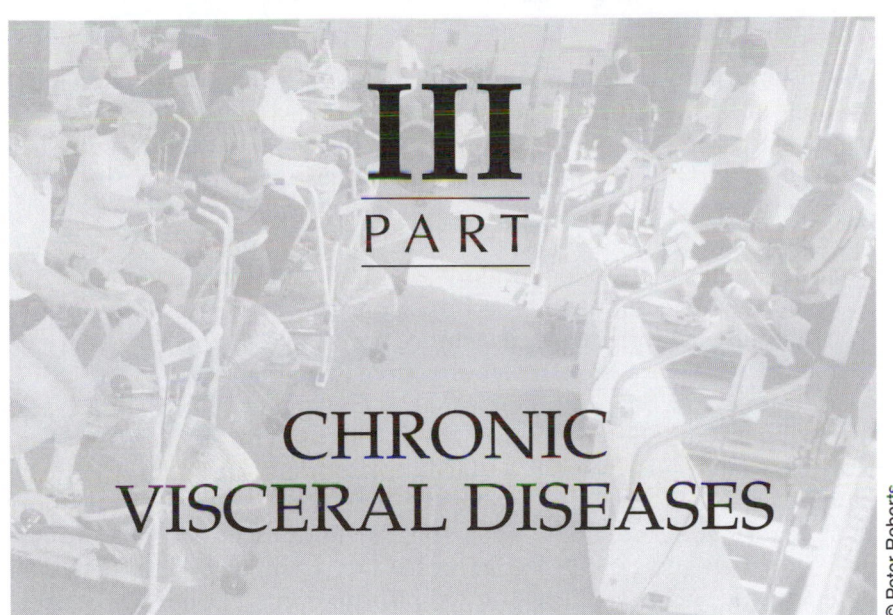

III PART

CHRONIC VISCERAL DISEASES

Coronary patients require a minimum level of strength for daily living, similar to persons without heart disease. Many cardiac patients lack the physical strength to perform common tasks such as yard work, carrying luggage, or opening windows. Of those patients who possess the requisite physical capacity, many lack the confidence to attempt activities involving even low levels of muscular exertion.

Several studies have demonstrated the safety and effectiveness of resistance training in selected coronary patients, especially those who previously participated in rehabilitative aerobic exercise training. These studies generally involved small numbers of low-risk male patients, 70 years or younger, with average to above-average aerobic fitness and normal or near-normal left ventricular function. However, the extent to which these applications can be extrapolated to other populations of coronary patients (e.g., older patients with low aerobic fitness and patients with severe left ventricular impairment) remains unclear. Accordingly, these patient subsets may require more careful progression and initial monitoring.

Mild-to-moderate resistance training can provide an effective method for improving strength and cardiovascular endurance, modifying coronary risk factors, and enhancing psychosocial well-being in clinically stable coronary patients. These adaptations should serve to maximize the crossover of training benefits to real-life situations, enabling the patient to better perform occupational and leisure-time activities.

Hypertension is a major public health problem in most Western industrialized countries. Control of hypertension remains a significant public health challenge in the United States, affecting an estimated 50 to

60 million Americans. Unfortunately, nearly 80% of hypertensive individuals do not receive adequate treatment, leaving many to suffer needlessly from stroke and heart disease. Resistance training with low resistances and high repetitions has proven safe and effective for *mildly* hypertensive patients. This form of training appears to be even more effective when done as a component of a comprehensive exercise program rather than independently. On the other hand, persons with more marked elevations in blood pressure (i.e., stage 2 or 3 hypertension) should add endurance/resistance training to their treatment regimen only after initiating antihypertensive drug therapy.

There are two types of strokes: ischemic and hemorrhagic. The former, involving thrombotic and embolic strokes, account for 80% of all strokes. Recent research studies suggest that, in appropriately functioning stroke patients, resistance training may be of benefit to both the affected and unaffected sides of the body. Nevertheless, there are no accepted guidelines on when and how to initiate resistance training post ischemic or hemorrhagic stroke. Until additional information is obtained, a conservative therapeutic approach is recommended.

Cardiac transplantation represents a viable alternative for nearly 3000 patients each year with end-stage heart failure. Despite surgery, these patients continue to experience exercise intolerance because of prolonged bed rest and convalescence, associated skeletal muscle anomalies, loss of muscle mass and strength, and the absence of autonomic cardiac innervation. Cardiac transplant patients should be encouraged to perform aerobic and progressive resistance exercise to counteract muscle wasting and other adverse side effects of immunosuppressive drug therapy, such as hyperlipidemia, hypertension, obesity, and diabetes. Moreover, resistance training has been shown to prevent glucocorticoid-induced myopathy in heart transplant recipients and restore fat-free mass to levels greater than before transplantation surgery. Gradual progression of low resistive workloads with relatively higher repetitions has been recommended for this patient population.

Finally, exercise training is a key component of rehabilitation programs for patients with respiratory diseases, including asthma, chronic obstructive pulmonary disease, and interstitial lung disease. Walking is strongly recommended because it is involved in most activities of daily living. However, some patients may require concomitant use of oxygen therapy to maintain adequate oxygenation during exercise. Traditional aerobic exercise should be complemented by resistance training of the upper and lower extremities. Typical exercises include high-repetition, low-resistive efforts of the arm and shoulder muscles. To reduce the likelihood of patients' becoming dyspneic when lifting, breathing should be appropriately coordinated; expiration generally occurs during the movement requiring the greatest effort.

12

Resistance Training in Patients With Coronary Heart Disease

Kerry J. Stewart, EdD
Johns Hopkins University

Barry A. Franklin, PhD
William Beaumont Hospital, Wayne State University,
and the University of Michigan

Ray W. Squires, PhD
Mayo Clinic

Introduction

Over the past 20 years, exercise training has become a standard of care in the therapeutic management of patients with coronary heart disease (CHD) (3). Patients who exercise improve their functional capacity and cardiac risk factor profiles, have fewer symptoms, and reduce their risk of cardiovascular mortality. A goal for most patients is to engage in as much physical activity as possible within their physiological and medical limitations, yet below the point of abnormal signs or symptoms—that is, angina, excessive blood pressure, myocardial ischemia, and left-ventricular dysfunction. Although the major focus has been on cardiovascular endurance fitness, the clinical application of resistance training for patients with CHD has increased in recent years. This chapter summarizes the health and fitness benefits of resistance training in patients with CHD, reviews indications for and contraindications to these programs, provides guidelines for resistance training exercise prescriptions, and details how these recommendations have evolved in recent years.

Rationale for Resistance Training

Traditionally, resistance training has been prescribed for health, fitness, and the prevention and rehabilitation of orthopedic problems. Physical activity and exercise guidelines from the American College of Sports Medicine (29), American Heart Association (18), American Association of Cardiovascular and Pulmonary Rehabilitation (2), the surgeon general's report on physical activity and health (46), and the NIH Consensus Development Panel on Physical Activity and Cardiovascular Health (34) all recommend resistance training as an integral component of a well-rounded physical conditioning program for healthy adults and patients with CHD. The rationale to support resistance training as an adjunct to cardiac rehabilitation stems from several lines of evidence (6, 7, 22, 28, 41-43, 45). These studies suggest that resistance training is safe and effective in improving muscular strength and endurance, aerobic fitness, and maintaining or increasing lean body mass. Resistance training may also favorably modify several risk factors for coronary disease, including hypertension, hyperlipidemia, glucose intolerance, and hyperinsulinemia (see table 12.1).

Strength Needs of Patients With Coronary Heart Disease

Patients with CHD have the same strength needs as other persons. Many patients will return to jobs that require muscular efforts and engage in activities that require muscular endurance, or both. Strength is important for leisure-time activities, preventing injury and maintaining good musculoskeletal health, increasing lean body mass, and preventing frailty in older persons (17, 21, 27). Also, sarcopenia, which refers to the age-related loss in muscle mass, may be delayed or offset by exercise-induced increases in muscle mass. Resistance training increases muscle mass and resting energy expenditure, which may also lead to reductions in body weight and fat stores (8, 12, 35, 40). Resistance forms of exercise can increase muscular strength and endurance in both men and women of all ages, with and without heart disease, by at least 25% (16). Other benefits of resistance training include increases in

TABLE 12.1   Effects of Resistance Exercise on Selected Health and Fitness Variables

Variable	Training adaptation
Bone mineral density	↑↑
Body composition	
% fat	↓
Lean body mass	↑↑
Glucose metabolism	
Insulin response to glucose challenge	↓↓
Basal insulin levels	↓
Insulin sensitivity	↑↑
Serum lipids	
HDL	↑↔
LDL	↓↔
Blood pressure at rest	
Systolic	↓↔
Diastolic	↓↔
Maximal oxygen uptake	↑↔
Endurance time	↑↑
Strength	↑↑↑
Physical function	↑↑↑
Basal metabolism	↑↑

↑ = increase; ↓ decrease; ↔ = unchanged; ↑ or ↓ = small effect; ↑↑ or ↓↓ = moderate effect; ↑↑↑ or ↓↓↓ = large effect; HDL = high-density lipoprotein cholesterol; LDL = low-density lipoprotein cholesterol.

Adapted from Pollock and Vincent 1996 (37).

bone mass, connective tissue thickness, muscle strength and endurance, and functional performance. Resistance training is also of value in the treatment of low back pain, osteoporosis, and orthopedic injury (37).

Some of the most dramatic improvements in response to resistance training have been reported in elderly persons. This is especially noteworthy since the Framingham Heart Study found that about half of women over age 65 cannot lift 10 lb (4.36 kg) (20). Perhaps the most striking example of resistance training benefits was an 8-week high-intensity strength training study of elderly men and women who ranged in age from 87 to 96 years (15). Nine of the 10 subjects who completed the resistance training program increased muscle strength by an average of 174%; walking speed by 48%; and midthigh muscle girth by 9%. The researchers concluded that resistance exercise enables dramatic strength gains even in very old and frail people.

Cardiovascular Fitness

Because of the principle of training specificity, resistance exercise programs alone do not provide a sufficient stimulus for optimal cardiovascular conditioning. Nevertheless, resistance training appears to contribute to improved cardiovascular responses to exercise. Following a resistance exercise program, heart rate and blood pressure responses are reduced when lifting any given load (33). Thus, resistance training can decrease cardiac demands during daily activities such as carrying groceries or lifting moderately heavy to heavy objects.

In one study (26), resistance training increased muscular endurance with modest to no improvement in aerobic capacity. Maximal oxygen uptake during treadmill and cycle ergometer testing remained essentially unchanged after 10 weeks of heavy resistance training; however, submaximal endurance time to exhaustion increased by 47% during cycling and 12% during treadmill running. Another study (1) reported that 12 weeks of resistance training improved submaximal walking time by 38%, whereas treadmill performance in a sedentary control group remained unchanged. These findings suggest that endurance is not a function of aerobic training alone, but can be enhanced by increased muscular strength.

Combined Aerobic and Resistance Training

Many cardiac rehabilitation programs have combined aerobic and resistance training for comprehensive cardiovascular and musculoskeletal conditioning. A widely used approach for the resistance component is circuit weight training (CWT). CWT consists of a series of lifting exercises using moderate loads and frequent repetitions. With CWT, the subject moves from one machine to another, using 8-12 different exercises, with work/rest intervals of 30-45 s and 30-60 s, respectively. A typical circuit will consist of 8-12 different exercises. Table 12.2 highlights some of key differences between CWT and a more conventional weightlifting approach; the latter typically employs barbells and involves heavier workloads and fewer repetitions. Conventional weight training is primarily an anaerobic activity, whereas CWT engages both anaerobic and aerobic metabolism. Because conventional weight training uses heavier loads and fewer repetitions, it has little effect on aerobic endurance. Because CWT involves sustained motion, it has the advantage of developing muscle strength and aerobic endurance simultaneously. Also, because of its moderate static load, CWT has gained greater clinical acceptance in persons with CHD compared with exercises that impose a high static load.

One of the first randomized studies of resistance training in patients with CHD (28) showed that CWT combined with aerobic training for 10 weeks, 3 days/week, increased cardiovascular endurance; in contrast, a

TABLE 12.2 Differences Between Conventional Resistance Training and Circuit Weight Training

Conventional resistance training	Circuit weight training
Primarily anaerobic	Anaerobic and aerobic metabolism
Improves strength	Improves muscular strength, endurance, and aerobic fitness
Heavy weight loads	Moderate loads
High static load	Moderate static load
Few repetitions	Frequent repetitions

control group performing only aerobic training remained unchanged. Both groups followed the same warm-up and 20 min walk/jog at 85% HR max, but the resistance group did an additional 20 min of CWT instead of volleyball. The addition of resistance training resulted in a 12% increase in cardiovascular endurance measured as treadmill duration compared with the aerobic training alone (see figure 12.1). Furthermore, the combined resistance and aerobic group improved muscular strength as measured by one-repetition maximum (1-RM) on 7 of 8 weightlifting exercises, whereas the aerobic training alone group improved on one strength exercise (table 12.3). Total strength, calculated as the sum of all 8 weightlifting exercises, increased by 24%. Those patients who continued combined resistance and aerobic training, with an average attendance of greater than 50% over the subsequent 3 years, had increases in both arm and leg strength compared to the aerobic training only group, who remained unchanged (see figure 12.2) (43).

Table 12.4 is a summary of six randomized controlled trials of resistance training in selected patients with CHD. Overall, these studies demonstrate that mild- to moderate-intensity resistance training resulted in consistent improvement in measures of muscular strength for both the upper and lower extremities. Most of these studies also found a substantial improvement in cardiovascular fitness for combined resistance and aerobic exercise compared with aerobic exercise only. None of these studies reported medical complications among the 174 patients who participated.

Safety Issues and Hemodynamic Responses to Resistance Training

In the early years of cardiac rehabilitation, most patients with CHD were told to avoid resistance training or lifting anything "heavy."

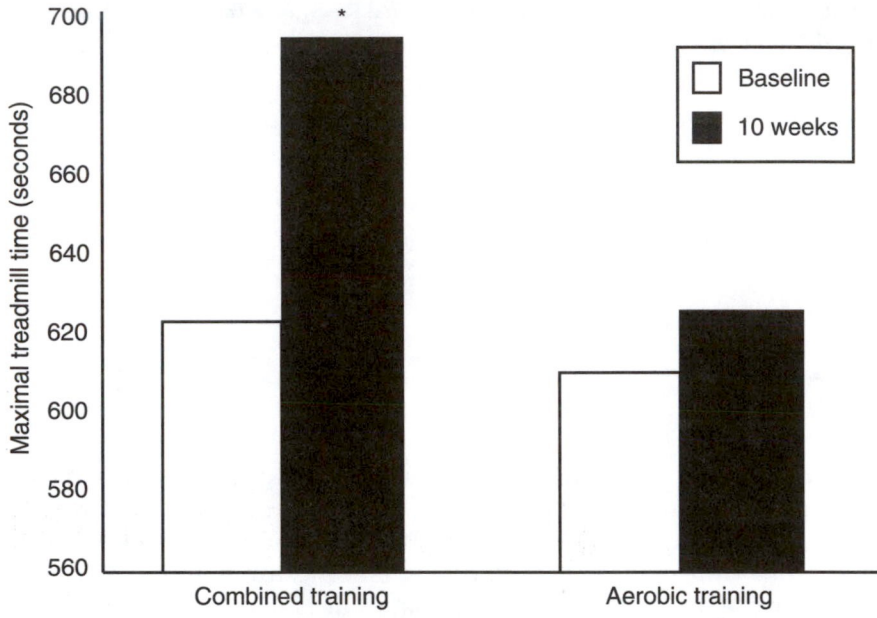

Figure 12.1 Combined resistance and aerobic training for 10 weeks resulted in a 12% increase in maximal treadmill time compared with aerobic training by itself; * $p < 0.05$ baseline versus 10 weeks of training.

Adapted from Kelemen et al. 1986 (28).

TABLE 12.3 Percent Change in Maximal Strength for 8 Different Weightlifting Exercises After 10 Weeks of Different Types of Training

Exercise	Combined resistance and aerobic training	Aerobic training alone
Vertical fly	26.9*	9.0
Arm curl	11.8*	0.0
Shoulder press	17.0*	7.0
Leg curl	27.0*	19.0*
High pulley	10.0	−4.0
Leg extension	52.0*	12.0
Low pulley	26.6*	13.0
Bench press	6.0*	−2.0

* $p < 0.05$ baseline versus 10 weeks

Adapted from Kelemen et al. 1986 (28).

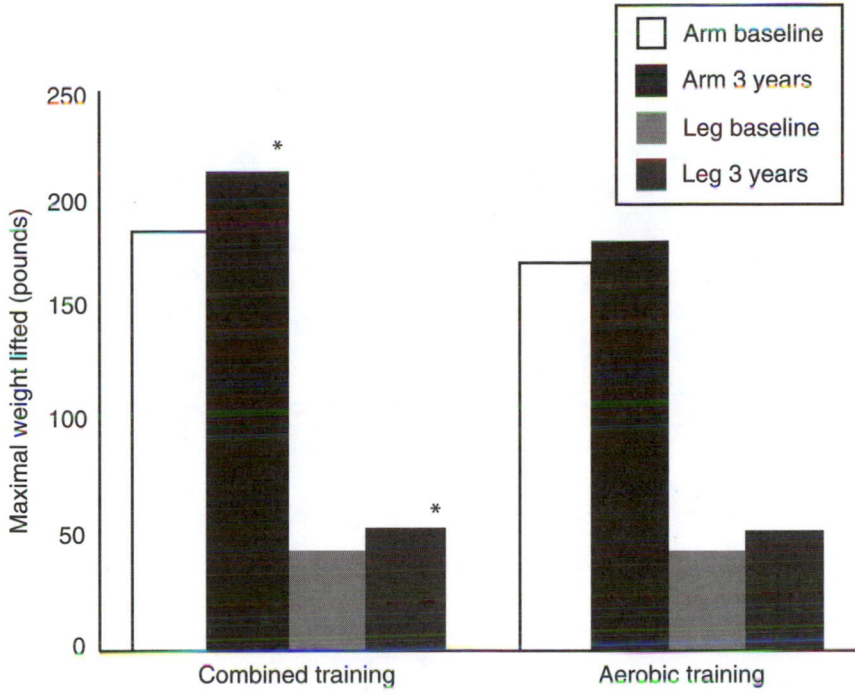

Figure 12.2 Mean values for maximal weight lifted for arm (total of 4 exercises) and leg (total of 2 exercises) strength in the combined training and aerobic training groups at baseline and 3 years. The combined group increased arm and leg strength, whereas the aerobic group did not change. * $p < 0.05$.

Adapted from Stewart et al. 1988 (43).

These recommendations were based on concerns about exaggerated heart rate and blood pressure responses and that resistance exercise had the potential to induce threatening arrhythmias, transient ventricular dysfunction, myocardial ischemia, or combinations of these. Another consideration was that most cardiac rehabilitation programs focused on aerobic conditioning, and the benefits of strength training were unclear. Prescribed exercise involved large muscle groups and rhythmic contractions with the avoidance of static exercises. Fortunately, in recent years, scientific information has accumulated on the acute and chronic responses to resistance training in high-risk patient groups (9, 38, 45), including recent reports on the safety and effectiveness of resistance training in selected patients with congestive heart failure (47).

Resistance training as compared with aerobic training at similar levels of metabolic work generally fails to elicit angina pectoris, ischemic ST-segment depression, or worrisome ventricular arrhythmias (5, 10, 30, 31,

TABLE 12.4 Comparison of Selected Randomized Controlled Trials of Resistance Training in Subjects With Coronary Artery Disease*

Study	N	Cardiac events	Weeks after event**	Training protocol	Fitness results
Keleman et al. (28)	40	MI/CABG/AP	>12	Exp: 20 min aerobic activity + 2 sets of 10-15 reps at 40% 1-RM (8 stations) 3 times/wk for 10 weeks Con: 20 min aerobic activity + 20 min game activity, 3 times/wk for 10 weeks	Exp: strength ↑ 24%, treadmill time ↑ 12% Con: strength ↑ 7%, treadmill time ↑ 2%
McCartney et al. (32)	24	MI/CABG/AP	>4	Exp: 35 min aerobic activity + 2 sets of 10-15 reps at 50% 1-RM (4 stations) 2 times/wk for 10 weeks Con: 35 min aerobic activity + 25 min game activity 2 times/wk for 10 weeks	Exp: strength ↑ 29%, peak cycle power ↑ 15% Con: strength ↑ 8%, peak cycle power ↑ 2%
Haennel et al. (23)	24	CABG	9-10	Exp: 3 sets 8-16 reps (6 stations) 3 times/wk for 8 weeks Aerobic: cycle 24 min 3 times/wk for 8 weeks Con: no exercise	Exp: strength ↑ 25%, $\dot{V}O_2$peak ↑ 11% Aerobic: strength ↑ 27%, $\dot{V}O_2$peak ↑ 20% Con: strength ↑ 9%, $\dot{V}O_2$peak ↑ 4%

Study	n	Population	Weeks after event**	Exercise protocol	Results
Butler et al. (7)	25	MI/CABG	>6	Exp: 2 sets 10 reps at 40% 1-RM (8 stations) + 15 min aerobic activity 3 times/wk for 12 weeks Con: 30 min aerobic activity 3 times/wk for 12 weeks	Exp: strength ↑ 22%, treadmill time ↑ 23% Con: strength ↑ 14%, treadmill time ↑ 30%
Stewart et al. (45)	23	MI	4-6	Exp: 2 sets of 10-15 reps at 40% 1-RM (6 stations) + 8 min aerobic activity 3 times/wk for 10 weeks Con: 25 min aerobic activity 3 times/wk for 10 weeks	Exp: strength ↑ 23%, $\dot{V}O_2$peak ↑ 14% Con: strength ↑ 10%, $\dot{V}O_2$peak ↑ 8%
Beniamini et al. (4)	29 (M) 9 (F)	MI/CABG/PTCA/AP	6-16	Exp: 3 sets of 8-12 reps at 50-80% 1-RM + 35 min aerobic activity 2 times/wk for 12 weeks Con: 35 min aerobic activity + flexibility exercises 2 times/wk for 12 weeks	Exp: strength ↑ 67%, treadmill time ↑ 28% Con: strength ↑ 9%, treadmill time ↑ 15%

MI = myocardial infarction; CABG = coronary artery bypass grafting; PTCA = percutaneous transluminal coronary angioplasty; AP = angina pectoris; Exp = experimental group performing resistance exercise; Con = control group; 1-RM = one-repetition maximum.

* No medical complications were reported in any of the studies.

** Weeks after event = time interval from cardiac event to start of resistance training.

39, 48). Blood pressure during weightlifting remains within a clinically acceptable range when lifting is performed at 40% of 1-RM (one-repetition maximum) (22, 25). Although the increase in the rate-pressure product, which reflects myocardial oxygen demand, may be similar to what occurs with aerobic exercise, the hemodynamic determinants are different. With resistance exercise, there is a higher blood pressure but lower heart rate response to increasing exercise workloads, as compared with aerobic exercise. One potential benefit of a lower heart rate combined with a higher blood pressure is enhanced coronary perfusion during diastole.

The clinical response to dynamic exercise with and without a resistance component was examined in patients with stable angina who routinely developed anginal symptoms, ischemic ST-segment depression, or both during treadmill testing (5). Patients performed trials of dynamic exercise that consisted of treadmill walking and trials of isodynamic exercise that consisted of walking while carrying weights. The treadmill speed was adjusted during isodynamic exercise so that the metabolic cost of work was the same as walking without weights. The dynamic work was done aerobically, while the isodynamic work was a combination of aerobic and resistance exercise. During dynamic exercise, the heart rate response was higher compared with the isodynamic exercise (figure 12.3). During isodynamic exercise, the blood pressure response was higher because of the superimposed resistance component. The resulting rate-pressure products, which reflect the work of the heart, were similar (table 12.5). However, isodynamic exercise produced less ST-segment depression compared with aerobic work. The likely mechanism for this response was increased coronary perfusion, secondary to a lower heart rate and elevated diastolic blood pressure.

Another safety concern is the effects of resistance training on left-ventricular function. A 1989 review of the literature (13) concluded that resistance training has no deleterious effects on left-ventricular diastolic function and no adverse effects on systolic left-ventricular function if the left-ventricular function is normal at rest. However, in patients with abnormal resting left-ventricular function, the recommendation was to avoid heavy forms of weightlifting to reduce the risk of exacerbating left-ventricular dysfunction. Nevertheless, a potential benefit from resistance training in patients with chronic heart failure is the resulting increased lean muscle mass that may counterbalance the muscle wasting that occurs with this syndrome.

In our recent clinical and research experience with patients with left-ventricular ejection fractions (LVEF) as low as 10%, the use of resistance exercise at 30-50% of maximal effort has produced no apparent adverse cardiovascular effects (47). Two recent pilot studies of resistance training in patients with chronic heart failure illustrate the potential benefits and

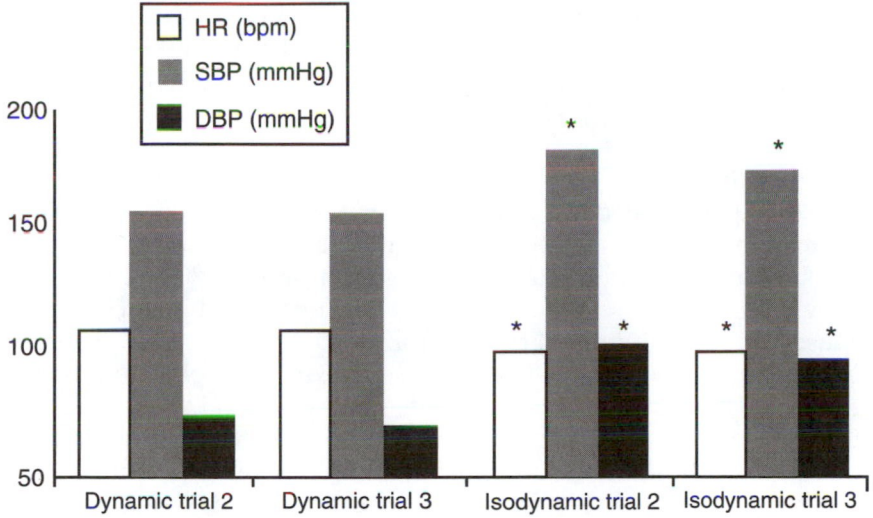

Figure 12.3 Hemodynamic responses to dynamic and isodynamic exercise. During dynamic exercise, the heart rate response was higher compared with the isodynamic exercise, whereas systolic and diastolic blood pressure responses were higher during isodynamic work that had a resistance component. * $p < 0.001$ dynamic versus isodynamic exercise.

Adapted from Bertagnoli et al. 1990 (5).

TABLE 12.5 Exercise With Resistance Component (Isodynamic) Produced Less ST-Segment Depression Compared With Dynamic Work (Aerobic) at Similar Rate Pressure Products

Exercise	*Rate pressure product (bpm × mmHg/100)*	*ST Δ (mm)*
Dynamic trial 1	182	−1.7
Dynamic trial 2	180	−1.4
Dynamic trial 3	180	−1.5
Isodynamic trial 2	185*	−0.4*
Isodynamic trial 3	184	−0.4*

* $p < 0.001$ isodynamic versus dynamic; bpm = beats per minute; mmHg = millimeters of mercury
Adapted from Bertagnoli et al. 1990 (5).

safety of such activity. In one of these studies (24), 9 men, with a stable, well-compensated heart failure and a mean LVEF of 26 ± 6%, participated in an 11-week CWT program. The patients performed up to 6 circuits of hydraulic resistance exercise (12-25 repetitions in 30 s) involving knee flexion and extension, chest press, and upright rowing, and 1-2 min of aerobic exercise between each set of resistance exercise. Muscle strength increased by 17-40%, whereas there was no change in aerobic capacity. The study was completed without any medical complications.

In the other study, 14 patients with left-ventricular dysfunction (LVEF $31 \pm 10\%$) participated in a 3 times per week, 6-month program (11). The exercise program consisted of 30 min of aerobic exercise at 60% of aerobic capacity, and 3 sets of 15 repetitions at 60-80% of 1-RM, on 6 weight pulley exercises involving lower- and upper-body muscle groups. Muscle strength improved by 14% for the knee extensors, and aerobic capacity increased by 10%. There were no medical complications during exercise. The New York Heart Association Functional Class improved from 2.7 to 1.5, on average, and there were no adverse changes in LVEF or end-diastolic diameter as determined by echocardiography.

A recent review of 12 different studies examined resistance testing or training in patients with CHD (49). CWT was generally added to the aerobic regimens of patients with CHD who had been aerobically trained, generally for 3 months or more. In all of these studies, and the studies cited previously (28, 43, 45, 47), the absence of signs or symptoms of myocardial ischemia, abnormal blood pressure responses, and untoward events suggests that resistance exercise is safe for selected patients. However, further research is needed before definitive recommendations can be made about the appropriate level of resistance training in patients with severe left-ventricular dysfunction.

Types of Equipment

The primary types of resistance equipment in structured programs are weight machines, free weights, weighted cuffs and hand weights, elastic tubes and bands, and wall pulleys. Light calisthenics can also be used when equipment is not available. In general, weight machines are relatively easy to use, safe, and may enhance compliance. The AACVPR *Guidelines for Cardiac Rehabilitation and Secondary Prevention* (2) recommends the use of weight machines in a circuit format as an optimal choice for comprehensive conditioning.

Multistation machines with 2-4 weight stacks allow more than one person to exercise at a time and provide a wide variety of upper- and lower-extremity exercises. One disadvantage of some machines is that the lowest weight may be too heavy for older and frail individuals. One strategy is to start these individuals with hand weights, wall pulleys, or elastic tubes and bands before progressing them to machines. Free weights are another option but require some degree of skill to assure proper technique and safety. Some patients struggle with free weights because they are difficult to balance, cumbersome to load and unload, and easy to drop.

Recommendations for Weight Training

In 1995, the AACVPR in its first edition of *Guidelines for Cardiac Rehabilitation Programs* (3) recommended weight training as a complementary format to aerobic training. The recommendation was that weight intensity be set at loads corresponding to 30-50% of maximum, and to perform 12-15 repetitions in 30-45 s, with rest periods of 30-45 s between exercises. However, patients should be permitted to take as much time as they need between stations, particularly older or markedly deconditioned persons who need to progress to these goals. It was also suggested that circuits include 8-12 exercises and 2-3 sets of each exercise, 3 days a week.

A recent review showed that performing one set of each exercise provides nearly the same improvements in muscular strength and endurance as multiple-set regimens (14). Consequently, for the average patient beginning a strength training regimen, single-set programs performed a minimum of 2 times per week are now recommended over multiple-set programs because they are highly effective and less time consuming. Such regimens should include 8-10 different exercises at a load that permits 8-15 repetitions per set for cardiac patients (figure 12.4). A summary of contemporary prescriptive guidelines for patients with cardiovascular disease is shown in table 12.6 (2, 18, 19, 36).

Musculoskeletal Considerations

Before beginning resistance training, the patient's musculoskeletal system should be evaluated, with emphasis on previous injuries, a history of orthopedic surgery, arthritis, or other causes of joint or muscle pain. When performing resistance exercise, patients should be encouraged to avoid limiting joint or muscle pain. Heart rate and blood pressure should be assessed during the first few sessions of resistance training to ensure appropriate responses. Baseline levels of muscle strength for the major muscle groups can be assessed by 1-RM or 3-RM testing.

Patient Selection Guidelines

In 1995, the AACVPR (3) recommended that patients wait at least 3 months after myocardial infarction or coronary bypass before beginning resistance training. In fact, it was suggested that weight training be delayed until phase III cardiac rehabilitation, which is typically 3 months past a cardiac event. It was also suggested that patients complete 2-3 months of aerobic training, and have an aerobic capacity of 6-7 METs before engaging in weightlifting exercises. This conservative

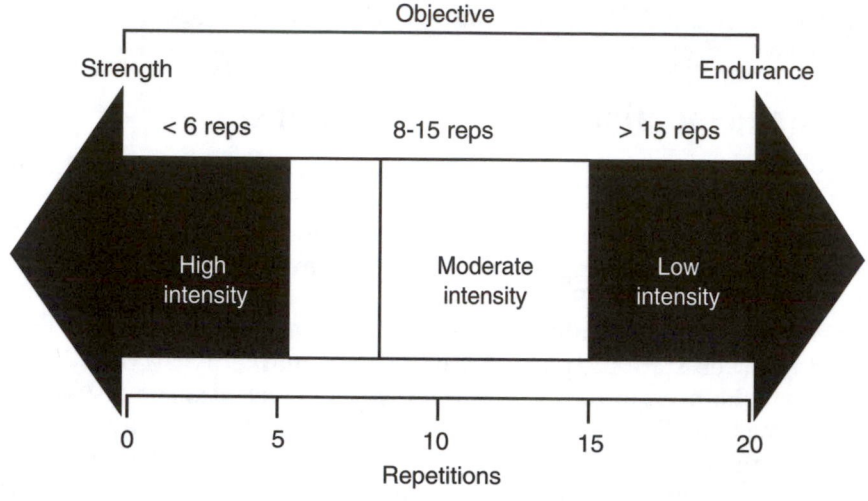

Figure 12.4 Classification of resistance training intensity. Using weight loads that permit 8-15 repetitions (reps) will generally facilitate improvements in muscular strength and endurance, regardless of age or health status.

TABLE 12.6 Contemporary Standards, Guidelines, and Position Statements Regarding Resistance Training for Patients With Cardiovascular Disease

Reference	Sets; reps	Stations/ devices*	Frequency
1995 AHA Exercise Standard (18)	1 set; 10-15 reps	8-10 exercises	2-3 d · wk⁻¹
1999 AACVPR guidelines (2)	1 set; 12-15 reps	8-10 exercises	2-3 d · wk⁻¹
2000 ACSM guidelines (19)	1 set; 10-15 reps	8-10 exercises	2-3 d · wk⁻¹
2000 AHA advisory (36)	1 set; 10-15 reps	8-10 exercises	2-3 d · wk⁻¹

AHA = American Heart Association; AACVPR = American Association of Cardiovascular and Pulmonary Rehabilitation; ACSM = American College of Sports Medicine; reps = repetitions

*Minimum one exercise per major muscle group: e.g., chest press, shoulder press, triceps extension, biceps curl, pull-down (upper back), lower back extension, abdominal crunch/curl, quadriceps extension or leg press, leg curls (hamstrings), calf raise

approach was based on the available data at the time. Based on increased clinical experience with weight training and the absence of reported cardiovascular events, the 1999 AACVPR guidelines (2) have taken a less conservative approach for starting weight training (table 12.7). However, major contraindications to resistance training remain unchanged and include symptomatic congestive heart failure, uncontrolled arrhythmias, severe valvular disease, and uncontrolled hypertension.

TABLE 12.7   American Association of Cardiovascular and Pulmonary Rehabilitation (AACVPR) Guidelines for Beginning Resistance Training

A minimum of 5 weeks after myocardial infarction, including 3 weeks of continuous participation in aerobic exercise

A minimum of 8 weeks after coronary artery bypass graft surgery, including 3 weeks of continuous participation in aerobic exercise

A minimum of 2 weeks of consistent participation in aerobic exercise following percutaneous transluminal coronary angioplasty

Adapted from AACVPR 1999 (2).

Resistance Training Soon After Myocardial Infarction

Although the 1999 AACVPR guidelines provide a basis for when to start resistance training, few data exist regarding the safety and efficacy of resistance training soon after myocardial infarction. While resistance training is widely prescribed in phases III and IV cardiac rehabilitation, it is often delayed in many phase II programs despite its potential benefit. In a recent study (45), combining resistance training and aerobic exercise as early as 4 weeks after uncomplicated myocardial infarction improved cardiorespiratory fitness and muscle strength more than aerobic exercise alone. The training protocol is shown in table 12.4. Maximal oxygen uptake increased 14% in the combined training group, whereas there were no significant improvements in patients that performed only aerobic training (figure 12.5). Arm and leg strength increased in each group. However, the improvements were greater for the combined training group—31% versus 16% for leg strength and 20% versus 10% for arm strength. The combined groups also demonstrated decreases in total and LDL cholesterol (44). The absence of signs or symptoms of myocardial ischemia, abnormal hemodynamic responses, evidence of adverse changes in left-ventricular function, and clinical complications suggests that incorporating weight training into cardiac rehabilitation is safe in selected patients.

Conclusion

Resistance training appears to be safe and effective in patients with CHD for developing cardiovascular fitness and muscular strength and endurance. Strength gains in the range of 20- 25% for most muscle groups can

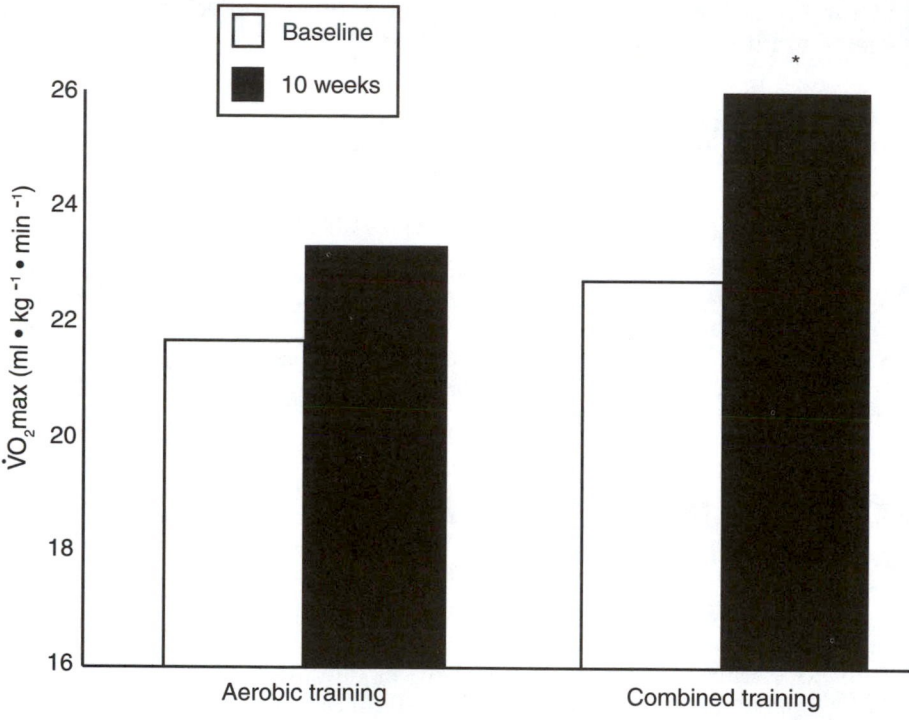

Figure 12.5 Mean values for maximal oxygen uptake for combined resistance and aerobic training and aerobic training only at baseline and 10 weeks. Exercise training started as early as 4 weeks after acute myocardial infarction; * $p < 0.01$ baseline versus 10 weeks.

Adapted from Stewart et al. 1998 (45).

be expected. When resistance training was combined with aerobic exercise, gains of 10-12% in maximal oxygen uptake and endurance performance beyond that produced by aerobic training have been demonstrated. Mild- to moderate-intensity resistance training is also effective for modifying coronary risk factors and enhancing psychosocial and physical well-being. Contemporary exercise guidelines have endorsed resistance training as part of the exercise prescription for most healthy adults and many patients with CHD. Further study is needed to determine the risks and benefits of resistance training in patients with more limiting cardiovascular disease and more extensive infarcts, and at higher risk for recurrent myocardial infarction.

References

1. Ades, P.A., D.L. Ballor, and T. Ashikaga. 1996. Weight training improves walking endurance in healthy elderly persons. *Annals of Internal Medicine* 124: 568-572.

2. American Association of Cardiovascular and Pulmonary Rehabilitation. 1999. *Guidelines for cardiac rehabilitation and secondary prevention.* 3d ed. Champaign, IL: Human Kinetics.
3. American Association of Cardiovascular and Pulmonary Rehabilitation. 1995. *Guidelines for cardiac rehabilitation programs.* 2d ed. Champaign, IL: Human Kinetics.
4. Beniamini, Y., J.J. Rubenstein, A.D. Faigenbaum, A.H. Lichtenstein, and M.C. Crim. 1998. High-intensity strength training of patients enrolled in an outpatient cardiac rehabilitation program. *Journal of Cardiopulmonary Rehabilitation* 19: 8-17.
5. Bertagnoli, K., P. Hanson, and A. Ward. 1990. Attenuation of exercise-induced ST depression during combined isometric and dynamic exercise in coronary artery disease. *American Journal of Cardiology* 65: 314-317.
6. Butler, R., G. Palmer, and F. Rogers. 1992. Circuit weight training in early cardiac rehabilitation. *Journal of American Osteopathy Association* 92: 77-89.
7. Butler, R.M., W.H. Beierwaites, and F. J. Rogers. 1987. The cardiovascular response to circuit weight training in patients with cardiac disease. *Journal of Cardiopulmonary Rehabilitation* 7: 402-409.
8. Campbell, W.W., M.C. Crim, V.R. Young, and W.J. Evans. 1994. Increased energy requirements and changes in body composition with resistance training in older adults. *American Journal of Clinical Nutrition* 60: 167-175.
9. Daub, W.D., G.P. Knapik, and W.R. Black. 1996. Strength training early after myocardial infarction. *Journal of Cardiopulmonary Rehabilitation* 16: 100-108.
10. DeBusk, R.F., R. Valdez, N. Houston, and W. Haskell. 1978. Cardiovascular responses to dynamic and static efforts soon after myocardial infarction. *Circulation* 58: 368-375.
11. Delagardelle, C., P. Feiereisen, R. Krecké, B. Essamri, and J. Beissel. 1999. Objective effects of a 6 months' endurance and strength training program in outpatients with congestive heart failure. *Medicine and Science in Sports and Exercise* 31: 1102-1107.
12. Dupler, T.L., and C. Cortes. 1993. Effects of a whole-body resistive training regimen in the elderly. *Gerontology* 39: 314-319.
13. Effron, M.B. 1989. Effects of resistive training on left ventricular function. *Medicine and Science in Sports and Exercise* 21: 694-697.
14. Feigenbaum, M.S., and M.L. Pollock. 1999. Prescription of resistance training for health and disease. *Medicine and Science in Sports and Exercise* 31: 38-45.
15. Fiatarone, M.A., E.C. Marks, N.D. Ryan, C.N. Meredith, L.A. Lipsitz, and W.J. Evans. 1990. High-intensity strength training in nonagenarians. Effects on skeletal muscle. *Journal of the American Medical Association* 263: 3029-3034.
16. Fleck, S.J., and W.J. Kraemer. 1997. *Designing resistance training programs.* 2d ed. Champaign, IL: Human Kinetics.
17. Fleg, J.L., and E.G. Lakatta. 1988. Role of muscle loss in the age-associated reduction in VO_2max in older men. *Journal of Applied Physiology* 68: 329-333.
18. Fletcher, G.F., G. Balady, V.F. Froelicher, L.H. Hartley, W.L. Haskell, and M.L. Pollock. 1995. Exercise standards: A statement for healthcare professionals from the American Heart Association. *Circulation* 91:580-615.
19. Franklin, B.A., E.T. Howley, and M.H. Whaley, eds. 2000. *ACSM's guidelines for exercise testing and prescription.* Philadelphia: Lippincott Williams & Wilkins.
20. Franklin, B.A., and F. Munnings. 1995. Rejuvenation through exercise. *Encyclopaedia Britannica 1996 Medical and Health Annual,* 263-268.
21. Gersten, J.W. 1991. Effect of exercise on muscle function decline with aging. *Western Journal of Medicine* 154: 579-582.
22. Ghilarducci, L.E., R.G. Holly, and E.A. Amsterdam. 1989. Effects of high resistance training in coronary artery disease. *American Journal of Cardiology* 64: 866-870.
23. Haennel, R.G., H.A. Quinney, and C.T. Kappagoda. 1991. Effects of hydraulic circuit training following coronary artery bypass surgery. *Medicine and Science in Sports and Exercise* 23: 158-165.

233

24. Hare, D.L., T.M. Ryan, S.E. Selig, A.M. Pellizzer, T.V. Wrigley, and H. Krum. 1999. Resistance exercise training increases muscle strength, endurance, and blood flow in patients with chronic heart failure. *American Journal of Cardiology* 83: 1674-1677.

25. Haslam, D., N. McCartney, and R. McKelvie. 1988. Direct measurement of arterial blood pressure during formal weight lifting in cardiac patients. *Journal of Cardiopulmonary Rehabilitation* 8: 213-225.

26. Hickson, R.C., M.A. Rosenkoette, and M.M. Brown. 1980. Strength training effects on aerobic power and short-term endurance. *Medicine and Science in Sports and Exercise* 12: 336-339.

27. Kallman, D.A., C. Plato, and J. Tobin. 1990. The role of muscle loss in age-related decline in grip strength: A cross-sectional and longitudinal analysis. *Journal of Gerontology* 45: M82-M88.

28. Kelemen, M.H., K.J. Stewart, and R.E. Gillilan. 1986. Circuit weight training in cardiac patients. *Journal of the American College of Cardiology* 7: 38-42.

29. Kenney, W.L. (ed). 1995. *ACSM's guidelines for exercise testing and prescription.* 5th ed. Media, PA: Williams & Wilkins.

30. Logan, R., and P. Burridge. 1981. Pre-discharge exercise testing involving weight carrying after myocardial infarction. *New Zealand Medical Journal* 93: 69-71.

31. Markiewicz, W., N. Houston, and R.A. DeBusk. 1979. A comparison of static and dynamic exercise after myocardial infarction. *Israeli Journal of Medicine and Science* 11: 984-987.

32. McCartney, N., R.S. McKelvie, D.R. Haslam, and N.L. Jones. 1991. Usefulness of weightlifting training in improving strength and maximal power output in coronary artery disease. *American Journal of Cardiology* 67: 939-945.

33. McCartney, N., R.S. McKelvie, and J. Martin. 1993. Weight-training-induced attenuation of the circulatory response of older males to weight lifting. *Journal of Applied Physiology* 74: 1056-1060.

34. NIH Consensus Development Panel on Physical Activity and Cardiovascular Health. 1996. Physical activity and cardiovascular health. *Journal of the American Medical Association* 276: 241-246.

35. Poehlman, E.T., A.W. Gardner, P.A. Ades, S.M. Katzman-Rooks, S.M. Montgomery, O.K. Atlas, D.L. Ballor, and R.S. Tyzbir. 1992. Resting energy metabolism and cardiovascular disease risk in resistance-trained and aerobically trained males. *Metabolism* 41: 1351-1360.

36. Pollock, M.L., B.A. Franklin, G. Balady, et al. 2000. Resistance exercise in individuals with and without cardiovascular disease: Benefits, rationale, safety, and prescription. *Circulation* 101: 828-833.

37. Pollock, M.L., and K.R. Vincent. 1996. *Resistance training for health.* Washington, DC: President's Council on Physical Fitness and Sports.

38. Schwartz, R.S., and V.A. Hirth. 1995. The effects of endurance and resistance training on blood pressure. *International Journal of Obesity and Related Metabolic Disorders* 19: S52-57.

39. Sheldahl, L.M., N.A. Wilke, F.E. Tristani, and J.H. Kalbfleisch. 1985. Response to repetitive static-dynamic exercise in patients with coronary artery disease. *Journal of Cardiac Rehabilitation* 5: 129-145.

40. Sipila, S., and H. Suominen. 1995. Effects of strength and endurance training on thigh and leg muscle mass and composition in elderly women. *Journal of Applied Physiology* 78: 334-340.

41. Sparling, P.B., J.D. Cantwell, C.M. Dolan, and R.K. Niederman. 1990. Strength training in a cardiac rehabilitation program: A six-month follow-up. *Archives of Physical Medicine and Rehabilitation* 71: 148-152.

42. Squires, R.W., A.J. Muri, L.J. Anderson, T.D. Miller, and G.T. Gau. 1991. Weight training during Phase II (early outpatient) cardiac rehabilitation: Heart rate and blood pressure responses. *Journal of Cardiopulmonary Rehabilitation* 11: 360-364.

43. Stewart, K., M. Mason, and M.H. Kelemen. 1988. Three-year participation in circuit weight training improves muscular strength and self-efficacy in cardiac patients. *Journal of Cardiovascular and Pulmonary Rehabilitation* 8: 292-296.

44. Stewart, K.J., L.D. McFarland, and J.J. Weinhofer. 1997. Incorporating weight training into cardiac rehabilitation soon after myocardial infarction: Effects on lipids. *Circulation* 96: I-733.

45. Stewart, K.J., L.D. McFarland, J.J. Weinhofer, E. Cottrell, C.S. Brown, and E.P. Shapiro. 1998. Safety and efficacy of weight training soon after acute myocardial infarction. *Journal of Cardiopulmonary Rehabilitation* 18: 37-44.

46. U.S. Department of Health and Human Services. *Physical activity and health: A report of the surgeon general.* 1996. Atlanta, GA: U.S. Department of Health and Human Services, Centers for Disease Control and Prevention, National Center for Chronic Disease Prevention and Health Promotion.

47. Vaitkevicius, P.V., C. Ebersold, Z. Haydar, K.J. Stewart, and J.L. Fleg. 1997. The utility of exercise training to improve functional capacity of elderly heart failure patients. *Circulation* 96: I-85.

48. Vander, L.B., B.A. Franklin, D. Wrisley, and M. Rubenfire. 1986. Acute cardiovascular responses to Nautilus exercise in cardiac patients: Implications for exercise training. *Annals of Sports Medicine* 2: 165-169.

49. Wenger, N.K., E.S. Froelicher, L.K. Smith, P.A. Ades, K. Berra, J.A. Blumenthal, C.M.E. Certo, A.M. Dattilo, D. Davis, R.F. DeBusk, J.P. Drozda Jr., B.J. Fletcher, B.A. Franklin, H. Gaston, P. Greenland, P.E. McBride, C.G.A. McGregor, N.B. Oldridge, J.C. Piscatella, and F.J. Rogers. 1995, October. *Cardiac rehabilitation. Clinical practice guideline no. 17.* Rockville, MD: U.S. Department of Health and Human Services, Public Health Service, Agency for Health Care Policy and Research and the National Heart, Lung, and Blood Institute. AHCPR Publication No. 96-0672.

13

CHAPTER

Resistance Training for Hypertension and Stroke Patients

Neil F. Gordon, MD, PhD, MPH
Ash Contractor, MBBS, MEd
Richard F. Leighton, MD
Saint Joseph's/Candler Health System

Hypertension is a major public health problem, affecting an estimated 15-30% of persons in most Western industrialized countries. In the United States, as many as 50 million individuals are estimated to have an elevated blood pressure or to be taking antihypertensive medication (25). According to the National Health and Nutrition Examination Survey III (NHANES III), conducted between 1988 and 1994, the estimated prevalence of hypertension for Americans aged 20-74 years is 24.4% for non-Hispanic white males, 19.3% for non-Hispanic white females, 35% for non-Hispanic African American males, 34.2% for non-Hispanic African American females, 25.2% for Mexican American males, and 22% for Mexican American females (8). Compared with whites, African Americans develop hypertension at an earlier age, and it is more severe among African Americans than whites at any decade of life (5, 8, 25).

The risk for nonfatal and fatal cardiovascular disease, renal disease, and all-cause mortality increases progressively with higher levels of systolic and diastolic blood pressure. The positive relationship between systolic and diastolic blood pressure and the risk for cardiovascular disease has long been recognized. This relationship has been shown to be strong, continuous, graded, consistent, independent, predictive, and etiologically significant for persons with and without known cardiovascular disease. In particular, hypertension constitutes a major risk factor for coronary heart disease and stroke, which remain the first and third leading causes of death, respectively, in the United States (5, 25).

In terms of mortality rates, coronary heart disease is the major cardiovascular sequel of hypertension. However, stroke also exacts an enormous burden. In the United States, there are an annual estimated 731,000 strokes and 4 million stroke survivors (20). On average, someone has a stroke every 53 s, and every 3.3 min someone dies from a stroke in the United States. Stroke is the leading cause of serious, long-term disability in the United States. It is estimated that annual direct and indirect costs for stroke care total $40 billion in this country (5, 20, 25).

Improving muscle strength through the inclusion of resistance exercise training has become an accepted component of comprehensive exercise programs for healthy persons as well as those with a variety of chronic diseases (1, 4). In this chapter, we discuss the potential benefits and cardiovascular risks of resistance training for persons with hypertension, and present guidelines for resistance training in hypertensive patients. Because hypertension is the most prevalent and modifiable risk factor for stroke, we also make reference to this specific patient population.

Brief Pathophysiological, Prevention, and Therapeutic Overview

Blood pressure is determined by the product of cardiac output and total peripheral resistance. Therefore, blood pressure can be elevated either as a result of elevated cardiac output, increased total peripheral resistance, or both. Hypertension is defined as a systolic blood pressure of 140 mmHg or greater or a diastolic blood pressure of 90 mmHg or greater. Table 13.1 provides the classification scheme of blood pressure for adults aged 18 years or older as advocated by the Sixth Report of the Joint National Committee on Prevention, Detection, Evaluation, and Treatment of High Blood Pressure (JNC VI) (25). Although stage 1 hypertension is the most common form of high blood pressure in the adult population, all stages are associated with an increased risk of nonfatal cardiovascular events and renal disease. Moreover, high-normal blood pressure (i.e., systolic blood pressure of 130-139 mmHg and/or diastolic blood pressure of 85-89 mmHg) is now known to be

TABLE 13.1   Classification of Blood Pressure for Adults Aged 18 Years and Older*

Category	Systolic BP, mmHg		Diastolic BP, mmHg
Optimal	<120	and	<80
Normal	120-129	and	80-84
High-normal	130-139	or	85-89
Hypertension**			
Stage 1	140-159	or	90-99
Stage 2	160-179	or	100-109
Stage 3	≥180	or	≥110

*Not taking antihypertensive drugs and not acutely ill. When systolic and diastolic blood pressures fall into different categories, the higher category should be selected to classify the individual's blood pressure status.
**Based on the average of two or more readings taken at each of two or more visits after an initial screening.
Abbreviations: BP = blood pressure
Reprinted from JNC VI 1997 (25).

associated with an accentuated risk for the development of hypertension and target organ damage (25).

Among hypertensive adults between the ages of 18 and 65 years who are seen in typical clinical practice, the hypertension of 95% has no identifiable cause (26). Their hypertension is defined as either primary, essential, or idiopathic. Although their cardiac output may be high initially, hypertension usually persists in these patients because of an increased peripheral resistance. Secondary (and possibly reversible) forms of hypertension include renal parenchymal disease, renal vascular hypertension, adrenal hyperfunction (pheochromocytoma, Cushing's syndrome, primary aldosteronism), and coarctation of the aorta. Persons who are elderly have a higher frequency of renal parenchymal disease and renovascular hypertension. Medications, including oral contraceptives, may elevate blood pressure (25, 26).

According to JNC VI, the goal of prevention and management of hypertension is to reduce morbidity and mortality by the least intrusive means possible (25). This may be accomplished by achieving and maintaining a systolic blood pressure below 140 mmHg and diastolic blood pressure below 90 mmHg and lower if tolerated, while controlling other cardiovascular disease risk factors. To accomplish this, the JNC VI recommends the following lifestyle modifications alone or with pharmacological treatment:

- Lose weight if overweight.
- Limit alcohol intake to no more than 1 oz (30 ml) of ethanol (e.g., 24 oz [720 ml] of beer, 10 oz [300 ml] of wine, or 2 oz [60 ml] of 100 proof

whiskey) per day or 0.5 oz (15 ml) ethanol per day for women and lighter-weight people.
- Increase aerobic physical activity (30-45 min most days of the week).
- Reduce sodium intake to no more than 100 mmol/day (2.4 g of sodium or 6 g of sodium chloride).
- Maintain adequate intake of dietary potassium (approximately 90 mmol/day).
- Maintain adequate intake of dietary calcium and magnesium for general health.
- Stop smoking and reduce intake of dietary saturated fat and cholesterol for overall cardiovascular health.

The decision to initiate pharmacological therapy requires consideration of several factors—in particular, the degree of blood pressure elevation, the presence of target organ damage, and the presence of clinical cardiovascular disease or other risk factors (see tables 13.2 and 13.3). As is evident from tables 13.2 and 13.3, patients who have previously suffered a transient ischemic attack or stroke should be considered for prompt pharmacological therapy if they have hypertension, or, for those with heart failure, renal insufficiency, or diabetes, if they have high-normal blood pressure. However, immediately after the occurrence of an ischemic stroke, it is appropriate to withhold antihypertensive treatment, unless blood pressure is very high, until the situation has stabilized (25).

TABLE 13.2 Risk Stratification and Treatment

Blood pressure stages (mmHg)	Risk group A (no risk factors; no TOD/CCD)	Risk group B (at least 1 risk factor, not including diabetes; no TOD/CCD)*	Risk group C (TOD/CCD and/or diabetes, with or without other risk factors)
High-normal (130-139/85-89)	Lifestyle modification	Lifestyle modification	Drug therapy**
Stage 1 (140-159/90-99)	Lifestyle modification (up to 12 months)	Lifestyle modification (up to 6 months)	Drug therapy
Stages 2 and 3 (≥160/≥100)	Drug therapy	Drug therapy	Drug therapy

*For patients with multiple risk factors, clinicians should consider drugs as initial therapy plus lifestyle modifications.
**For those with heart failure, renal insufficiency, or diabetes.
Abbreviations: TOD/CCD indicates target organ disease/clinical cardiovascular disease (see table 13.3)
Reprinted from JNC VI 1997 (25).

TABLE 13.3   Components of Cardiovascular Risk Stratification in Patients With Hypertension

MAJOR RISK FACTORS*

- Smoking
- Dyslipidemia
- Diabetes mellitus
- Age >60 years
- Sex (men and postmenopausal women)
- Family history of cardiovascular disease: women <65 years or men <55 years

TARGET ORGAN DAMAGE (TOD)/CLINICAL CARDIOVASCULAR DISEASE (CCD)

Heart diseases
  - Left-ventricular hypertrophy
  - Angina or prior myocardial infarction
  - Prior coronary revascularization
  - Heart failure

Stroke or transient ischemic attack

Nephropathy

Peripheral arterial disease

Retinopathy

Note: Although not originally included in the JNC VI categorization, a sedentary lifestyle and obesity should be considered as major risk factors.

Reprinted from JNC VI 1997 (25).

There are two major types of strokes: ischemic and hemorrhagic. Ischemic strokes account for approximately 80% of all strokes. There are two major types of ischemic strokes: thrombotic and embolic. Thrombotic ischemic strokes account for approximately 60% of all strokes and are most commonly precipitated by atherosclerosis. Embolic ischemic strokes account for approximately 20% of all strokes and are most commonly precipitated by underlying cardiac disease, including atrial fibrillation, valvular heart disease, and coronary heart disease.

Hemorrhagic strokes account for approximately 20% of all strokes. There are two major types of hemorrhagic strokes: those that result from intracerebral hemorrhage and those that result from subarachnoid hemorrhage. Most intracerebral hemorrhages are related to hypertension. The most common cause of a subarachnoid hemorrhage is a ruptured aneurysm, which is often precipitated by hypertension. Hemorrhagic strokes are less common than ischemic strokes, but they are more likely to be fatal. However, survivors of hemorrhagic strokes are less likely to be severely disabled than survivors of ischemic strokes.

Benefits and Cardiovascular Risks of Resistance Training

A single session of aerobic exercise usually evokes a normal rise in systolic blood pressure from baseline levels in unmedicated persons with hypertension, although the response may be exaggerated or diminished in certain individuals. However, because of an elevated baseline level, the absolute level of systolic blood pressure attained during dynamic exercise is usually higher in persons with hypertension. In addition, their diastolic blood pressure may not change, or even may slightly rise, during dynamic exercise, probably as a result of an impaired vasodilatory response (19).

The acute cardiovascular responses to resistance exercise differ from those of aerobic exercise in several fundamental ways. In particular, heavy resistance exercise elicits a pressor response that involves only moderate increases in heart rate and cardiac output relative to aerobic exercise, but a greater elevation in systolic and diastolic blood pressure. For example, in a study by MacDougall et al. in which blood pressures were directly recorded by means of a capacitance transducer connected to a catheter in the brachial artery, the mean value during a double-leg press performed by five experienced bodybuilders was 302/250 mmHg, with pressures in one subject exceeding 480/350 mmHg (28).

Traditionally, hypertensive patients have been discouraged from performing any type of resistance training for fear of precipitating a cerebrovascular event or placing an excessive demand on a myocardium that may already display left-ventricular dysfunction. Such fears have arisen primarily as a result of the marked pressor response elicited during an acute bout of heavy resistance exercise (18).

Contrary to what might be expected, studies investigating the impact of long-term participation in resistance training on resting blood pressure have generally failed to document a deleterious effect. Indeed, longitudinal training studies have shown that chronic resistance training may modify resting blood pressures in a favorable manner (18).

In a study by Hurley et al. of the effects of 16 weeks of high-intensity resistance training in 11 normotensive males, supine diastolic blood pressure decreased from 84 ± 7 mmHg before training to 79 ± 6 mmHg after training ($p < 0.05$), while supine systolic blood pressure remained essentially unaltered (24). Similarly, whereas seated systolic blood pressures were not significantly modified in a study by Harris and Holly of 10 men with mild hypertension who participated in 9 weeks of circuit weight training, seated diastolic blood pressures fell from 96 ± 20 to 91 ± 25 mmHg ($p < 0.05$) (23). In both of these studies, no significant blood pressure changes were noted in the sedentary control groups (23, 24).

Hagberg et al. have further demonstrated that adolescents with mild systolic hypertension who lower their systolic blood pressures with aerobic exercise training are able to maintain the reductions or even reduce their blood pressures further by subsequently replacing aerobic training with resistance training (21). In their study, the decrease in blood pressure with aerobic training was not associated with significant decreases in either cardiac output or total peripheral resistance. However, maintenance of the decreased blood pressure with resistance training was associated with a decreased total peripheral resistance. With the cessation of all forms of training, total peripheral resistance and systolic blood pressure returned to initial levels.

Gilders et al. studied the effects of a high-intensity resistance training program in normotensive women (16). They found impressive increases in strength and in average cross-sectional muscle fiber area, but no changes in casual or ambulatory 24 h blood pressure readings. Regarding the latter, Hardy and Tucker recently evaluated the effect of a single bout of resistance training on ambulatory blood pressure levels in 24 mildly hypertensive men (22). In their study, a 45 min single bout of resistance training was found to lower systolic and, especially, diastolic blood pressures for at least 1 h postexercise.

Thus, while considerable further research is needed to fully clarify the situation, preliminary evidence suggests that resistance training performed on a long-term basis does not result in elevated resting blood pressures and might, in fact, elicit favorable decreases. The benefits of resistance exercise in lowering blood pressure appear to be most marked with circuit resistance training. While the beneficial influence of resistance training on blood pressure and other cardiovascular disease risk factors is less than with traditional endurance exercise training, resistance training is still of potential importance for hypertensive individuals in maintaining and enhancing strength. Additional benefits include positive effects on bone density, energy metabolism, and functional status.

The above-mentioned studies, however, do not provide sufficient data on the cardiovascular safety of an acute bout of resistance exercise. These studies also do not serve to allay fears that chronic resistance exercise may adversely affect the structural integrity of the cerebral blood vessels and left ventricle, which may already have been impaired by years of hypertension.

We have previously reported on the cardiovascular safety of maximal strength testing performed by 6653 men ($n = 5460$) and women ($n = 1193$) under uniform circumstances at a single facility (Cooper Clinic, Dallas, Texas) (17). All participants underwent a comprehensive preventive medical examination and subsequently performed a series of maximal strength evaluations. This included 4 maximal-effort unilateral isokinetic knee extensions and flexions at an angular velocity of 60°/s with the right and then the left leg, and determination of the maximum weight that could be used to complete one repetition (i.e., one-repetition maximum [1-RM]) on a variable-resistance, universal supine bench press and seated leg-press machine. The mean age was 42 ± 9 years for the men and 40 ± 10 years for the women (range = 20-69 years). A substantial number of the participants had major risk factors for cardiovascular disease, but only a small percentage of the men (1.4%) and women (1%) had a previous diagnosis of cardiac disease. Resting systolic blood pressure was in the high-normal range (130-139 mmHg) in 12% of the men and 5% of the women, and elevated (≥140 mmHg) in 7% of the men and 2% of the women. Resting diastolic blood pressure was in the high-normal range (85-89 mmHg) in 8% of the men and 5% of the women, and elevated (≥90 mmHg) in 16% of the men and 6% of the women. No participant experienced a clinically significant nonfatal (i.e., requiring medical consultation or intervention) or fatal cardiovascular event in association with maximal strength testing. Our observations are corroborated by data on 4500 individuals aged 18 to 93 years who completed approximately 20,000 maximal strength tests at another center without any nonfatal or fatal cardiovascular events (17). Collectively, these data suggest that a single bout of strenuous resistance exercise may be safer from a cardiac standpoint than previously believed. Although additional studies are needed, this may be related to a variety of factors, including increases in subendocardial perfusion.

Experimental evidence on the chronic effects of resistance training on the risk for cerebrovascular complications in humans with hypertension is unavailable at present. To determine whether chronic resistance training would result in a higher incidence of cerebrovascular lesions in animals, Tipton et al. investigated 40 stroke-prone hypertensive rats using an elegant study design (32). The rats were trained to perform resistance training over an electrical grid. During the 21-week study, resistance training was performed 4-5 times per week, and each session involved 1-3 sets of 6-10 repetitions performed with a hang time of 7-10 s per hang, while gradually increasing the amount of weight supported. The procedure for chronic forelimb hanging enabled the rats to increase their strength by 115%, but did not result in an elevation in resting blood pressure. Moreover, when the brains of the rats were histologically examined by a veterinarian pathologist on completion of the study, 4 of the animals in the nonhanging control group had evidence of previous strokes, whereas only 1 of the resistance-trained animals exhibited similar lesions. Although considerable further research is needed before the findings of this study can be extrapolated to humans with hypertension, they suggest that resistance training may not necessarily accentuate the risk of the hypertensive patient for cerebrovascular complications. In contrast, a review by Tipton et al. documented an increased vulnerability of endurance-trained stroke-prone hypertensive rats to cerebrovascular lesions (31).

Myocardial hypertrophy is an adaptive mechanism that develops in response to increased hemodynamic loading of the heart. Depending on the specific cause, the increase in cardiac mass that occurs with myocardial hypertrophy is associated with characteristic alterations in the volume of the cardiac cavities and in the thickness of their walls. On the basis of these changes, myocardial hypertrophy can be classified anatomically as being either concentric (i.e., hearts with thick walls and small cavities) or eccentric (i.e., hearts with walls that are thicker than normal, but relatively thin due to cavities that are larger than normal). In contrast to volume overloading, which is associated with eccentric hypertrophy, the pressure overloading that results from chronic hypertension is associated with concentric hypertrophy (34). In hypertensive patients, concentric hypertrophy of the left ventricle is associated with an increased risk of major cardiovascular events even in the absence of any of the conventional cardiovascular risk factors (10). Theoretically, chronic resistance training, which also results in pressure overloading of the left ventricle, could be expected to contribute further to concentric hypertrophy in hypertensive patients and thereby accentuate their risk for cardiovascular morbidity and mortality.

However, although additional studies are needed to refute this possibility, several reviews of the cardiovascular adaptations to resistance training have concluded that while resistance training may increase left-ventricular wall thickness, there is little or no change in left-ventricular internal dimensions and either no effect or a slight enhancement of systolic function at rest (13, 15, 17). Moreover, whereas the pathological hypertrophy due to hypertension produces abnormalities in left-ventricular diastolic function, resistance training is characterized by normal diastolic function. It should also be noted that in the earlier mentioned study of stroke-prone hypertensive rats, resistance training in fact was not sufficient to stimulate further myocardial hypertrophy (13, 15).

Thus, although the eccentric hypertrophy that often results from the volume overloading induced by aerobic exercise training is physiologically more desirable than the concentric hypertrophy that may result from resistance training, neither form of exercise-induced hypertrophy appears to produce any untoward changes in left-ventricular function. Indeed, it is now postulated that both types of exercise-induced hypertrophy may be associated with an increase in myocyte vascularity that is commensurate with the degree of hypertrophy of the myocytes themselves and may thereby improve myocardial function and assure myocyte health (34). It is also of some interest that circuit resistance training can even be performed with a high level of safety by select patients with coronary artery disease (1, 33).

The clinical manifestations of a stroke include impaired motor control characterized by muscle weakness, altered muscle tone, and abnormal movement patterns. These impairments often limit the ability to perform functional activities of daily living such as walking, stair climbing, and self-care. Recovery generally continues for 6 months after a stroke, with most of the spontaneous recovery occurring in the first 30 days after the stroke (11).

Muscle weakness is one of the most prominent consequences of stroke. Recent studies have shown that the weakness of the affected side of stroke survivors is attributable not only to a decrease in maximum force generated, but also to a disorganized profile of force generation (9). A study by Sunnerhagen et al. has further demonstrated that the nonaffected side of stroke survivors is weaker than that of healthy persons when evaluated 6-24 months poststroke (30). While this observation could be explained by deconditioning, it is believed that neuroanatomic factors also play a role because approximately 10% of the descending motor pathway does not cross over to the other side of the body (30).

The implications of the above studies are that, in appropriately functioning stroke patients, resistance training may be of benefit to both the affected and unaffected sides of the body. However, resistance training has not been widely used in stroke rehabilitation because it has been hypothesized to interfere with coordination and timing in motor control (6). This hypothesis has not been substantiated by recent studies (7, 12, 14, 29). Although additional studies are needed, the results of recent research suggest that stroke patients can derive substantial increases in strength by participating in a resistance training program (12, 14, 27).

Resistance Training Guidelines

The American College of Sports Medicine (ACSM) does not recommend resistance training as the primary form of exercise for hypertensive individuals. Rather, resistance training is recommended as a component of a well-rounded exercise program (3).

Resistance training may span a continuum of devices (e.g., light hand-held weights, elastic bands, progressively heavier free weights, and various types of resistance training machines) and resistance loads. To assist with risk stratification prior to the initiation of a resistance training program, a distinction should be drawn between lower-load and higher-load resistance programs. In their guidelines for cardiac patients, the American Association of Cardiovascular and Pulmonary Rehabilitation

(AACVPR) categorizes loads of 50% or greater of 1-RM as higher-load resistance training (1). Although there are no widely accepted guidelines on screening of individuals prior to resistance training, it appears prudent to extrapolate the guidelines of the ACSM, which are intended for endurance exercise training, to resistance training (4). When doing so, one approach is to categorize vigorous exercise as higher-load resistance training involving loads of 50% or greater of 1-RM and/or eliciting a perceived exertion rating of 12 or higher using the Borg 6-20 scale (2). Thus, prior to participation by hypertensive individuals in higher-load resistance training, a medical examination and graded exercise test with electrocardiographic monitoring would be recommended for persons with symptoms of or known cardiac, pulmonary, or metabolic disease; men $\geq$45 years and women $\geq$55 years; and, irrespective of age, persons with additional coronary artery disease risk factors.

As is the case for endurance exercise training, persons with a systolic blood pressure above 179 mmHg and/or diastolic blood pressure above 109 mmHg should not participate in higher-load resistance training until their blood pressure is under better control (18). Provided there are none of the other generally accepted contraindications to exercise, hypertensive individuals without cardiac disease may follow the guidelines of the ACSM for resistance training for the average healthy adult (2). However, it may be prudent to recommend 10-15 repetitions for each set of exercises rather than 8-12 repetitions (i.e., higher repetitions with lower loads). Thus, a minimum of 1 set of 10-15 repetitions to near fatigue of at least 8-10 exercises involving the major muscle groups (arms, shoulders, chest, abdomen, back, hips, and legs) should be performed 2-3 days per week (2). For hypertensive patients with cardiac disease, the guidelines of the AACVPR are more appropriate and are listed in tables 13.4 and 13.5 (1).

The American College of Cardiology in collaboration with the ACSM have published recommendations for determining eligibility for competition in athletes with cardiovascular abnormalities (27). For these recommendations, exercise is divided into two broad categories: static and dynamic. Competitive weightlifting is classified as a sport involving high static and low dynamic components (class 3A). Competitive bodybuilding is classified as a sport involving high static and moderate dynamic components (class 3B). The following recommendations are made for hypertensive adults (ages 18 years and older):

- The presence of stage 1 or stage 2 hypertension (see table 13.1) in the absence of target organ damage or concomitant heart disease (see table 13.3) should not limit the eligibility for any competitive sports. However, the hypertensive athlete should have blood pressure measured every 2-4 months, or more frequently if indicated.

TABLE 13.4 Guidelines of the American Association of Cardiovascular and Pulmonary Rehabilitation: Patient Considerations for Higher-Load (50% or Greater of 1-RM) Resistance Exercise Programming*

Although there are data documenting the safety of resistance training after MI, CABGS, or PTCA, certain precautions should be taken. Care must be taken to avoid problems associated with sternal wound healing (CABGS) and femoral arterial puncture site (PTCA). In addition, avoidance of excessive myocardial work in post-MI patients is essential soon after (< 6-8 weeks) the acute cardiac event.

For all cardiac patients, there should be no evidence of
- symptomatic congestive heart failure,
- uncontrolled arrhythmias,
- severe valvular disease,
- unstable symptoms, and
- uncontrolled hypertension. Patients with moderate hypertension (SBP $\geq$ 160 mmHg or DBP $\geq$ 100 mmHg) should be referred to appropriate management; however, moderate hypertension is not an absolute contraindication for participation in a resistance training program.

Participation in resistance training may begin following
- a minimum of 5 weeks post-MI including 3 weeks of continuous aerobic program participation;
- a minimum of 8 weeks post-CABGS including 3 weeks of continuous aerobic program participation; and
- a minimum of 2 weeks of consistent aerobic participation post-PTCA.

---

*A resistance exercise program, for the purposes of this table, is defined as one in which patients lift weights corresponding to 50% or greater of 1-RM. The use of elastic bands, 1-3 lb hand weights, and light free weights may be initiated in a progressive fashion at immediate outpatient program entry, provided there are no other contraindications.

Abbreviations: 1-RM = one-repetition maximum; MI = myocardial infarction; CABGS = coronary artery bypass graft surgery; PTCA = percutaneous transluminal coronary angioplasty; SBP = systolic blood pressure; DBP = diastolic blood pressure.

Adapted from AACVPR 1999 (1).

TABLE 13.5 Guidelines of the American Association of Cardiovascular and Pulmonary Rehabilitation: Resistance Training

---

To prevent soreness and minimize the risk of injury, the initial load should allow 12-15 repetitions comfortably. If a 1-RM pretraining evaluation is used, this load would be approximately 30-50% 1-RM. Low-risk-stratified, aerobically trained patients may be progressed to higher relative loads, depending on program goals.

Perform 1 set of up to 8-10 exercises (major muscle groups), 2-3 days per week. Additional sets may be added, but incremental gains are not proportionate.

Specific considerations:
- a. Exercise large muscle groups before small muscle groups.
- b. Increase loads by 5-10 lb when 12-15 repetitions can be comfortably lifted.
- c. Raise weights with slow, controlled movements; emphasize complete extension of the limbs when lifting.

d. Exhale (blow out) during the exertion phase of the lift (e.g., exhale when pushing a weight stack overhead and inhale when lowering it).

e. Sustained, tight gripping may evoke an excessive blood pressure response to lifting.

f. Minimize rest periods between exercises to maximize muscular endurance, as tolerable.

g. Avoid straining. An RPE rating of 11 (fairly light) to 13 (somewhat hard) may be used as a subjective guide to effort.

h. Stop exercise in the event of warning signs or symptoms, especially dizziness, arrhythmias, unusual shortness of breath, and/or anginal discomfort.

Abbreviations: 1-RM = one-repetition maximum; RPE = rating of perceived exertion (6-20 scale).
Adapted from AACVPR 1999 (1).

- Athletes with stage 3 hypertension (see table 13.1) should be restricted, particularly from high static sports (classes 3A to 3C), until their hypertension is controlled by either lifestyle modification or drug therapy (and in the absence of evidence of target organ damage).
- When hypertension coexists with other cardiovascular diseases, eligibility for participation in competitive athletics is usually based on the type and severity of the other associated conditions.

Currently, there are no accepted guidelines on when and how to initiate resistance training post ischemic or hemorrhagic stroke. Until such guidelines are available, it may be prudent to follow guidelines similar to those for postmyocardial infarction patients. As emphasized by the AACVPR, a guiding principle should be development of a resistance training program that does not supersede the physiological limit set for the endurance training component, is progressive in nature, and is safe. Until there is a broader knowledge base, a conservative approach is recommended (1).

References

1. American Association of Cardiovascular and Pulmonary Rehabilitation. 1999. *Guidelines for cardiac rehabilitation and secondary prevention programs*. 3d ed. Champaign, IL: Human Kinetics.

2. American College of Sports Medicine. 1998. The recommended quantity and quality of exercise for developing and maintaining cardiorespiratory and muscular fitness, and flexibility in healthy adults. *Medicine and Science in Sports and Exercise* 30: 975-991.

3. American College of Sports Medicine. 1993. Physical activity, physical fitness, and hypertension. *Medicine and Science in Sports and Exercise* 25 (10): i-x.

4. American College of Sports Medicine. 2000. *ACSM's guidelines for exercise testing and prescription*. 6th ed. Baltimore: Lippincott Williams & Wilkins.

5. American Heart Association. 1998. *1999 Heart and stroke statistical update*. Dallas: American Heart Association.

6. Bobath, B. 1998. *Adult hemiplegia: Evaluation and treatment*. 2d ed. London: Heinemann.

7. Brown, D.A., and S.A. Kautz. 1998. Increased workload enhances force output during pedaling exercise in persons with poststroke hemiplegia. *Stroke* 29: 598-606.

8. Burt, V.L., P. Wheiton, E.J. Roccella, C. Brown, J.A. Cutler, M. Higgins, M.J. Horan, and D. Labarthe. 1995. Prevalence of hypertension in the U.S. adult population. Results from the Third National Health and Nutrition Examination Survey, 1988-1991. *Hypertension* 25: 305-313.

9. Canning, C.G., L. Ada, and N. O'Dwyer. 1999. Slowness to develop force contributes to weakness after stroke. *Archives of Physical Medicine and Rehabilitation* 80: 66-70.

10. DiPette, D.J., and E.D. Frohlich. 1988. Cardiac involvement in hypertension. *American Journal of Cardiology* 61: 67H-72H.

11. Duncan, P.W., and S.M. Lai. 1997. Stroke recovery. *Topics in Stroke Rehabilitation* 4: 51-58.

12. Duncan, P., L. Richards, D. Wallace, J. Stoker-Yates, P. Pohl, C. Luchies, A. Ogle, and S. Studenski. 1998. A randomized, controlled pilot study of a home-based exercise program for individuals with mild and moderate stroke. *Stroke* 29: 2055-2060.

13. Effron, M.B. 1989. Effects of resistive training on left ventricular function. *Medicine and Science in Sports and Exercise* 21: 694-697.

14. Engardt, M., E. Knutsson, M. Jonsson, and M. Stemhag. 1995. Dynamic muscle strength training in stroke patients: Effects on knee extension torque, electromyographic activity, and motor function. *Archives of Physical Medicine and Rehabilitation* 76: 419-425.

15. Fleck, S. J. 1988. Cardiovascular adaptations to resistance training. *Medicine and Science in Sports and Exercise* 20: S146-S151.

16. Gilders, R.M, E.S. Malicky, J.E. Falkel, R.S. Staron, and G.A. Dudley. 1991. The effect of resistance training on blood pressure in normotensive women. *Clinical Physiology* 11: 307-314.

17. Gordon, N.F., H.W. Kohl, M.L. Pollock, H. Vaandrager, L.W. Gibbons, and S.N. Blair. 1995. Cardiovascular safety of maximal strength testing in healthy adults. *American Journal of Cardiology* 76: 851-853.

18. Gordon, N.F. 1997. Hypertension. In *ACSM's exercise management for persons with chronic diseases and disabilities*, 59-63. Champaign, IL: Human Kinetics.

19. Gordon, N.F., C.B. Scott, W.J. Wilkinson, J.J. Duncan, and S.N. Blair. 1990. Exercise and mild essential hypertension. Recommendations for adults. *Sports Medicine* 10 (6): 390-394.

20. Gorelick, P.B., R.L. Sacco, D.B. Smith, M. Alberts, L. Mustone-Alexander, D. Rader, J. Ross, E. Raps, M. Ozer, L. Brass, M. Malone, S. Goldberg, J. Booss, D. Hanley, J. Toole, N. Greengold, and D. Rhew. 1999. Prevention of a first stroke. A review of guidelines and a multidisciplinary consensus statement from the National Stroke Association. *Journal of the American Medical Association* 281: 1112-1120.

21. Hagberg, J.M., D. Goldring, A.A. Ehsani, et al. 1983. Effect of exercise training on the blood pressure and hemodynamic features of hypertensive adolescents. *American Journal of Physiology* 63: 270-276.

22. Hardy, D.O., and L.A. Tucker. 1998. The effects of a single bout of strength training on ambulatory blood pressure levels in 24 mildly hypertensive men. *American Journal of Health Promotion* 13 (2): 69-72.

23. Harris, K.A., and R.G. Holly. 1987. Physiological response to circuit weight training in borderline hypertensive subjects. *Medicine and Science in Sports and Exercise* 19: 246-252.

24. Hurley, B.F., J.M. Hagberg, A.P. Goldberg, D.R. Seals, A.A. Ehsani, R.E. Brennan, and J.O. Holloszy. 1988. Resistive training can reduce coronary risk factors without altering VO_2max or percent body fat. *Medicine and Science in Sports and Exercise* 20: 150-154.

25. Joint National Committee on Prevention, Detection, Evaluation, and Treatment of High Blood Pressure. 1997. The Sixth Report of the Joint National Committee on Prevention, Detection, Evaluation, and Treatment of High Blood Pressure. *Archives of Internal Medicine* 157: 2413-2446.

26. Kaplan, N.M. 1997. Systemic hypertension: Mechanisms and diagnosis. In *Heart disease: A textbook of cardiovascular medicine*, edited by E. Braunwald, 807-839. Philadelphia: Saunders.

27. Kaplan, N.M., R.B. Deveraux, and H.S. Miller. 1994. Task force 4: Systemic hypertension. *Journal of the American College of Cardiology* 24: 885-888.

28. MacDougall, J.D., D. Tuxen, D.G. Sale, et al. 1985. Arterial blood pressure response to heavy resistance exercise. *Journal of Applied Physiology* 58: 785-790.

29. Sharp, S.A., and B.J. Brouwer. 1997. Isokinetic strength training of the hemiparetic knee: Effects on function and spasticity. *Archives of Physical Medicine and Rehabilitation* 78: 1231-1236.

30. Sunnerhagen, K.S., U. Svantesson, L. Lonn, M. Krotkiewski, and G. Grimby. 1999. Upper motor neuron lesions: Their effect on muscle performance and appearance in stroke patients with minor motor impairment. *Archives of Physical Medicine and Rehabilitation* 80: 155-161.

31. Tipton, C.M. 1984. Exercise, training, and hypertension. *Exercise and Sport Science Reviews* 12: 245-307.

32. Tipton, C.M., S. McMahon, E.M. Youmans, et al. 1988. Response of hypertensive rats to acute and chronic conditions of static exercise. *American Journal of Physiology* 254: H592-H598.

33. Verrill, D.E., and P.M. Ribisl. 1996. Resistive exercise training in cardiac rehabilitation: An update. *Sports Medicine* 21: 347-383.

34. Weber, J.R. 1988. Left ventricular hypertrophy. Its prime importance as a controllable risk factor. *American Heart Journal* 116: 272-279.

14
CHAPTER

Resistance Training for Organ Transplant Recipients

Randy W. Braith, PhD
Peter M. Magyari, MS
University of Florida—Gainesville

Introduction

In little more than two decades, organ transplantation has evolved from an experimental and rarely performed procedure to an accepted life-extending therapy for end-stage organ failure. Nearly 330,000 patients have received transplanted organs over the past 20+ years, and the number continues to rise, with recent annual figures approaching 21,000 procedures in the United States (43) and surpassing 35,000 procedures worldwide (26). In the early years, organ transplantation was associated with low survival rates, but since 1990 the reported 1- and 5-year survival rates have increased to ~80% and ~70%, respectively. Dramatic improvements in organ preservation, surgical procedures, and immunosuppressive drug management continue to reduce morbidity and improve survival.

Short-term survival, however, is no longer the pivotal issue for most organ transplant recipients (OTR). Rather, a return to functional lifestyle with good quality of life is now the desired procedural outcome. To achieve this outcome, aggressive exercise rehabilitation is essential. Before transplantation, most OTR have suffered from chronic debilitating illness and may have required prolonged hospitalization for mechanical support or an assist device. Prolonged bed rest causes peak oxygen consumption ($\dot{V}O_2$peak) to regress approximately 26% within the first 1-3 weeks (35), and similar regressions are observed in skeletal muscle structure and function (cross-sectional area [CSA]) (3, 4, 17, 25, 38, 40). After transplantation, OTR must also contend with de novo Cushingoid symptoms conferred by the catabolic side effects of glucocorticoid immunosuppression regimens. Most notably, chronic glucocorticoid therapy causes osteoporosis and skeletal muscle myopathy.

Until recently, resistance training was excluded from OTR rehabilitation regimens because of concerns about the heightened risk of musculoskeletal injury in patients receiving bolus glucocorticoids. Provocative recent evidence, however, indicates that the anabolic benefits of resistance exercise in OTR greatly outweigh the risks. Indeed, there is growing clinical consensus that resistance training is essential to achieve optimal outcomes in the postoperative management of OTR. The first portion of this chapter will present rationale for including resistance training in rehabilitation programs designed for OTR. The second portion of the chapter will review the available research involving resistance training with OTR. The chapter will conclude with recommendations for implementation of a resistance training program for this new and expanding patient population.

Indications for Resistance Training in Transplant Recipients

Transplant recipients are typically severely deconditioned prior to transplant. Resistance training is an effective therapy for restoring functional capacity. In addition, resistance training can attenuate some of the negative side effects of immunosuppresive drug treatment required for organ acceptance in transplant recipients.

Pretransplant Skeletal Muscle Atrophy

Organ failure invites a "spectrum of disuse" in skeletal muscle. Deficits in the volume of muscle tissue, muscle strength, and slow-to-fast fiber transformation are a consistent and nondiscriminant finding in heart (4, 25, 40), lung (17, 38), liver (9), and kidney (36) transplant candidates. Skeletal muscle atrophy is reported in up to 70% of transplant candidates, and leg fatigue, rather than central mechanisms, is a primary factor limiting exercise tolerance (15, 17, 20, 25).

Morphological Abnormalities

Morphological data from biopsy studies in organ failure patients reveal that there is a pronounced and selective atrophy in highly oxidative, fatigue resistant, type I muscle fibers, resulting in a shift in fiber-type distribution toward the glycolytic, less fatigue resistant, type II muscle fibers (11, 15, 37, 42). One laboratory has reported a significant correlation between the percent distribution of the three myosin heavy chain (MHC) isoforms in the gastrocnemius, the severity of organ failure, and $\dot{V}O_2$peak (MHC1 = slow aerobic; MHC2a = fast oxidative; MHC2b = fast glycolytic) (45).

Enzymatic Abnormalities

Enzymatic reserve is also altered and becomes shifted toward less fatigue resistance. Significant reductions in the oxidative enzymes succinate dehydrogenase, citrate synthase, and cytochrome oxidase have been reported (32, 37, 41, 42). Mitochondria volume and the surface density of mitochondrial cristae are also significantly diminished (11). In contrast, the anaerobic enzyme lactate dehydrogenase is significantly increased (37). Studies using ^{31}P-NMR spectroscopy and in-magnet protocols corroborate the biopsy data and report increased depletion of phosphocreatine (PCr), lower muscle pH at submaximal workloads, and less rapid resynthesis of PCr, which is an indicator of mitochondrial phosphorylation in organ failure patients (21). The available evidence suggests that intrinsic intramuscular abnormalities exist in organ failure patients that are unrelated to blood flow (10, 11). Reductions in skeletal muscle mass (13-15%) and aerobic enzyme activity, and an increased percentage of fast-twitch type IIb fibers all act in concert to induce early anaerobic metabolism during exercise. Early onset of anaerobic metabolism, in turn, limits exercise tolerance in organ failure patients (30).

Diminished Aerobic Capacity

Diminished $\dot{V}O_2$peak is a common manifestation of OTR (4, 8, 23). The concept of a single factor limiting $\dot{V}O_2$peak in OTR is now obsolete; the mechanisms responsible for attenuated $\dot{V}O_2$peak are diverse, including reduced cardiac index, reduced pulmonary ventilatory and diffusion capacity, impaired peripheral vasodilation, and depressed oxidative capacity of skeletal muscle. However, muscle atrophy is a particularly important determinant of exercise capacity in OTR. In fact, skeletal muscle weakness may preclude objective measurement of OTR because of the fact that treadmill and cycle ergometer testing devices make enormous demands on peripheral leg strength en route to eliciting peak cardiovascular performance. For example, heart transplant recipients consistently achieve $\dot{V}O_2$peak values that are only 60-70% of age-matched norms, and this impairment in $\dot{V}O_2$peak is routinely ascribed to chronotropic incompetence and diastolic dysfunction (4, 7, 19). However, one-repetition maximum (1-RM) knee extension strength values (normalized for lean body mass) in heart transplant recipients are only 60-70% of values achieved by age-matched control subjects (4). More importantly, Braith et al. have shown that knee extension strength is highly correlated ($r = 0.92$) with $\dot{V}O_2$peak in heart transplant recipients, when compared with normal control subjects ($r = 0.65$) (figure 14.1) (4, 5).

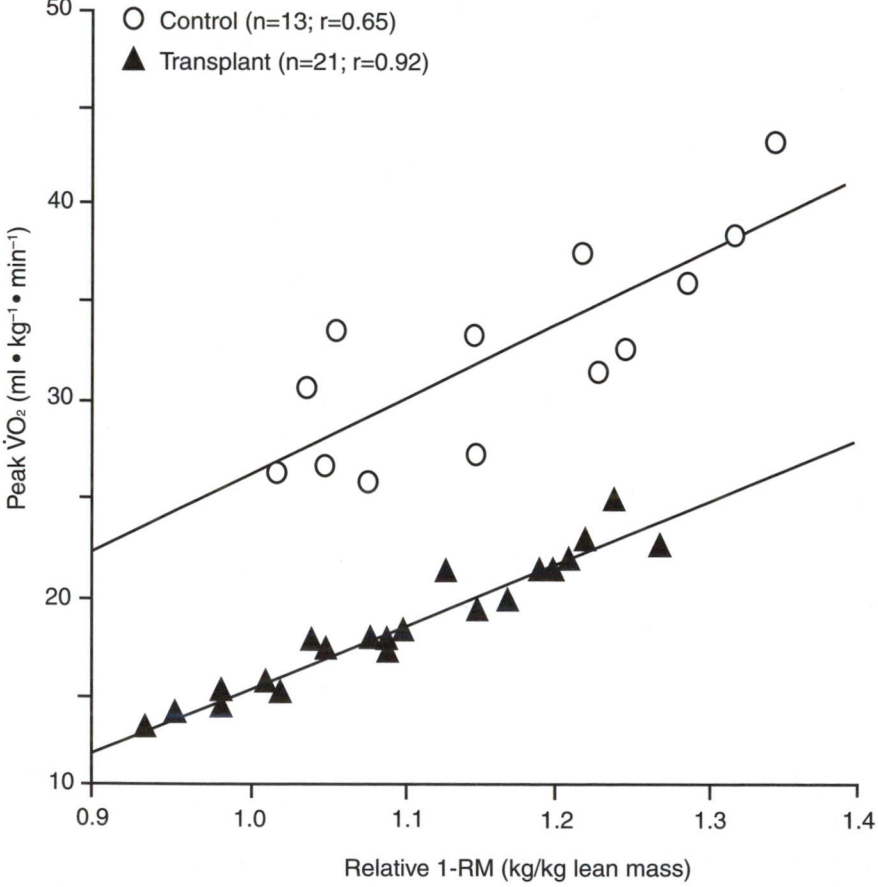

Figure 14.1 The relationship between one-repetition maximum (1-RM) strength of the knee extensors, corrected for lean body mass, and peak oxygen consumption ($\dot{V}O_2$peak) in heart transplant recipients and age-matched normal control subjects. Adapted from Braith et al. 1993 (4).

These correlational data support the hypothesis that $\dot{V}O_2$peak in subjects with normal leg strength is restricted by cardiovascular function. In contrast, skeletal muscle atrophy in OTR appears to be a primary factor limiting aerobic power. We speculate that training-induced improvements in $\dot{V}O_2$peak, treadmill time to exhaustion, and peak heart rate in OTR are a function of increased leg strength.

Glucocorticoid-Induced Muscle Myopathy

As discussed above, skeletal muscle myopathy originates before transplantation and is observed in most organ failure patients. The preoperative muscle abnormalities are not immediately resolved by organ transplantation and contribute to exercise intolerance in OTR indefinitely (4, 8, 16, 40). After transplantation, skeletal muscle function is further altered by immunosuppression regimens that include glucocorticoids (prednisone, methylprednisolone). Long-term treatment with exogenous glucocorticoids promotes atrophy, particularly in type II fibers, by increasing the rate of protein catabolism and amino acid efflux while simultaneously decreasing the rate of protein synthesis (8). In aggregate, skeletal muscle in an OTR has undergone preoperative shifts away from type I toward type IIb fibers, and postoperative steroid-induced atrophy of type II fibers occurs. The consequences of both preoperative and postoperative transformations in skeletal muscle in OTR are not clearly understood. Horber et al. reported significant decrements in thigh muscle mass in both male (45%) and female (20%) kidney transplant recipients up to 18 months posttransplantation (13). Braith et al. found that knee extension strength (normalized for lean body mass) in heart transplant recipients at 18 months after transplantation was only 60-70% of values achieved by age-matched control subjects (4). At 3, 12, and 15 months after heart transplantation, no significant changes in fiber type are observed, PCr depletion remains elevated, and PCr resynthesis rate remains diminished, indicating a sustained emphasis on anaerobic bioenergetic pathways (8, 40). In addition, capillary density and capillary/fiber ratio in skeletal muscle remain significantly reduced below age-matched norms (24% and 27%, respectively) in OTR late after transplantation (2, 23).

Glucocorticoid-Induced Osteoporosis

Bone loss is another clinically significant Cushingoid symptom that occurs coincident with the administration of glucocorticoids. Glucocorticoids have multiple well-documented deleterious effects on the skeleton, including

1. suppression of osteoblast number, function, and recruitment, which inhibits new bone growth;

2. activation of osteoclasts, which increases bone resorption;
3. suppression of gastrointestinal absorption of calcium and phosphate, independent of vitamin D status; and
4. increased renal excretion of calcium, resulting in negative calcium balance (24).

Osteoporosis is documented in nearly 100% of OTR (6, 18, 24, 27, 29, 33, 39). Trabecular or cancellous bone of the axial skeleton is lost more rapidly than cortical bone mass from the long bones. The lumbar vertebra are particularly susceptible to osteoporosis in OTR, with bone losses of 10-20% observed only 60 days after transplantation (6, 12, 18, 27, 28, 39). Skeletal demineralization is accompanied by a high incidence of nontraumatic fractures, with radiological evidence of spontaneous long-bone fractures present in up to 44% of OTR early in the postoperative period (33). More important clinically, however, is the alarming incidence of lumbar compression fractures in up to 50% of OTR (34, 39). Additionally, OTR receiving long-term glucocorticoids have an increased incidence of aseptic necrosis of bone in the hip and knee joints, resulting in total joint replacement (24).

Pharmacological Therapy for Osteoporosis

The rapid and significant loss of trabecular bone observed early in the postoperative period begins to stabilize and plateau at approximately 6 months after transplantation, coincident with the tapering of glucocorticoids (6). However, regional bone mineral density does not return to pretransplantation levels (6, 18, 29). Calcium supplementation, bisphosphonate agents, estrogenic and androgenic hormones, and calcitonin have all been used to prevent glucocorticoid-induced osteoporosis, but at best they attenuate further bone loss rather than restore new bone growth (29, 31, 44). Bone mineral density in OTR remains significantly below age-matched norms, and bone mineral levels do not recover toward preoperative levels in patients up to 36 months after transplantation (6, 29, 39, 44).

Summary

In summary, skeletal muscle myopathy is a consistent and nondiscriminant finding in nearly all end-stage organ failure patients who become candidates for transplantation. After successful organ transplantation, OTR must also contend with de novo Cushingoid symptoms caused by chronic glucocorticoid immunosuppression regimens. Most notably, long-term glucocorticoid therapy causes osteoporosis and skeletal muscle myopathy. Because steroid-induced myopathy and osteoporosis can be crippling complications after transplantation, it is appropriate to look for effective prophylactic treatments to attenuate or prevent the catabolic effects of glucocorticoids. Recent reports indicate that resistance exercise is both osteogenic and myogenic if initiated early after heart transplantation. In the following portion of the chapter we will review the available experience with resistance training in OTR.

Resistance Training Studies With Transplant Recipients

The inclusion of resistance training as an adjunct therapy in the postoperative recovery of OTR is a relatively new approach to restoring functional quality to patients in this clinical population. The majority of controlled and standardized studies are from the laboratory of Dr. Randy Braith at the University of Florida or Dr. Fritz Horber's lab at the University of Berne, Switzerland (table 14.1). Although the total number of investigations implementing resistance training in OTR is small and the studies were single-center, initial findings are provocative and encourage larger, multicenter trials.

The Effects of Resistance Exercise on Glucocorticoid-Induced Muscle Myopathy

Glucocorticoid-induced muscle myopathy results in a loss of muscle mass and skeletal muscle functional capacity in organ transplant recipients. Resistance training helps restore these detrimental side effects of glucocorticoids.

Muscle Mass
Both variable-resistance (5) and isokinetic-resistance (13, 14, 16) training regimens have elicited significant increases in muscle mass in OTR. Horber and coworkers assessed thigh muscle mass using computed tomography (CT) in 12 clinically stable kidney transplant recipients before and after 7 weeks of isokinetic resistance exercise (14). Training consisted of 8-10 sets of 8 maximal flexions and extensions of the knee at 60°/s with 30 s rest between sets, followed by (after a 3 min rest) 4 sets to failure at 180°/s with 45 s of rest between sets. Only the left leg was trained, while the right leg was used as a nonexercise control. Before training, midthigh CT scans showed that the muscle area of both legs was significantly below that of age-matched norms. After 7 weeks of isokinetic exercise, muscle mass was restored to normal values in the trained leg only.

In a comprehensive resistance training study conducted by Braith et al., 14 male heart transplant recipients were randomized into either a 6-month training group ($n = 7$) or a control group ($n = 7$) (5). The training regimen consisted of two components: lumbar-extension training 1 day/week on a MedX Lumbar Extension Machine and upper- and lower-body resistance training 2 days/week using Nautilus and MedX variable-resistance

TABLE 14.1 Selected Data From Studies Investigating Resistance Training in Organ Transplant Recipients

Investigator	Type of organ transplant	Number studied	Description of training		
			Mean time posttransplant	Length of training	Frequency of training
Braith et al. 1996 (6)	Heart	$N = 16$ Tx controls	2 months	6 months	2/week
Braith et al. 1998 (5)	Heart	$N = 14$ Tx controls	2 months	6 months	2/week
Horber et al. 1985 (13)	Kidney	$N = 12^*$ Non-Tx controls	>6 months	7 weeks	3/week
Horber et al. 1985 (14)	Kidney	$N = 24^*$ Non-Tx controls	>6 months	7 weeks	3/week
Horber et al. 1987 (16)	Kidney	$N = 18$ Non-Tx controls	>16 months	7 weeks	3/week
Kobashigawa et al. 1999 (22)	Heart	$N = 27$ Tx controls	2 weeks	6 months	1-3/week

*Contralateral leg also used as a control.
Tx = transplant, FFM = fat-free mass,
MVF = maximal volitional fatigue, BMD = bone mineral density, $\uparrow$ = increase, > = greater than.
All increases ($\uparrow$) were significant: p 0.05.

		Results of training		
Type of resistance training	Muscle size	Muscle function	Ultrastructural adaptations	Bone mineral density
Variable-resistance machines, 1 set 10-15 reps to MVF				Restored BMD to pre-Tx levels; no change in controls
Variable-resistance machines, 1 set 10-15 reps to MVF	FFM > controls at 3 months and > pre-Tx at 6 months	↑ in knee extension, bench press, and lumbar strength was 4-6× that of controls		
1 leg isokinetic knee flexion/ extension, 60°/s and 180°/s, multiple sets to MVF	↑ in midthigh muscle area of both trained and untrained legs	Peak torque and total work output were restored in trained leg only vs. normal controls		
1 leg isokinetic knee flexion/ extension, 60°/s and 180°/s, multiple sets to MVF	Midthigh muscle area restored to normal control values	Peak torque and total work output were restored in trained leg only vs. normal controls		
1 leg isokinetic knee flexion/ extension, 60°/s and 180°/s, multiple sets to MVF		Power output/ muscle mass ↑ similar to controls	↑ mitochondrial density, capillary density, and volume of sarcoplasm	
Calisthenic-type strengthening and aerobic exercises		↑ in sit-to-stand rate was ~3× > in exercise group vs. control		

machines incorporating each of the major muscle groups of the body (see table 14.2). A single set of 10-15 repetitions was performed for each exercise. Initial training weights were set at 50% of 1-RM. When the subject was able to complete 15 repetitions prior to reaching volitional muscle fatigue, resistance was increased by 5-10% at the subsequent training session. Body composition was assessed using a dual-energy X-ray absorptiometer (Lunar Corp.) prior to transplantation, 2 months posttransplantation, and after 3 and 6 months of the resistance exercise program (figure 14.2). Fat-free mass (FFM) was significantly decreased from pretransplant levels in both groups at only 60 days after transplant. FFM was decreased further after 3 and 6 months in the control group despite participation in home-based walking programs. After 3 months of resistance training, subjects had restored FFM to pretransplant levels, and after 6 months of training FFM was significantly greater than before transplantation. In absolute terms, the control group lost 4 kg of FFM in 8 months following transplantation, while the resistance training group increased FFM by 2.2 kg, when compared with pretransplant values.

Muscle Strength

Muscular strength was also assessed in both of the studies mentioned earlier. Braith et al. found significant strength increases in both the resistance-trained heart transplant recipients and nontrained control patients at completion of the study (5). However, the magnitude of improvement in skeletal muscle strength in the training group was 4-6 times greater than in the control group (see figures 14.3 and 14.4).

Horber et al. found peak torque and total work output to be significantly reduced in kidney transplant recipients compared with nontransplant controls at >6 months posttransplant (14). After 7 weeks of isokinetic resistance training, peak torque and total work output values for the trained leg in kidney transplant recipients recovered to values comparable to nontransplant controls, while peak torque and total work output values remained significantly depressed for the nontrained leg.

TABLE 14.2   Resistance Exercises Performed by Heart Transplant Recipients

1. Lumbar extension	6. Triceps extension
2. Duo-decline chest press	7. Biceps flexion
3. Knee extension	8. Shoulder press
4. Pullover	
5. Knee flexion	9. Abdominals

Heart transplant recipients performed this regimen of resistance exercises in order 2 times per week. Lumbar extension exercise was performed only 1 time per week. Subjects used the greatest resistance possible to complete a single set consisting of 10-15 repetitions for each exercise. We strove to have the subjects attain momentary volitional failure during the last repetition in each set. This regimen was effective as part of a strategy to prevent steroid-induced osteoporosis and steroid myopathy in heart transplant recipients (5, 6).

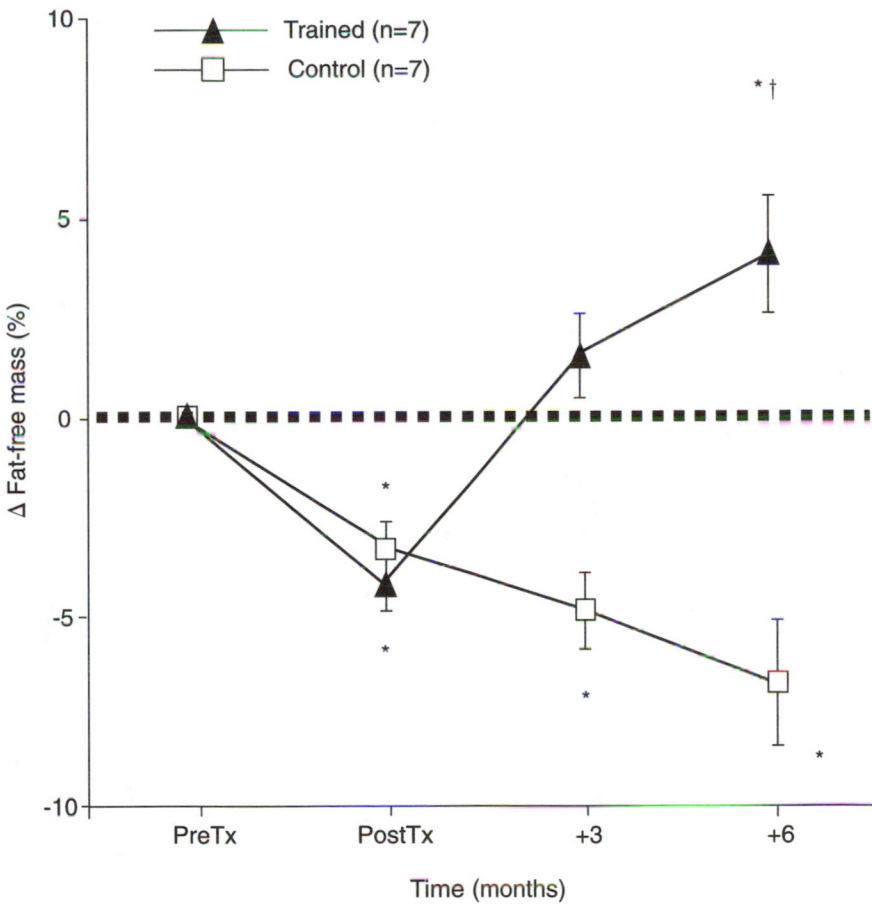

Figure 14.2 Changes in fat-free mass (FFM) at 2 months after heart transplantation, and after 3 and 6 months of a resistance exercise program or control period. Data are mean ± SEM; * $p \leq 0.05$ versus pretransplantation value; † $p \leq 0.05$ trained group versus control group.

Adapted from Braith et al. 1998 (5).

Muscle Ultrastructure

The only study to assess the effects of resistance training on skeletal muscle ultrastructure in OTR was conducted by Horber et al. in kidney transplant recipients ($N = 18$) (16). Muscle biopsies were obtained from the vastus lateralis muscle at midthigh level, using the Bergstrom technique (1, p. 11-12), before and after 7 weeks of isokinetic resistance training. Training resulted in similar increases in what the authors called "muscle efficiency" (power output/muscle mass) in kidney transplant recipients ($n = 9$) and nontransplant controls ($n = 9$).

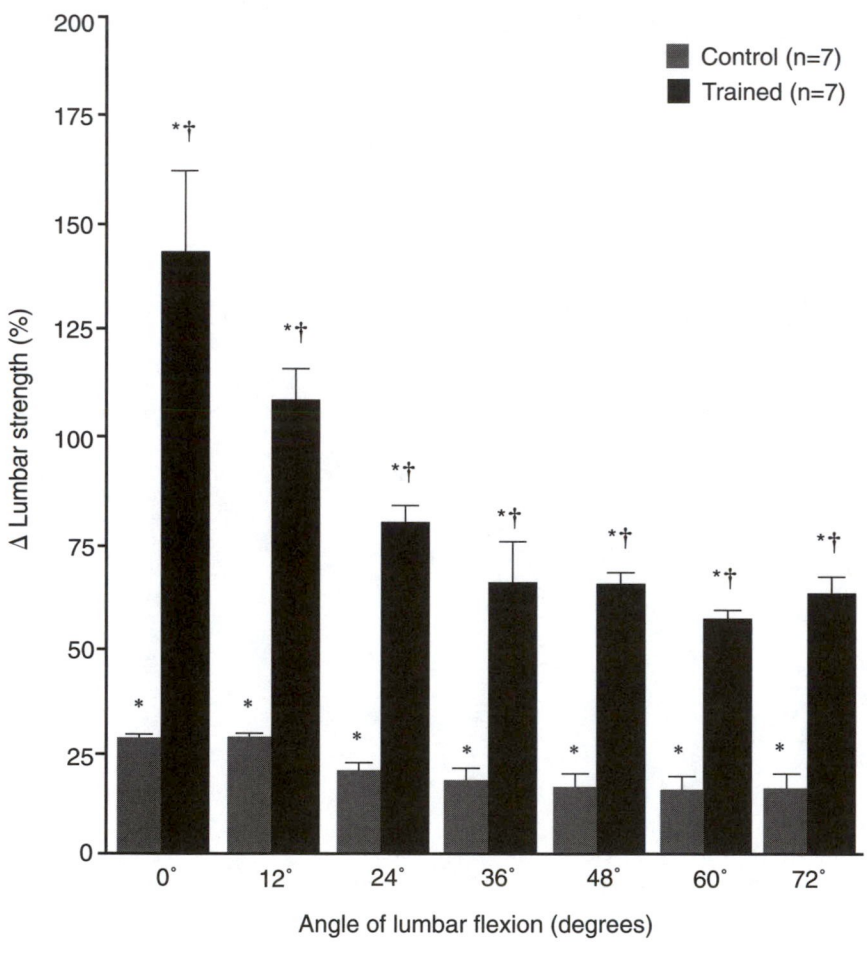

Figure 14.3 Changes in lumbar extensor strength after 6 months of a resistance exercise program or control period. Data are mean ± SEM; * $p \leq 0.05$ versus posttransplantation baseline value; † $p \leq 0.05$ trained group versus control group. Adapted from Braith et al. 1998 (5).

The increase in muscle efficiency in nontransplant controls after resistance training was associated with significant increases in the volume of sarcoplasm. The ultrastructural changes that accompanied the increase in muscle efficiency in kidney transplant patients included increases in both capillary and mitochondrial density as well as an increase in the volume of sarcoplasm. These ultrastructural adaptations demonstrate that resistance training can elicit anabolic remodeling in transplant recipients, despite chronic glucocorticoid therapy.

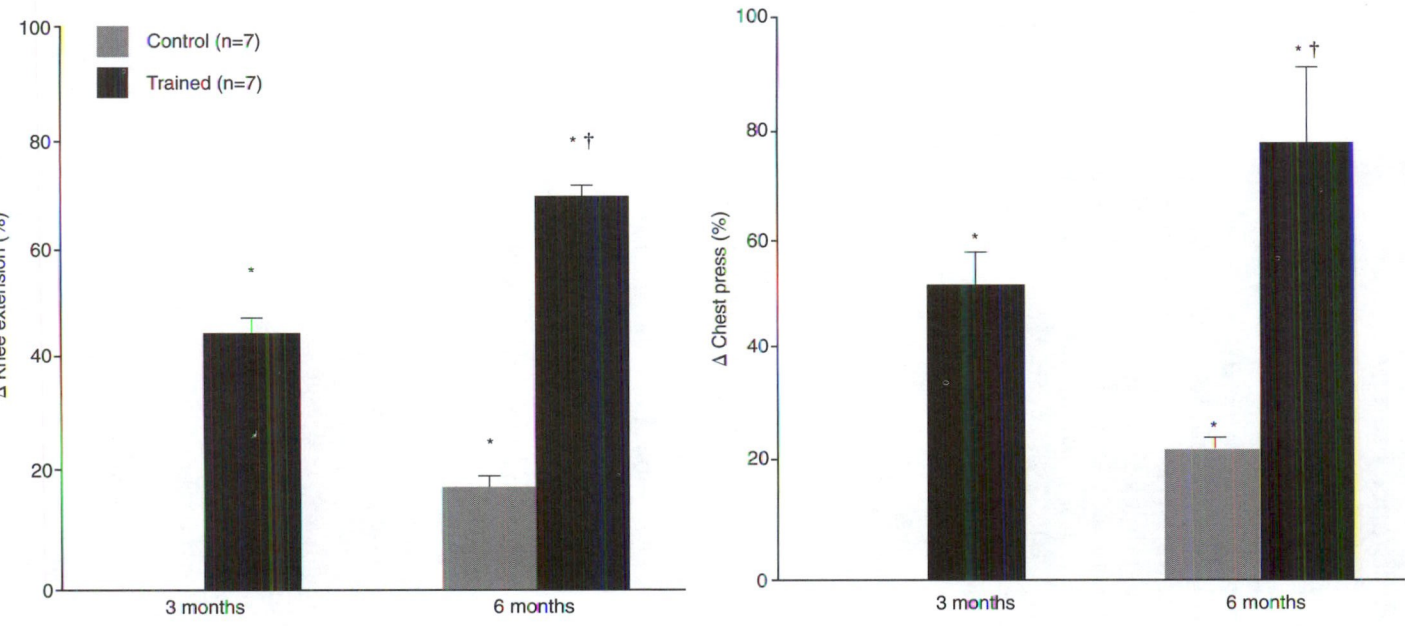

Figure 14.4 Changes in bilateral knee-extension strength and chest-press strength after 3 and 6 months of a resistance exercise program or control period. Data are mean ± SEM; control = did not train and were not tested at 3 months; * $p \leq 0.05$ versus posttransplantation baseline value; † $p \leq 0.05$ trained group versus control group.

Adapted from Braith et al. 1998 (5).

The Effects of Resistance Exercise
on Glucocorticoid-Induced Osteoporosis

Braith et al. conducted the first prospective controlled study to determine the efficacy of resistance exercise training as a therapy for defective bone metabolism in OTR (6). Sixteen ($N = 16$) consecutive male patients listed with the United Network for Organ Sharing (UNOS) as heart transplant candidates were recruited. The patients were randomly assigned either to a training group that would participate in a program of resistance exercise after transplantation ($n = 8$; 56 ± 6 years of age; 21 ± 13 weeks UNOS list) or to a control group that would not perform resistance exercise ($n = 8$; 52 ± 10 years of age; 26 ± 17 weeks UNOS list). Changes in bone mineral density (BMD) of the axial and appendicular skeleton were determined by dual-energy X-ray absorptiometry performed before transplantation, 2 months after transplantation, and after 3 and 6 months of a resistance training program or a control period. Resistance exercise training was initiated at 2 months after transplantation and consisted of two components: (1) lumbar-extensor exercise 1 day/week on a MedX Lumbar Extension Machine; and (2) upper- and lower-body resistance training 2 days/week using MedX variable-resistance machines. Subjects used the greatest resistance possible to complete a single set consisting of 10-15 repetitions for each exercise. The last repetition was considered volitional failure. The specific resistance exercises are outlined in table 14.2, and the results of the study are presented in figure 14.5. Significant bone loss occurred within only 2 months after heart transplantation and was characterized by a rapid early phase and a plateau phase after ~5 months. BMD losses from regions of the axial skeleton composed of trabecular bone, such as the lumbar vertebra and femur neck, were proportionately greater than BMD losses from regions of the appendicular skeleton composed of cortical bone. BMD losses in the lumbar vertebra were 12.2% and 14.9% in the control and training groups, respectively, at only 2 months after transplantation. The main finding of this study was that a 6-month program of variable-resistance exercise was osteogenic and restored BMD to pretransplantation levels in heart transplant recipients despite continued immunosuppression with glucocorticoids. In contrast, regional BMD in the control group did not show any statistically significant recovery toward preoperative levels by 8 months after transplantation.

Unpublished data by Braith et al. at the University of Florida have identified similar dramatic losses in bone mass in adult liver and lung transplant recipients early in the postoperative period. Resistance training studies involving both transplant groups are currently in progress. Nevertheless, this problem is not confined to adult OTR. Pediatric heart

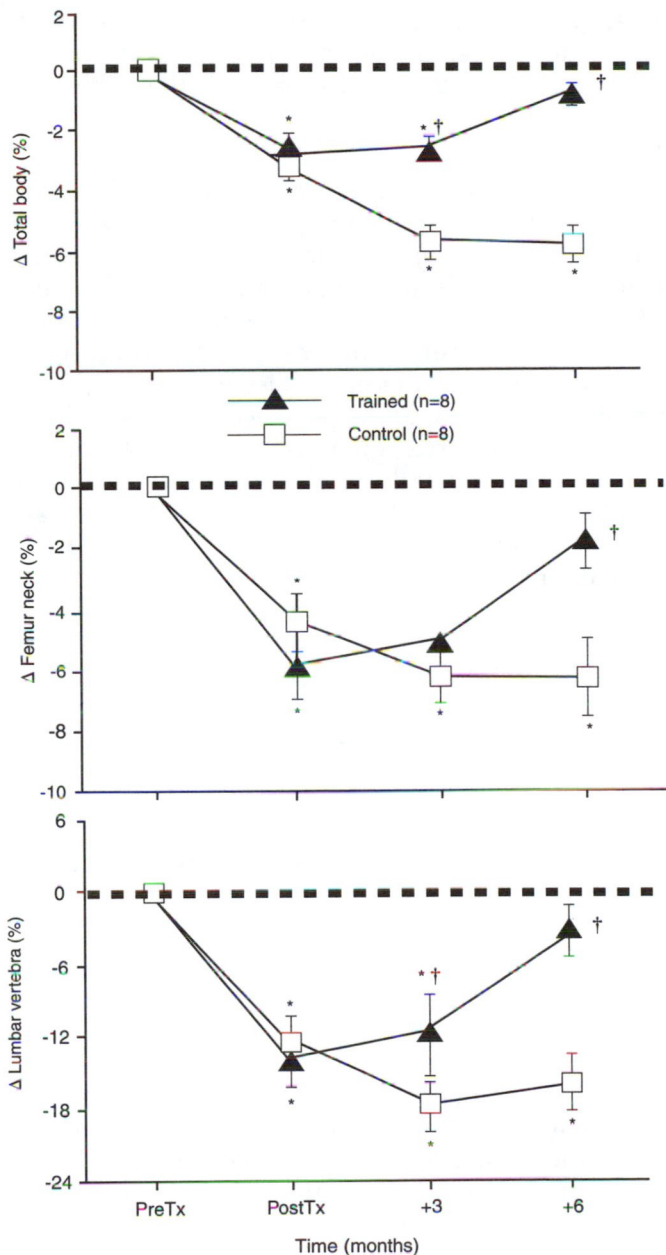

Figure 14.5 Changes in bone mineral density of the total body, femur neck, and lumbar vertebra at 2 months after heart transplantation (PostTx) and after 3 and 6 months of a resistance exercise program or a control period. Data are mean ± SEM; * $p \leq 0.05$ versus pretransplantation (PreTx) value; † $p \leq 0.05$ trained group versus control group.

Adapted from Braith et al. 1996 (6).

transplant recipients studied in our laboratory have regional BMD that is ~85% of age-matched control values (unpublished data). These young patients appear to be at extreme risk for osteoporotic morbidity later in life.

Summary

In the absence of a resistance training program, muscle mass continues to decline in OTR after transplantation. Short-term (7 weeks) resistance training programs have demonstrated the effectiveness of resistance training in restoring muscle mass to pretransplant levels, whereas long-term (6 months) resistance training programs have significantly increased muscle mass beyond pretransplant values. Muscle strength improves in OTR who do not receive resistance training as part of their postoperative therapy, even in the presence of continued muscle atrophy, but the magnitude of strength improvement is 4-6 times greater in OTR who participate in resistance training. In addition to the myogenic effects of resistance training in OTR, resistance training has also elicited significant osteogenic effects in this osteoporosis-prone population. The tangible benefits of resistance training in OTR include increased muscle and bone mass and improved function. The intangible benefits for skeletal muscle of incorporating resistance training into the postoperative rehabilitation program are substantiated by the enhanced quality of life that these benefits afford OTR.

Resistance Training Guidelines for Organ Transplant Recipients

Research clearly indicates that resistance training benefits organ transplant recipients. The following guidelines are recommended.

Exercise Prescription

When developing resistance training programs for OTR, rehabilitation staff must consider the diminished physical capacity of these patients. A relatively small resistance training stimulus is capable of eliciting significant myogenic and osteogenic responses in this population. Therefore, a low-volume program consisting of 1 set of 10-15 repetitions for each major muscle group of the body (8-10 exercises), 2-3 days per week is recommended. Conservative initial resistance and gradual progression is essential in this clinical population. The resistance training program for OTR should include the components shown in table 14.3.

Resistance training is only one facet of an effective exercise program in this clinical population. Low-volume resistance training programs (1 set/body part) afford patients both the time and energy to incorporate cardiopulmonary and stretching exercises into their exercise program. This becomes an important consideration, because time and energy

TABLE 14.3   Exercise Prescription for Organ Transplant Recipients

---

ORIENTATION

Day 1   Instruction on proper lifting and breathing techniques with little or no resistance. The instruction is designed to familiarize the patient with the exercise equipment.

Days 2-3   One set of 10-15 repetitions of each exercise using minimal resistance. This allows the patient to practice proper lifting and breathing techniques and gradually introduces the musculoskeletal system to the stress of resistance training.

STRENGTH TESTING

Day 4   One-repetition maximum (1-RM) tests used to determine initial training resistance.

INITIAL RESISTANCE

Following this orientation period, initial training weights should be set at 40-50% of 1-RM.

PROGRESSION

When the patient is capable of completing >15 repetitions prior to reaching volitional muscle fatigue, resistance should be increased by 5-10% at the subsequent training session.

---

constraints are often cited as primary factors limiting adherence and compliance to exercise rehabilitation programs.

Safety Precautions

Organ transplant recipients have unique health problems that must be considered when prescribing resistance exercises. Risk of organ rejection, advanced osteoporosis, and transient hypotension in heart transplant recipients are examples of such health problems.

Rejection

Exercise training should be discontinued during acute allograft rejection that requires enhanced glucocorticoid immunosuppression. The possibility of a coronary event is heightened during bolus administration of glucocorticoids, and the catabolic influence of the glucocorticoids on bone and skeletal muscle supersedes the beneficial effects of exercise.

Advanced Osteoporosis

Subjects with BMD deficits greater than 2 SDs (standard deviations) from the norm are at great risk for fractures, and resistance training may be contraindicated. If OTR with severe established osteoporosis participate in resistance exercise programs, they must be carefully managed with conservative initial resistances and very gradual progressions of resistance loads.

Exercise Intensity
It is difficult to use heart rate (% of heart rate reserve) in prescribing exercise intensity in some OTR. For example, heart transplant patients have abnormal heart rate responsiveness to exercise due to autonomic sympathetic denervation. Lung transplant recipients are often limited by dyspnea, but their heart rate at the dyspnea threshold may not be reproducible. Therefore, a general guideline adopted by many programs responsible for exercise rehabilitation of OTR is to restrict exercise intensity to a level that elicits a heart rate ~20 beats greater than resting values.

Hypotension
Most OTR are mildly hypertensive due to side effects of immunosuppressive drugs and/or organ denervation. Heart transplant recipients, however, present a unique challenge during resistance training. Problems typically encountered with coronary patients in cardiac rehabilitation programs are associated with cardiac work and myocardial ischemia. In contrast, heart transplant recipients are not limited by coronary underperfusion, provided they are free from acute rejection or allograft vascular disease. Rather, the rehabilitation staff must take special precautions to ensure adequate maintenance of systemic blood pressure. We found that approximately 25% of heart transplant recipients experience transient hypotension during resistance exercise, and this problem was exaggerated when the exercise required lifting above the level of the heart (e.g., shoulder press). This hemodynamic problem is likely a consequence of autonomic sympathetic denervation. The denervated transplanted heart is almost entirely dependent on preload and the Frank-Starling mechanism for increasing cardiac output and systemic blood pressure.

We used the following maneuvers to help sustain venous return and prevent blood pooling in patients who experienced hypotension:

- Upper-body exercises were alternated with lower-body exercises in an attempt to prevent blood pooling.
- Symptomatic subjects walked 2 min between exercises or performed standing calf raises.
- All subjects concluded each training session with a 5 min cool-down walk at low intensity on the treadmill.

Conclusion

Achieving good outcomes after organ transplantation requires a carefully planned physical rehabilitation program based on a clear understanding of the exercise physiology of OTR. Patients can be taught proper lifting and breathing techniques that may partially compensate for the attenuated heart rate response and reduced pulmonary capacity. The limited experience with resistance training in OTR indicates that this intervention is safe and not associated with any increase in rejection. Most importantly, recent reports indicate that resistance exercise therapy, as part of a treatment strategy to prevent steroid-induced bone loss and skeletal muscle myopathy, is both osteogenic and myogenic if initiated early after heart transplantation.

The seriousness of steroid-induced health problems in OTR is highlighted by the fact that many transplant institutions currently exclude patients with established osteoporosis from organ transplantation, thereby denying some patients this life-extending alternative. These difficult decisions are based on the well-documented ineffectiveness of standard pharmacological therapies to reverse steroid-induced osteoporosis. Therapeutic alternatives, such as resistance training, are urgently needed to effectively prevent radical bone loss early in the postoperative period and stimulate new bone growth late after transplantation while improving muscle mass and strength in OTR.

References

1. Bergstrom, J. 1962. Muscle electrolytes in man determined by neutron activation analysis on needle biopsy specimen: A study in normal subjects, kidney patients, and patients with chronic diarrhoea. *Scandanavian Journal of Laboratory Investigations* 14 (suppl. 68): 1-110.
2. Biring, M., M. Fournier, D. Ross, and M. Lewis. 1998. Cellular adaptations of skeletal muscle to cyclosporine. *Journal of Applied Physiology* 84: 1967-1975.
3. Bloomfield, S.A. 1997. Changes in musculoskeletal structure and function with prolonged bed rest. *Medicine and Science in Sports and Exercise* 29: 197-206.
4. Braith, R.W., M.C. Limacher, S.H. Leggett, and M.L. Pollock. 1993. Skeletal muscle strength in heart transplant recipients. *Journal of Heart and Lung Transplant* 12: 1018-1023.
5. Braith, R., M. Welch, R. Mills, J. Keller, and M. Pollock. 1998. Resistance training prevents glucocorticoid-induced myopathy in heart transplant recipients. *Medicine and Science in Sports and Exercise* 30 (4): 483-489.
6. Braith, R., R. Mills, M. Welch, J. Keller, and M. Pollock. 1996. Resistance exercise training restores bone mineral density in heart transplant recipients. *Journal of American College of Cardiology* 28: 1471-1477.
7. Bussieres, L.M., P.W. Pflughelder, A.H. Menkes, R.J. Novick, F.N. McKenzie, A.W. Taylor, and W.J. Kostuk. 1995. Basis for aerobic impairment in patients after heart transplantation. *Journal of Heart and Lung Transplant* 14: 1073-1080.
8. Bussieres, L.M., P.W. Pflugfelder, A.W. Taylor, E.G. Noble, and W.J. Kostuk. 1997. Changes in skeletal muscle morphology and biochemistry after cardiac transplantation. *American Journal of Cardiology* 79: 630-634.
9. Campellone, J.V., D. Lacomis, D.J. Kramer, A.C. Van Cott, and M.J. Giuliani. 1998. Acute myopathy after liver transplantation. *Neurology* 50 (1): 46-53.
10. Clark, A.L., P.A. Poole-Wilson, and A.J. Coats. 1996. Exercise limitation in chronic heart failure: Central role of the periphery. *Journal of the American College of Cardiology* 28: 1092-1102.

11. Drexler, H., U. Reide, T. Munzel, H. Konig, E. Funke, and H. Just. 1992. Alterations of skeletal muscle in chronic heart failure. *Circulation* 85: 1751-1759.

12. Horber, F.F., J.P. Casez, U. Steiger, A. Czerniak, A. Montandon, and P. Jaeger. 1994. Changes in bone mass early after kidney transplantation. *Journal of Bone and Mineral Research* 9: 1-9.

13. Horber F.F., J.R. Scheidegger, B.E. Grunig, and F.J. Frey. 1985. Thigh muscle mass and function in patients treated with glucocorticoids. *European Journal of Clinical Investigation* 15: 302-307.

14. Horber F.F., J.R. Scheidegger, B.E. Grunig, and F.J. Frey. 1985. Evidence that prednisone induced myopathy is reversed by physical training. *Journal of Clinical Endocrinology and Metabolism* 61 (1): 83-88.

15. Horber, F.F., H. Hoopeler, J.R. Scheidegger, D. Herren, H. Claassen, H. Howald, C. Gerber, and F.J. Frey. 1986. Altered skeletal muscle ultrastructure in renal transplant patients on prednisone. *Kidney International* 30: 411-416.

16. Horber, F.F., H. Hoopeler, J.R. Scheidegger, B.E. Grunig, H. Howald, and F.J. Frey. 1987. Impact of physical training on the ultrastructure of midthigh muscle in normal subjects and in patients treated with glucocorticoids. *Journal of Clinical Investigation* 71: 1181-1190.

17. Jobin, J., F. Maltais, J.F. Doyon, P. Leblanc, P.M. Simard, A.A. Simard, and C. Simard. 1998. Chronic obstructive pulmonary disease: Capillarity and fiber-type characteristics of skeletal muscle. *Journal of Cardiopulmonary Rehabilitation* 18: 432-436.

18. Julian, B.A., D.A. Laskow, J. Dubovsky, E.V. Dubovsky, J.J. Curtis, and L.D. Quarles. 1991. Rapid loss of vertebral bone density after renal transplantation. *New England Journal of Medicine* 325: 544-550.

19. Kavanagh, T., M. Yacoub, D. Mertens, J. Kennedy, R. Campbell, and P. Sawyer. 1988. Cardiorespiratory responses to exercise training after orthotopic cardiac transplantation. *Circulation* 77: 162-171.

20. Killian, K.J., P. Leblanc, D.H. Martin, E. Summers, N.L. Jones, and E.J.M. Campbell. 1992. Exercise capacity and ventilatory, circulatory, and symptom limitation in patients with airflow limitation. *American Review of Respiratory Disease* 146: 935-940.

21. Kluess, H.A., M.A. Welsch, A.M. Properzio, et al. 1996. Accelerated skeletal muscle metabolic recovery following exercise training in heart failure. *Circulation* 94: I-192.

22. Kobashigawa, J., D. Leaf, N. Lee, M. Gleeson, H. Liu, M. Hamilton, J. Moriguchi, N. Kawata, K. Einhorn, E. Herlihy, and H. Laks. 1999. A controlled trial of exercise rehabilitation after heart transplantation. *New England Journal of Medicine* 340 (4): 272-277.

23. Lampert, E., S. Oyono-Enguéllé, B. Mettauer, H. Freund, and J. Lonsdorfer. 1996. Short endurance training improves lactate removal in patients with heart transplants. *Medicine and Science in Sports and Exercise* 28: 801-807.

24. Lukert, B. 1996. Glucocorticoid-induced osteoporosis. In *Osteoporosis*, edited by R. Marcus, D. Feldman, and J. Kelsey. San Diego: Academic Press, 801-831.

25. Mancini, D., G. Walter, N. Reichek, R. Lenkinski, K. McCully, J. Mullen, and J. Wilson. 1992. Contribution of skeletal muscle atrophy to exercise intolerance and altered metabolism in heart failure. *Circulation* 85: 1364-1373.

26. Matesanz, R., and B. Miranda. 1996. International figures on organ donation and transplantation activities 1989-1995. *Transplant Newsletter* 1: 1-2.

27. Meys, E., E. Fontanges, N. Fourcade, A. Thomasson, M. Pouyet, and P.D. Delmas. 1994. Bone loss after orthotopic liver transplantation. *American Journal of Medicine* 97: 445-450.

28. Muchmore, J.S., D.K. Cooper, Y. Ye, V.T. Schiegel, and N. Zuhdi. 1991. Loss of vertebral bone density in heart transplant patients. *Transplantation Proceedings* 23: 1184-1185.

29. Muchmore, J.S., D.K. Cooper, Y. Ye, V.T. Schiegel, and N. Zuhdi. 1992. Prevention of loss of vertebral bone density in heart transplant recipients. *Journal of Heart and Lung Transplantation* 11: 959-964.

30. Okita, K., K. Yonezawa, H. Nishijima, A. Hanada, M. Ohtsubo, T. Kohya, T. Murakami, and A. Kitabatake. 1998. Skeletal muscle metabolism limits exercise capacity in patients with chronic heart failure. *Circulation* 98: 1886-1891.

31. Porayko, M.K., R.H. Wiesner, J.E. Hay, R.A. Krom, E.R. Dickson, S. Beaver, and L. Schwerman. 1991. Bone disease in liver transplant recipients: Incidence, timing, and risk factors. *Transplantation Proceedings* 23:1462-1465.

32. Ralston, M., A. Merola, and C. Leier. 1991. Depressed aerobic enzyme activity of skeletal muscle in severe chronic heart failure. *Journal of Laboratory and Clinical Medicine* 117: 370-372.

33. Rich, G.M., G.H. Mudge, G.L. Laffel, and M.S. LeBoff. 1992. Cyclosporine A and prednisone associated osteoporosis in heart transplant recipients. *Journal of Heart and Lung Transplantation* 11: 950-958.

34. Rivas, M., T.S. Kim, R.S. Sharon, J.P. Bilezikian, and E. Shane. 1992. Bone loss and fractures occur within 6 months of heart transplantation [abstract]. *Journal of Bone Mineral Research* 7: 358a.

35. Saltin, B., B. Blomqvist, J.H. Mitchell, R.L. Johnson, K. Wildenthal, and C.B. Chapman. 1968. Response to submaximal and maximal exercise after bed rest and training. *Circulation* 38 (5 suppl.): VII 1-78.

36. Saxenhofer, H., J. Scheidegger, C. Descoeudres, P. Jaeger, and F.F. Horber. 1992. Impact of dialysis modality on body composition in patients with end-stage renal disease. *Clinical Nephrology* 38 (4): 219-223.

37. Schaufelberger, M., B. Erikson, G. Grimby, P. Held, and K. Swedberg. 1997. Skeletal muscle alterations in patients with chronic heart failure. *European Heart Journal* 18: 971-980.

38. Serres, I., M. Hayot, C. Prefaut, and J. Mercier. 1998. Skeletal muscle abnormalities in patients with COPD: Contribution to exercise intolerance. *Medicine and Science in Sports and Exercise* 30: 1019-1027.

39. Shane, E., S.J. Silverberg, D. Donovan, A. Papadopoulos, B.B. Staron, V. Addesso, B. Jorgesen, C. McGregor, and L. Schulman. 1996. Osteoporosis in lung transplantation candidates with end-stage pulmonary disease. *American Journal of Medicine* 101: 262-269.

40. Stratton, J., G. Kemp, R. Daily, M. Yacoub, and B. Rajagopalan. 1994. Effects of cardiac transplantation on bioenergetic abnormalities of skeletal muscle in congestive heart failure. *Circulation* 89: 1624-1631.

41. Sullivan, M.J., H. Green, and F. Cobb. 1991. Altered skeletal muscle metabolic response to exercise in chronic heart failure. *Circulation* 84: 1597-1607.

42. Sullivan, M.J., H. Green, and F. Cobb. 1990. Skeletal muscle biochemistry and histology in ambulatory patients with long-term heart failure. *Circulation* 81 (2): 518-527.

43. United Network of Organ Sharing (UNOS). 1999. Scientific Registry Data.

44. Van Cleemput, J., W. Daenen, P. Geusens, J. Dequeker, F. Van De Werf, and J. Vanhaecke. 1996. Prevention of bone loss in cardiac transplant recipients. *Transplantation* 61: 1495-1499.

45. Vescovo, G., F. Serafini, L. Dalla Libera, et al. 1998. Skeletal muscle myosin heavy chain composition in CHF: Correlation between the magnitude of the isoenzymatic shift, exercise capacity, and gas exchange measurements. *American Heart Journal* 135: 130-137.

15
CHAPTER

Resistance Training and Chronic Obstructive Pulmonary Disease

Michael J. Berry, PhD
Wake Forest University

Definition

Chronic obstructive pulmonary disease (COPD) is defined by the American Thoracic Society as a disease characterized by airflow obstruction due to either chronic bronchitis or emphysema (4, 5). Other characteristics of COPD include that the airway obstruction is progressive, there may be airway hyperactivity, and the airflow obstruction may be partially reversible. Chronic bronchitis is a clinical diagnosis for patients with chronic cough and sputum production. It is formally defined as the presence of a productive cough most days during three consecutive months in each of two successive years (5, 71). Emphysema is a pathological diagnosis defined by abnormal permanent enlargement of the air spaces distal to the terminal bronchioles. It is accompanied by destruction of the airspace walls without obvious fibrosis (71, 72, 78). Both chronic bronchitis and emphysema patients exhibit exacerbations, or periods of worsening symptoms, with their disease. The World Health Organization's International Classification of Disease (ICD) codes used by nosologists to classify COPD are 490, 491, 492, 494, 495, and 496.

Asthma (ICD code 493) has at times been subsumed under the rubric of COPD. It is characterized by inflammation and hyperresponsiveness of the tracheobronchial tree to a variety of stimuli (4). Additionally, asthma is characterized by episodes of reversible airway narrowing. Asthma patients experience exacerbations or attacks interspersed with symptom-free periods. In contrast, most patients with chronic bronchitis do not exhibit significant reversibility of their airway narrowing and have residual symptoms between exacerbations. While patients with COPD and asthma have similar clinical characteristics, the pathology of the two syndromes differs considerably, suggesting that they are different diseases (45). There is accumulating evidence to suggest that COPD is a multi-organ system disease, with muscle dysfunction being a contributor to the exercise intolerance seen in COPD patients (6). Because of the differences between COPD and asthma, they should be considered separately with respect to exercise prescription. Therefore, this chapter will focus on resistance training with COPD patients and not asthma patients.

Epidemiology

COPD is a major cause of morbidity and mortality and the fourth leading cause of death in the United States (5). It was estimated that in 1995 15.7 million Americans were diagnosed with COPD (53). Of all decedents from 1979 to 1993, 8.2% had a diagnosis of obstructive lung disease on their death certificates (48). In 1991, there were 85,544 deaths due to COPD, with an age-adjusted death rate of 18.6 per 100,000 persons (5). In 1996, there were 106,027 deaths due to COPD, and the age-adjusted death rate was 21 deaths per 100,000 (58). Whereas the death rate from other chronic diseases is decreasing, death rates from COPD are increasing (53).

In addition to being a major cause of mortality in the United States, COPD is a major health care cost and cause of morbidity and disability. In 1995, there were 553,000 hospitalizations where COPD was given as the diagnosis at the time of discharge. The average length of stay was 6.3 days, and the mean cost of each of these hospitalizations was $10,684 (1, 53). In 1995, there were 16,087,000 physician office visits that were attributable to COPD. Between 1990 and 1992, 800,000 Americans reported that emphysema resulted in activity limitation (53). In addition to emphysema limiting patient activity, COPD patients have lower levels of physical activity than age-matched controls, as reported by Serres et al. (65).

Pathophysiology

A number of anatomical, physiological, and pathological changes occur with COPD that can result in debilitation for the COPD patient. The primary cause of COPD is cigarette smoking. Because of the direct insult cigarette smoke has on the lungs, it has long been thought that the lungs were the primary organs affected by COPD. However, recent research suggests that the disease process itself or certain aspects of the disease process may also affect skeletal muscle.

Cigarette smoking affects the large airways (bronchi), the small airways (bronchioles), and the pulmonary parenchyma. The pathophysiological sequelae are a result of the effects of cigarette smoke on each of these structures and the degree of airway reactivity of each individual patient. Within the large airways, cigarette smoke causes enlargement of the bronchial mucus glands and dilation of the gland ducts. These factors result in excessive cough and sputum production, which are the characteristic symptoms of chronic bronchitis (77). The alterations that occur in the large airways have little effect on airflow or spirometry. It is not until there are additional changes to the small airways and the lung parenchyma that airflow obstruction occurs. Within the smaller airways, cigarette smoke causes mucus plugging, inflammation, and an increase in the smooth muscle. These all contribute to a decrease in the cross-sectional area of the airways that can have a profound effect on airflow and the COPD patients' spirometry (77). The expiratory flow rates—including the forced expiratory volume in one second ($FEV_{1.0}$), the $FEV_{1.0}$/forced vital capacity (FVC) ratio, and the midexpiratory flow rates—are all reduced.

Emphysema results in destructive changes to the alveolar walls. The net effect of these changes is twofold. First, loss of the alveolar walls results in a loss of the tethering effect the alveoli have on the smaller airways. That is, the alveoli help to support and keep the smaller airways open. Without this alveolar support, the smaller airways are more likely to collapse during expiration, adding further to airway obstruction. Secondly, destruction of the alveolar walls reduces the elastic recoil of the lungs. The reduced elastic recoil of the lungs decreases the force that drives air out of the lungs. The combination of these two effects results in a further reduction in airflow and an increase in the amount of work the respiratory muscles must do to meet the ventilatory demands of the body.

The combined effect of the airway obstruction and the reduced expiratory driving force results in a prolonged expiratory time. If expiratory time is insufficient, then the normal end-expiratory lung volume is not reached. The net result is an increase in the functional residual capacity and a hyperinflation of the lungs that will result in the diaphragm assuming a shorter, more flattened position. The diaphragm is a skeletal muscle and, as such, operates according to the length-tension relationship (50). This relationship describes the property whereby the tension developed by skeletal muscle is a function of its resting length. As a muscle is shortened or lengthened beyond its optimal length, the tension developed will decrease (29). Because of these geometric changes in the diaphragm with hyperinflation and the length-tension relationship in skeletal muscle, the shorter, flattened diaphragm has less force-generating potential (17, 59, 69). There is some evidence to suggest that the diaphragm may adapt to these chronic changes by shortening the optimal length of its fibers whereby each fiber generates its maximal tension at its new length (25, 67). Despite these adaptive changes, there is still evidence of a decreased diaphragmatic pressure-generating capacity in COPD patients.

During moderate exercise by normal healthy individuals, there is a reduction in end-expiratory lung volume of approximately 200-400 ml (34, 66). In contrast, patients with COPD demonstrate an increased end-expiratory lung volume during exercise, causing dynamic hyper-inflation of the lungs (73). This results in further diaphragm weakness that may contribute to dyspnea and a reduced exercise tolerance. It has been hypothesized that because the diaphragm is a skeletal muscle, positive adaptations may result from resistance training of this muscle (41).

In addition to the effect of COPD on the lungs, there is accumulating evidence that COPD patients have skeletal muscle dysfunction, and this may contribute to their exercise intolerance. Decreases in peripheral muscle strength have been reported in COPD patients (10, 19, 30, 32). When compared with age-matched normal subjects, COPD patients have a 20-30% reduction in quadriceps strength (19, 30, 32). These decreases in strength have been shown to be accompanied by a reduction in muscle cross-sectional area (10). Other studies have also reported decreases in muscle mass in patients with COPD (22, 64, 85). Presently, it is unclear which fiber type is most affected by the disease. An analysis of muscle biopsies from patients with moderate disease showed no changes in the proportions of fiber types; however, there was significant atrophy of type II fibers that was correlated with weight loss (36). In contrast, other studies with patients with advanced COPD have reported a reduction in the proportion of type I fibers when compared with control subjects (37, 83). This finding is consistent with the report of reduced oxidative enzyme activities in these patients (47). Additionally, this reduction in type I fibers has been shown to be accompanied by a corresponding increase in type IIb fibers (83). Both chronic hypoxemia (35) and chronic inactivity (83) have been suggested as contributors to the changes in fiber types, while steroid use has been suggested as a mediator of the muscle weakness (18, 19). Other possible contributors to the skeletal muscle abnormalities seen in COPD patients include chronic hypercapnia, inflammation, nutritional depletion, and comorbid conditions that may also affect skeletal muscle function (6).

Functional Impact of Respiratory and Peripheral Skeletal Muscle Dysfunction on Exercise Tolerance

Two common complaints of COPD patients are dyspnea, or shortness of breath, and a reduced exercise capacity. While the origin of the sensation of breathlessness is multifactorial, it is thought that respiratory muscle weakness may contribute to dyspnea (38, 46) and the associated reduced exercise tolerance (84). Additionally, it has been suggested that improving ventilatory muscle strength and endurance may help reduce dyspnea (54, 56) and increase exercise capacity (40).

In addition to the diaphragm muscle, accessory muscles aid in inspiration during certain conditions, such as increased ventilation during exercise. These accessory muscles of inspiration include the scalene, sternocleidomastoid (21), and the serratus anterior (61). In COPD patients, unsupported arm exercise results in greater levels of dyspnea as compared with lower-extremity exercise at reduced workloads (14). It was hypothesized that the arm exercise decreased participation of the accessory muscles in ventilation and thereby increased the work of the diaphragm. This may help explain why patients with COPD complain of dyspnea when performing activities of daily living with their upper extremities (74). Strategies aimed at improving the function of these accessory muscles of inspiration, such as resistance training, should prove beneficial to COPD patients.

Skeletal muscle dysfunction may contribute to the reduced exercise capacity found in COPD patients (39). Muscle strength has been reported to be a significant contributor to symptom intensity and work capacity in COPD patients (32). Additionally, quadriceps muscle strength has been shown to be positively correlated with 6 min walk distance and maximal oxygen consumption in these patients (30, 32). Based on the preceding observations, it appears that resistance training may be beneficial in the rehabilitation of patients with COPD.

Ventilatory Muscle Training

Ventilatory muscle training in COPD patients has been used to increase ventilatory muscle strength and endurance, with the goal of augmenting exercise capacity, relieving symptoms of dyspnea, and improving the health-related quality of life. Three strategies have been used to train the ventilatory muscles, including

1. voluntary isocapnic hyperpnea,
2. inspiratory resistive loading, and
3. inspiratory threshold loading.

With voluntary isocapnic hyperpnea, the patient breathes at as high a level of minute ventilation as possible for 10-15 min periods. Because the subject is hyperventilating, a rebreathing circuit must be used to maintain isocapnia. This rebreathing circuit is complex, is not portable, and requires monitoring. As a result of these problems, this type of training has not been used or studied extensively. With inspiratory resistive loading, the patient breathes through inspiratory orifices of smaller and smaller diameter while attempting to maintain a normal breathing pattern. A potential problem with this device is that the patient may slow his/her breathing frequency in an attempt to reduce the sensation of effort. This change in breathing pattern reduces the load on the inspiratory muscles such that a training response may not occur. With inspiratory threshold loading, the patient breathes through a device that permits airflow through it only when a certain inspiratory pressure has been achieved. Inspiratory threshold loading devices are small, do not require supervision, and avoid the problems associated with changing breathing patterns. Because of the challenges associated with voluntary isocapnic hyperpnea ventilatory muscle training, studies that have utilized this type of training will not be reviewed, nor will recommendations be given regarding this type of training.

Results from studies examining the efficacy of ventilatory muscle training in COPD patients are equivocal. Randomized controlled clinical trials examining the effects of inspiratory resistive loading and inspiratory threshold loading are shown in table 15.1. Of the 18 studies listed, 9 found increases in inspiratory muscle strength, and 10 reported increases in inspiratory muscle endurance. While most of the studies that found increases in inspiratory muscle strength and endurance also showed increases in exercise performance, these results have not been conclusively demonstrated. Goldstein et al. (28) and Chen et al. (15) compared the effects of inspiratory muscle training coupled with general exercise conditioning with those from general exercise conditioning alone. Both studies found inspiratory muscle training to improve inspiratory muscle strength and/or endurance. However, when the exercise capacity of those that combined inspiratory muscle training and general exercise conditioning was compared with the capacity of those that did only general exercise conditioning, no differences were found. These results suggest that inspiratory muscle training does not add significantly to a program of general exercise conditioning in patients with COPD.

TABLE 15.1 Results of Randomized Clinical Trials Examining the Efficacy of Ventilatory Muscle Training

Reference	Type training	Outcomes (as compared to a control group)
Belman & Shadmehr (8)	Resistive loading	Improved inspiratory muscle strength and endurance
Berry et al. (12)	Threshold loading coupled with general exercise conditioning	No change in inspiratory muscle strength No change in 12 min walk distance No change in dyspnea ratings
Bjerre-Jepsen et al. (13)	Resistive loading	No change in inspiratory muscle endurance No change in exercise tolerance
Chen et al. (15)	Resistive loading coupled with standard pulmonary rehabilitation	Improved inspiratory muscle endurance Improved inspiratory muscle strength No change in maximal or constant load cycle exercise
Dekhuijzen et al. (20)	Resistive loading coupled with standard pulmonary rehabilitation	Improved inspiratory muscle strength No improvement in maximal work capacity Increased 12 min walk distance
Falk et al. (24)	Resistive loading	Decreased dyspnea Improved submaximal exercise time
Goldstein et al. (28)	Threshold loading coupled with standard pulmonary rehabilitation	Improved inspiratory muscle endurance No change in inspiratory muscle strength No change in exercise tolerance
Guyatt et al. (31)	Resistive loading	No improvement in inspiratory muscle strength or endurance No improvement in 6 min walk distance No improvement in health-related quality of life
Harver et al. (33)	Resistive loading	Improved inspiratory muscle strength Decreased dyspnea

(continued)

TABLE 15.1 *(continued)*

Reference	Type training	Outcomes (as compared to a control group)
Larson et al. (40)	Threshold loading	Improved inspiratory muscle strength Improved inspiratory muscle endurance Improved 12 min walk distance No improvement in health-related quality of life
Lisboa et al. (42)	Threshold loading	Improved inspiratory muscle strength and endurance Decreased dyspnea Increased 6 min walk distance
Lisboa et al. (43)	Threshold loading	Decreased dyspnea Improved 6 min walk distance
McKeon et al. (52)	Resistive loading	No change in inspiratory muscle strength Increased inspiratory muscle endurance No increase in maximal cycle exercise, 12 min walk distance, or treadmill walking
Noseda et al. (55)	Resistive loading	Increased inspiratory muscle endurance No change in maximal or constant load cycle exercise
Pardy et al. (57)	Resistive loading	Improved 12 min walk distance Improved submaximal exercise endurance
Preusser et al. (60)	Threshold loading	Improved inspiratory muscle strength and endurance Improved 12 min walk distance
Wanke et al. (81)	Threshold loading coupled with general exercise conditioning	Improved inspiratory muscle strength and endurance Improved maximal exercise capacity
Weiner et al. (82)	Threshold loading coupled with general exercise conditioning	Improved inspiratory muscle strength and endurance Improved 12 min walk distance Improved submaximal exercise time

From the results of a meta-analysis on inspiratory muscle training, Smith et al. reported a moderate treatment effect for increased exercise capacity in those studies that showed improvements in inspiratory strength or endurance (70). The findings of Smith et al. emphasize the importance of the training stimulus. When Smith et al. examined the overall effects of inspiratory muscle training on inspiratory muscle strength and endurance, they found the effect to be small and specific to the training regimen. Overall, they found little evidence of important effects from inspiratory muscle training on clinically important outcomes such as functional exercise capacity and quality of life. Despite these primary findings, results from a secondary analysis suggest that the breathing pattern adopted by COPD patients undergoing inspiratory muscle training may effect outcomes. More specifically, Smith et al. concluded that increases in inspiratory muscle strength and endurance might result in clinically important improvements in functional status when the breathing pattern is controlled, a finding first suggested by Belman et al. (9).

Recently, the American College of Chest Physicians (ACCP) and the American Association of Cardiovascular and Pulmonary Rehabilitation (AACVPR) released evidence-based guidelines for pulmonary rehabilitation (2). In this document, recommendations for pulmonary rehabilitation were made, and the scientific evidence supporting the recommendation was reviewed. Inspiratory muscle training received a grade of B, suggesting that the scientific evidence from both observational and controlled clinical trials provided inconsistent results. Because of this grade, the recommendation was that inspiratory muscle training not be considered an essential component of pulmonary rehabilitation. However, it may still be used in patients who have decreased respiratory muscle strength and breathlessness, and who remain symptomatic despite optimal therapy.

Specific recommendations for inspiratory muscle training with respect to the intensity, frequency, or duration of training have not been developed. Most studies that have reported improvements in inspiratory muscle function have had patients perform inspiratory muscle training at a minimum of 30% of their maximal inspiratory pressure. The duration of this training is for 15 min, and the frequency is at least 3 times per week. These appear to be the minimal requisites of an exercise prescription if inspiratory muscle function is to be improved.

Recently, researchers have begun to investigate the various responses to using different training devices and techniques. Belman et al. have now shown that there are qualitative differences in ventilatory muscle loading when using different devices and breathing strategies (7). Tzelepis et al. have demonstrated, in normal healthy subjects, that the greatest increases in inspiratory muscle strength occur when training at low lung volumes (80). Additionally, Tzelepis and colleagues have shown that high inspiratory pressure training will increase inspiratory muscle strength, whereas high inspiratory flow training will increase flow performance (79). These results suggest that the concept of specificity of training that applies to peripheral skeletal muscle also applies to respiratory skeletal muscle. Despite these recent advances, the optimal stimulus for training the ventilatory muscles has not been clearly defined. Future studies are needed that will not only provide a comprehensive evaluation of important outcomes but also identify the load placed on the respiratory muscles.

Upper-Extremity Resistance Training

The use of upper-extremity resistance training has been advocated as a training modality to help reduce dyspnea in COPD patients. It has been suggested that COPD patients who perform upper-extremity exercise may experience ventilatory muscle fatigue because of the added work that the accessory muscles of inspiration must perform in supporting the arms (14). Only three studies have specifically examined the efficacy of upper-extremity resistance training in COPD patients. A summary of these studies is shown in table 15.2. In addition, there are studies that have examined the use of arm ergometer exercise, but these are outside of the scope of this chapter and will not be reviewed here. For those interested, the AACVPR has recently published a review of these studies (2).

The results from the studies investigating the efficacy of upper-extremity resistance training show that this type of training will bring about improvements in tasks that are specific to the training modality. This finding should not be surprising since previous research with normal healthy subjects has shown that training is specific to the task and the muscles trained (27, 44, 63). Additionally, several of the studies showed that training resulted in lower levels of oxygen consumption when subjects performed arm exercise following the training (16, 49). These lower levels of oxygen consumption would be expected to result in lower dyspnea levels when subjects are performing activities with the upper extremities. However, this has not been substantiated.

Ries and colleagues compared the effects of two upper-extremity resistance training programs (62). Following training, patients improved their performance on tests specific to the training performed. There were no changes in simulated activities of daily living tests following training. The investigators did, however, report that many of the patients in their study had subjective improvements in their ability to perform activities of daily living with their arms.

From these studies, it appears that patients with COPD can tolerate and benefit from a training program consisting of upper-extremity resistance exercise. While it has not been conclusively demonstrated

TABLE 15.2 Results of Trials Examining the Efficacy of Upper-Extremity Resistance Training

Reference	Type training	Outcomes
Couser et al. (16)	Arm ergometry at 60% of maximal workload. Unsupported arm exercise that consisted of bilateral shoulder abduction and extension for 2 min. Weight was added as tolerated. Both groups performed leg cycle ergometry at 60% of maximal workload.	Following training, minute ventilation and oxygen consumption were lower during arm elevation. Respiratory muscle strength did not change following training. No differences were reported between the two groups.
Martinez et al. (49)	Arm ergometry at a workload that engendered an RPE of 12-14 and an RPD of 3. Unsupported arm exercise that consisted of 5 shoulder and upper-arm exercises for up to 3½ min. Weight was added as tolerated. Both groups performed leg cycle ergometry at a workload that engendered an RPE of 12-14 and an RPD of 3 and inspiratory muscle training.	No difference in improvements in 12 min walk, cycle ergometer test, or respiratory muscle function. Task-specific unsupported arm exercise tests improved in the group that performed unsupported arm exercise. Decreased oxygen consumption in unsupported arm exercise tests in the group that performed unsupported arm exercise.
Ries et al. (62)	Gravity resistance exercises that included 5 low-resistance, high-repetition exercises to improve arm and shoulder endurance. Proprioceptive neuromuscular facilitation that included lower-frequency progressive resistance training with weights to improve arm and shoulder strength and endurance. Both groups participated in standard pulmonary rehabilitation that included walking.	Compared to a control group, both training groups improved on training test specific to the exercise modality. Patients reported subjective improvement in ability to perform activities of daily living using the upper extremities. No change in performance of cycle ergometry tests, simulated activities of daily living tests, or ventilatory muscle endurance tests.

RPE = rating of perceived exertion; RPD = rating of perceived dyspnea that this strategy will improve activities of daily living or physical function, preliminary results provide support for recommending that upper-extremity resistance training be included as part of a comprehensive rehabilitation program (2). These preliminary studies do not provide clear recommendations on the specific exercises that would benefit this population or on the resistance or number of repetitions that will provide the optimal benefits for these patients. Based on hypothetical considerations, the exercises should be ones that involve the accessory muscles of inspiration and include shoulder elevation. With respect to the amount of resistance used and number of sets and repetitions to be completed, the American College of Sports Medicine guidelines for "The Recommended Quantity and Quality of Exercise for Developing and Maintaining Cardiorespiratory and Muscular Fitness, and Flexibility in Healthy Adults" (3) and the recommendations of Evans (23) should be followed. A brief synopsis of these recommendations is presented in table 15.3.

Whole-Body Resistance Training

Whole-body resistance training has been advocated as a means of ameliorating the sequelae associated with the skeletal muscle dysfunction seen in COPD patients. Resistance training in normal healthy

TABLE 15.3 General Recommendations for Skeletal Muscle Resistance Training in Older Adults

Exercise prescription component	Recommendation
Intensity or repetitions	The intensity should be such that fatigue results after 8-15 repetitions. For more frail persons, the higher end of this range should be used. Resistance should be increased as strength increases. Each repetition should consist of 2-3 s of a concentric contraction (lifting) and 4-6 s of an eccentric contraction (lowering).
Sets	One set should be performed. There is no strong evidence to suggest a greater number of sets will yield greater increases in strength (26).
Frequency	Optimal frequency appears to be dependent on the muscle group being exercised. For the spine, 1-2 days per week will yield optimal results. For the upper and lower extremities, 2-3 times per week will yield optimal results.

individuals results in increases in the cross-sectional area of both type I and type II fibers, with the greatest increases in contractile proteins occurring in the latter fibers (75). Additionally, research has shown that it may be possible to selectively hypertrophy type I or type II fibers depending on the training strategy. Powerlifters who train with high resistance and low repetitions have greater fiber areas in type II fibers. In comparison, bodybuilders who train with lower resistance and higher repetitions have a lower percentage of type II fibers, and selective type II fiber hypertrophy is not evident (76). Evans has reported that high-intensity resistance training in older adults results in increases in both type I and type II fibers, with the greatest increases occurring in type I fibers. Additionally, he has reported that lower-body maximal oxygen consumption increases significantly, suggesting that the increased muscle mass may be responsible (23).

Because of the atrophy of type I and type II fibers and the decreases in strength reported in patients with COPD, it appears that resistance training may be beneficial for patients with COPD. Despite a strong rationale for resistance training in COPD patients, there is a dearth of knowledge regarding the efficacy of resistance training in these patients. To date, only two studies have systematically investigated the effects of resistance training programs in patients with COPD.

Simpson et al. randomized 34 patients with COPD to either a resistance training group or a control group (68). Those randomized to the resistance training group completed 3 sets of 10 repetitions of single-arm curls, single-leg extensions, and single-leg presses. The resistance was progressively increased from 50% of the one-repetition maximum (1-RM) during the first week of training to 85% during the eighth and final week of training. Significant increases in muscular strength and cycling endurance time were found in the experimental group. Responses to the chronic respiratory disease questionnaire, a measure of health-related quality of life, showed improvements in dyspnea and mastery of activities of daily living.

More recently, Bernard et al. evaluated whether the addition of resistance training to a 12-week program of aerobic training resulted in additional benefit for patients with COPD (11). The resistance training program consisted of one upper-extremity and three lower-extremity exercises. The program started with 2 sets of 8-10 repetitions at 60% of the 1-RM and progressed to 3 sets of 8-10 repetitions at 80% of the 1-RM. Patients in the resistance training program demonstrated significant increases in muscular strength and muscle mass. However, changes in peak work rate, distance walked in 6 min, and quality of life were comparable in the two groups. As a result, the investigators concluded that the addition of resistance training to an aerobic training program did not translate into additional improvements in exercise capacity or quality of life. While this study did not provide direct support for the use of resistance training in COPD patients, it did confirm that peripheral muscles in COPD patients show structural adaptations to resistance training. It should be noted that the strength and muscular deficiencies seen in the COPD patients in this investigation were not completely corrected with the training regimen used. Thus, it may be that a more intense training program or a longer period of training is needed in order to recognize the potential benefits of resistance training in these patients.

Based on the preliminary results of the studies that have evaluated upper-, lower-, and whole-body resistance training in COPD patients, it appears that resistance training may offer distinct advantages over other forms of exercise training for these patients. Consequently, it should be included in a comprehensive exercise rehabilitation program. Presently there are no clear recommendations for the optimal training prescriptions that should be used with COPD patients. As such, it is recommended that these patients adhere to existing recommendations for resistance training in older adults (see table 15.3) (3, 23).

Future Research

Because of the lack of information defining the optimal resistance training prescription for patients with COPD, additional research is needed in this area. Specific questions that need to be addressed include the following:

1. What is the role of ventilatory muscle resistance training, and which patients would benefit the most from this type of training?
2. What is the optimal training intensity, duration, and frequency for ventilatory muscle resistance training?
3. Should COPD patients work on developing muscular strength, muscular endurance, or a combination of the two?
4. Are different training strategies needed for the upper extremities than for the lower extremities?
5. What is the optimal training intensity, duration, and frequency for upper- and lower-extremity resistance training?
6. What are the effects of resistance training on measures of quality of life and on activities of daily living?
7. What effect does resistance training have on bone density, a potential consequence of long-term corticosteroid use among patients with COPD (51)?

References

1. Agency for Health Care Policy and Research. 1999. *Clinical Classifications for Health Policy Research: Hospital Inpatient Statistics, 1995.* HCUP-3 Research Note. Rockville, MD: Agency for Health Care Policy and Research.

2. ACCP/AACVPR Pulmonary Rehabilitation Guidelines Panel. 1997. Pulmonary rehabilitation: Joint ACCP/AACVPR evidence-based guidelines. *Chest* 112: 1363-1396.
3. American College of Sports Medicine. 1998. The recommended quantity and quality of exercise for developing and maintaining cardiorespiratory and muscular fitness, and flexibility in healthy adults. *Medicine and Science in Sports and Exercise* 30: 975-991.
4. American Thoracic Society. 1987. Standards for the diagnosis and care of patients with chronic obstructive pulmonary disease (COPD) and asthma. *American Review of Respiratory Disease* 136: 225-244.
5. American Thoracic Society. 1995. Standards for diagnosis and care of patients with chronic obstructive pulmonary disease. *American Journal of Respiratory and Critical Care Medicine* 152: S77-S152.
6. American Thoracic Society and European Respiratory Society. 1999. Skeletal muscle dysfunction in chronic obstructive pulmonary disease. *American Journal of Respiratory and Critical Care Medicine* 159: S1-S40.
7. Belman, M.J., W.C. Botnick, S.D. Nathan, and K.H. Chon. 1994. Ventilatory load characteristics during ventilatory muscle training. *American Journal of Respiratory and Critical Care Medicine* 149: 925-929.
8. Belman, M.J., and R. Shadmehr. 1988. Targeted resistive ventilatory muscle training in chronic obstructive pulmonary disease. *Journal of Applied Physiology* 65: 2726-2735.
9. Belman, M.J., S.G. Thomas, and M.I. Lewis. 1986. Resistive breathing training in patients with chronic obstructive pulmonary disease. *Chest* 90: 662-669.
10. Bernard, S., P. Leblanc, F. Whittom, G. Carrier, J. Jobin, R. Belleau, and F. Maltais. 1998. Peripheral muscle weakness in patients with chronic obstructive pulmonary disease. *American Journal of Respiratory and Critical Care Medicine* 158: 629-634.
11. Bernard, S., F. Whittom, P. Leblanc, J. Jobin, R. Belleau, C. Berube, G. Carrier, and F. Maltais. 1999. Aerobic and strength training in patients with chronic obstructive pulmonary disease. *American Journal of Respiratory and Critical Care Medicine* 159: 896-901.
12. Berry, M.J., N.E. Adair, K.S. Sevensky, A. Quinby, and H.M. Lever. 1996. Inspiratory muscle training and whole-body reconditioning in chronic obstructive pulmonary disease. *American Journal of Respiratory and Critical Care Medicine* 153: 1812-1816.
13. Bjerre-Jepsen, K., N.H. Secher, and A. Kok-Jensen. 1981. Inspiratory resistance training in severe chronic obstructive pulmonary disease. *European Journal of Respiratory Diseases* 62: 405-411.
14. Celli, B.R., J. Rassulo, and B.J. Make. 1986. Dyssynchronous breathing during arm but not leg exercise in patients with chronic airflow obstruction. *New England Journal of Medicine* 314: 1485-1490.
15. Chen, H., R. Dukes, and B.J. Martin. 1985. Inspiratory muscle training in patients with chronic obstructive pulmonary disease. *American Review of Respiratory Disease* 131: 251-255.
16. Couser, J.I., F.J. Martinez, and B. Celli. 1993. Pulmonary rehabilitation that includes arm exercise reduces metabolic and ventilatory requirements for simple arm elevation. *Chest* 103: 37-41.
17. Danon, J., W.S. Druz, N.B. Goldberg, and J.T. Sharp. 1979. Function of the isolated paced diaphragm and the cervical accessory muscles in C1 quadriplegics. *American Review of Respiratory Disease* 119: 909-919.
18. DeCramer, M., V. de Bock, and R. Dom. 1996. Functional and histologic picture of steroid-induced myopathy in chronic obstructive pulmonary disease. *American Journal of Respiratory and Critical Care Medicine* 153: 1958-1964.
19. DeCramer, M., L.M. Lacquet, R. Fagard, and P. Rogiers. 1994. Corticosteroids contribute to muscle weakness in chronic airflow obstruction. *American Journal of Respiratory and Critical Care Medicine* 150: 11-16.

289

20. Dekhuijzen, P.N., H.T. Folgering, and H.C. Van. 1991. Target-flow inspiratory muscle training during pulmonary rehabilitation in patients with COPD. *Chest* 99: 128-133.

21. Druz, W.S., and J.T. Sharp. 1981. Activity of respiratory muscles in upright and recumbent humans. *Journal of Applied Physiology* 51: 1552-1561.

22. Engelen, M.P., A.M. Schols, W.C. Baken, G.J. Wesseling, and E.F. Wouters. 1994. Nutritional depletion in relation to respiratory and peripheral skeletal muscle function in out-patients with COPD. *European Respiratory Journal* 7: 1793-1797.

23. Evans, W.J. 1999. Exercise training guidelines for the elderly. *Medicine and Science in Sports and Exercise* 31: 12-17.

24. Falk, P., A.M. Eriksen, K. Kolliker, and J.B. Andersen. 1985. Relieving dyspnea with an inexpensive and simple method in patients with severe chronic airflow limitation. *European Journal of Respiratory Diseases* 66: 181-186.

25. Farkas, G.A., and C. Roussos. 1982. Adaptability of the hamster diaphragm to exercise and/or emphysema. *Journal of Applied Physiology* 53: 1263-1272.

26. Feigenbaum, M.S., and M.L. Pollock. 1999. Prescription of resistance training for health and disease. *Medicine and Science in Sports and Exercise* 31: 38-45.

27. Gergley, T.J., W.D. McArdle, P. DeJesus, M.M. Toner, S. Jacobowitz, and R.J. Spina. 1984. Specificity of arm training on aerobic power during swimming and running. *Medicine and Science in Sports and Exercise* 16: 349-354.

28. Goldstein, R., J. De Rosie, S. Long, T. Dolmage, and M.A. Avendano. 1989. Applicability of a threshold loading device for inspiratory muscle testing and training in patients with COPD. *Chest* 96: 564-571.

29. Gordon, A.M., A.F. Huxley, and F.J. Julian. 1966. The variation in isometric tension with sarcomere length in vertebrate muscle fibres. *Journal of Physiology (London)* 184: 170-192.

30. Gosselink, R., T. Troosters, and M. DeCramer. 1996. Peripheral muscle weakness contributes to exercise limitation in COPD. *American Journal of Respiratory and Critical Care Medicine* 153: 976-980.

31. Guyatt, G., J. Keller, J. Singer, S. Halcrow, and M. Newhouse. 1992. Controlled trial of respiratory muscle training in chronic airflow limitation. *Thorax* 47: 598-602.

32. Hamilton, A.L., K.J. Killian, E. Summers, and N.L. Jones. 1995. Muscle strength, symptom intensity, and exercise capacity in patients with cardiorespiratory disorders. *American Journal of Respiratory and Critical Care Medicine* 152: 2021-2031.

33. Harver, A., D.A. Mahler, and J.A. Daubenspeck. 1989. Targeted inspiratory muscle training improves respiratory muscle function and reduces dyspnea in patients with chronic obstructive pulmonary disease. *Annals of Internal Medicine* 111: 117-124.

34. Henke, K.G., M. Sharratt, D. Pegelow, and J.A. Dempsey. 1988. Regulation of end-expiratory lung volume during exercise. *Journal of Applied Physiology* 64: 135-146.

35. Hildebrand, I.L., C. Sylven, M. Esbjornsson, K. Hellstrom, and E. Jansson. 1991. Does chronic hypoxaemia induce transformations of fibre types? *Acta Physiologica Scandinavica* 141: 435-439.

36. Hughes, R.L., H. Katz, V. Sahgal, J.A. Campbell, R. Hartz, and T.W. Shields. 1983. Fiber size and energy metabolites in five separate muscles from patients with chronic obstructive lung diseases. *Respiration* 44: 321-328.

37. Jakobsson, P., L. Jorfeldt, and A. Brundin. 1990. Skeletal muscle metabolites and fibre types in patients with advanced chronic obstructive pulmonary disease (COPD), with and without chronic respiratory failure. *European Respiratory Journal* 3: 192-196.

38. Killian, K.J., and N.L. Jones. 1988. Respiratory muscles and dyspnea. *Clinics in Chest Medicine* 9: 237-248.

39. Killian, K.J., P. Leblanc, D.H. Martin, E. Summers, N.L. Jones, and E.J. Campbell. 1992. Exercise capacity and ventilatory, circulatory, and symptom limitation in patients with chronic airflow limitation. *American Review of Respiratory Disease* 146: 935-940.

40. Larson, J.L., M.J. Kim, J.T. Sharp, and D.A. Larson. 1988. Inspiratory muscle training with a pressure threshold breathing device in patients with chronic obstructive pulmonary disease. *American Review of Respiratory Disease* 138: 689-696.

41. Leith, D.E., and M. Bradley. 1976. Ventilatory muscle strength and endurance training. *Journal of Applied Physiology* 41: 508-516.

42. Lisboa, C., V. Munoz, T. Beroiza, A. Leiva, and E. Cruz. 1994. Inspiratory muscle training in chronic airflow limitation: Comparison of two different training loads with a threshold device. *European Respiratory Journal* 7: 1266-1274.

43. Lisboa, C., C. Villafranca, A. Leiva, E. Cruz, J. Pertuze, and G. Borzone. 1997. Inspiratory muscle training in chronic airflow limitation: Effect on exercise performance. *European Respiratory Journal* 10: 537-542.

44. Magel, J.R., W.D. McArdle, M. Toner, and D.J. Delio. 1978. Metabolic and cardiovascular adjustment to arm training. *Journal of Applied Physiology* 45: 75-79.

45. Magnussen, H., K. Richter, and C. Taube. 1998. Are chronic obstructive pulmonary disease (COPD) and asthma different diseases? *Clinical and Experimental Allergy* 28 (suppl. 5): 187-194.

46. Mahler, D.A., and C.K. Wells. 1988. Evaluation of clinical methods for rating dyspnea. *Chest* 93: 580-586.

47. Maltais, F., A.A. Simard, C. Simard, J. Jobin, P. Desgagnes, and P. Leblanc. 1996. Oxidative capacity of the skeletal muscle and lactic acid kinetics during exercise in normal subjects and in patients with COPD. *American Journal of Respiratory and Critical Care Medicine* 153: 288-293.

48. Mannino, D.M., C. Brown, and G.A. Giovino. 1997. Obstructive lung disease deaths in the United States from 1979 through 1993. An analysis using multiple-cause mortality data. *American Journal of Respiratory and Critical Care Medicine* 156: 814-818.

49. Martinez, F.J., P.D. Vogel, D.N. Dupont, I. Stanopoulos, A. Gray, and J.F. Beamis. 1993. Supported arm exercise vs unsupported arm exercise in the rehabilitation of patients with severe chronic airflow obstruction. *Chest* 103: 1397-1402.

50. McCully, K.K., and J.A. Faulkner. 1983. Length-tension relationship of mammalian diaphragm muscles. *Journal of Applied Physiology* 54: 1681-1686.

51. McEvoy, C.E., K.E. Ensrud, E. Bender, H.K. Genant, W. Yu, J.M. Griffith, and D.E. Niewoehner. 1998. Association between corticosteroid use and vertebral fractures in older men with chronic obstructive pulmonary disease. *American Journal of Respiratory and Critical Care Medicine* 157: 704-709.

52. McKeon, J.L., J. Turner, C. Kelly, A. Dent, and P.V. Zimmerman. 1986. The effect of inspiratory resistive training on exercise capacity in optimally treated patients with severe chronic airflow limitation. *Australian and New Zealand Journal of Medicine* 16: 648-652.

53. National Heart, Lung, and Blood Institute. 1998. *Morbidity and Mortality: 1998 Chartbook on Cardiovascular, Lung, and Blood Diseases*, 1-128. Bethesda, MD: National Institutes of Health.

54. Nield, M.A. 1999. Inspiratory muscle training protocol using a pressure threshold device: Effect on dyspnea in chronic obstructive pulmonary disease. *Archives of Physical Medicine and Rehabilitation* 80: 100-102.

55. Noseda, A., J.P. Carpiaux, W. Vandeput, T. Prigogine, and J. Schmerber. 1987. Resistive inspiratory muscle training and exercise performance in COPD patients: A comparative study with conventional breathing retraining. *Bulletin of European Physiopathology and Respiration* 23: 457-463.

56. O'Donnell, D.E., M. McGuire, L. Samis, and K.A. Webb. 1995. The impact of exercise reconditioning on breathlessness in severe chronic airflow limitation. *American Journal of Respiratory and Critical Care Medicine* 152: 2005-2013.

57. Pardy, R.L., R.N. Rivington, P.J. Despas, and P.T. Macklem. 1981. Inspiratory muscle training compared with physiotherapy in patients with chronic airflow limitation. *American Review of Respiratory Disease* 123: 421-425.

291

58. Peters, K.D., K.D. Kochanek, and S.L. Murphy. 1998. Deaths: Final data for 1996. *National Vital Statistics Report* 47: 1-99.
59. Polkey, M.I., D. Kyroussis, C.H. Hamnegard, G.H. Mills, M. Green, and J. Moxham. 1996. Diaphragm strength in chronic obstructive pulmonary disease. *American Journal of Respiratory and Critical Care Medicine* 154: 1310-1317.
60. Preusser, B.A., M.L. Winningham, and T.L. Clanton. 1994. High- vs low-intensity inspiratory muscle interval training in patients with COPD. *Chest* 106: 110-117.
61. Reid, D.C., J. Bowden, and P. Lynne-Davies. 1976. Role of selected muscles of respiration as influenced by posture and tidal volume. *Chest* 70: 636-640.
62. Ries, A.L., B. Ellis, and R.W. Hawkins. 1988. Upper extremity exercise training in chronic obstructive pulmonary disease. *Chest* 93: 688-692.
63. Saltin, B., K. Nazar, D.L. Costill, E. Stein, E. Jansson, B. Essen, and D. Gollnick. 1976. The nature of the training response; peripheral and central adaptations of one-legged exercise. *Acta Physiologica Scandinavica* 96: 289-305.
64. Schols, A.M., P.B. Soeters, A.M. Dingemans, R. Mostert, P.J. Frantzen, and E.F. Wouters. 1993. Prevalence and characteristics of nutritional depletion in patients with stable COPD eligible for pulmonary rehabilitation. *American Review of Respiratory Disease* 147: 1151-1156.
65. Serres, I., V. Gautier, A. Varray, and C. Prefaut. 1998. Impaired skeletal muscle endurance related to physical inactivity and altered lung function in COPD patients. *Chest* 113: 900-905.
66. Sharratt, M.T., K.G. Henke, E.A. Aaron, D.F. Pegelow, and J.A. Dempsey. 1987. Exercise-induced changes in functional residual capacity. *Respiration Physiology* 70: 313-326.
67. Similowski, T., S. Yan, A.P. Gauthier, P.T. Macklem, and F. Bellemare. 1991. Contractile properties of the human diaphragm during chronic hyperinflation. *New England Journal of Medicine* 325: 917-923.
68. Simpson, K., K. Killian, N. McCartney, D.G. Stubbing, and N.L. Jones. 1992. Randomised controlled trial of weightlifting exercise in patients with chronic airflow limitation. *Thorax* 74: 70-75.
69. Smith, J., and F. Bellemare. 1987. Effect of lung volume on in vivo contraction characteristics of human diaphragm. *Journal of Applied Physiology* 62: 1893-1900.
70. Smith, K., D. Cook, G.H. Guyatt, J. Madhaven, and A.D. Oxman. 1992. Respiratory muscle training in chronic air flow limitation: A meta-analysis. *American Review of Respiratory Disease* 145: 533-539.
71. Snider, G.L. 1989. Chronic obstructive pulmonary disease: A definition and implications of structural determinants of airflow obstruction for epidemiology. *American Review of Respiratory Disease* 140: S3-S8.
72. Snider, G.L., J. Kleinerman, W.M. Thurlbeck, and Z.K. Bengali. 1985. The definition of emphysema. Report of a National Heart, Lung, and Blood Institute, Division of Lung Diseases workshop. *American Review of Respiratory Disease* 132: 182-185.
73. Stubbing, D.G., L.D. Pengelly, J.L. Morse, and N.L. Jones. 1980. Pulmonary mechanics during exercise in subjects with chronic airflow obstruction. *Journal of Applied Physiology* 49: 511-515.
74. Tangri, S., and C.R. Woolf. 1973. The breathing pattern in chronic obstructive lung disease during the performance of some common daily activities. *Chest* 63: 126-127.
75. Tesch, P.A. 1988. Skeletal muscle adaptations consequent to long-term heavy resistance exercise. *Medicine and Science in Sports and Exercise* 20: S132-S134.
76. Tesch, P.A., and L. Larsson. 1982. Muscle hypertrophy in bodybuilders. *European Journal of Applied Physiology* 49: 301-306.
77. Thurlbeck, W.M. 1990. Pathophysiology of chronic obstructive pulmonary disease. *Clinics in Chest Medicine* 11: 389-403.
78. Thurlbeck, W.M., and N.L. Muller. 1994. Emphysema: Definition, imaging, and quantification. *American Journal of Roentgenology, Radium Therapy, and Nuclear Medicine* 163: 1017-1025.

79. Tzelepis, G.E., D.L. Vega, M.E. Cohen, A.M. Fulambarker, K.K. Patel, and F.D. McCool. 1994. Pressure-flow specificity of inspiratory muscle training. *Journal of Applied Physiology* 77: 795-801.
80. Tzelepis, G.E., D.L. Vega, M.E. Cohen, and F.D. McCool. 1994. Lung volume specificity of inspiratory muscle training. *Journal of Applied Physiology* 77: 789-794.
81. Wanke, T., D. Formanek, H. Lahrmann, H. Brath, M. Wild, C. Wagner, and H. Zwick. 1994. Effects of combined inspiratory muscle and cycle ergometer training on exercise performance in patients with COPD. *European Respiratory Journal* 7: 2205-2211.
82. Weiner, P., Y. Azgad, and R. Ganam. 1992. Inspiratory muscle training combined with general exercise reconditioning in patients with COPD. *Chest* 102: 1351-1356.
83. Whittom, F., J. Jobin, P.M. Simard, P. Leblanc, C. Simard, S. Bernard, R. Belleau, and F. Maltais. 1998. Histochemical and morphological characteristics of the vastus lateralis muscle in patients with chronic obstructive pulmonary disease. *Medicine and Science in Sports and Exercise* 30: 1467-1474.
84. Wijkstra, P.J., E.M. TenVergert, T.W. van der Mark, D.S. Postma, R.V. Altena, and G.H. Koeter. 1994. Relation of lung function, maximal inspiratory pressure, dyspnoea, and quality of life with exercise capacity in patients with chronic obstructive pulmonary disease. *Thorax* 49: 468-472.
85. Wuyam, B., J.F. Payen, P. Levy, H. Bensaidane, H. Reutenauer, J.F. Le Bas, and A.L. Benabid. 1992. Metabolism and aerobic capacity of skeletal muscle in chronic respiratory failure related to chronic obstructive pulmonary disease. *European Respiratory Journal* 5: 157-162.

16

CHAPTER

Resistance Exercise for Patients With Diabetes Mellitus

Otto A. Sánchez, MD
Arthur S. Leon, MD
University of Minnesota

Disease Prevalence

Diabetes mellitus (DM) is defined by the American Diabetes Association as a heterogeneous group of metabolic diseases characterized by hyperglycemia, caused by either defects in insulin secretion, insulin action, or both. The resulting chronic hyperglycemia is associated with dysfunction, damage, and ultimately failure of various organs, especially the eyes, kidneys, nerves, and cardiovascular system (27).

DM affects 5.1% of the American population over 20 years of age, or about 16 million persons, half of whom are unaware they have the condition. In addition, the prevalence of impaired fasting glucose, a precursor of DM, is about 7%. That makes the combined prevalence of these two conditions to be around 29 million persons (39). The prevalence of diabetes varies greatly among ethnic and racial groups. For example, the age-adjusted prevalence of diabetes in white Hispanics is twice as high as in non-Hispanic whites in the United States (11), while non-Hispanic blacks have a still higher prevalence of DM than Hispanic whites (39). The observed differences in prevalence of diabetes by race and ethnicity probably represent an expression of both genetic and cultural habits in the etiology of DM.

Rates of DM increase with age. At age 40-49 years, its prevalence is 2.3%, and by age 60-74 years it increases to 10.8% (39). With the growing percentage of the population over age 65 and a progressively longer life expectancy, substantially higher rates of DM and its complications are expected during the next decade unless preventive measures are improved (54).

DM is a major risk factor for premature cardiovascular disease (CVD), including heart attacks, stroke, and peripheral vascular disease. It is also the major cause in the United States of end-stage kidney disease, requiring chronic dialysis or renal transplant, and is responsible for more then half of all nontraumatic lower-leg amputations. In 1994, 56,692 deaths, or 19.5 per 100,000, were attributed to DM, making it the seventh leading cause of mortality in the United States (10). However, this figure does not reflect its true public health impact, since the majority of deaths in people with diabetes are secondary to CVD or end-stage renal disease. A more realistic figure for the actual number of deaths directly or indirectly related to DM was more likely over 180,000 in 1994 (10). These figures highlight the importance of DM as a public health problem.

Classification and Clinical Presentation

There are two major types of diabetes, commonly labeled type 1 and type 2. Type 1 DM results from an insulin-deficiency state, generally due to autoimmune destruction of the pancreatic β-cells, and is strongly associated with specific types of histocompatibility leucocyte antigen (HLA) complexes (28). Type 1 DM usually becomes clinically evident before age 30. The insulin-deficient state results in hyperglycemia due to both reduced cell glucose uptake and excess glucose release from the liver. When blood glucose excretion exceeds the reabsorption threshold for glucose in the kidney, glucose is lost in the urine (glycosuria), along with increased water (polyuria). The increase in the volume of urine may result in dehydration, stimulating thirst (polydipsia). Weight loss results from excessive protein and fat catabolism to compensate for the inability to use carbohydrate as fuel, which are direct consequences of both insulin insufficiency and increased activity of the counter-regulatory hormones. These four symptoms—weight loss, glycosuria, polyuria, and polydipsia—are the cardinal clinical manifestations of DM. Increased activity of hormone-sensitive lipase in the adipocytes, also associated with insulin deficiency and increased counter-regulatory hormonal activity, results in an excess presentation of fatty acids to the liver. This leads to excess ketone body formation and ketoacidosis, which can be a fatal complication in the absence of insulin-replacement therapy.

Type 2 DM accounts for 90-95 % of all cases of DM in the United States. It usually begins later in life than type 1 diabetes (generally after age 40). This type of diabetes primarily results from an insulin-resistant state with a relative insulin deficiency despite normal or elevated blood levels. In contrast to type 1 DM, most people with type 2 DM are obese and/or have increased subcutaneous and visceral fat in the abdominal region. Although type 2 diabetic patients also may present with glycosuria, polyuria, and polydipsia, usually the disease onset is accompanied only by nonspecific symptoms, such as blurred vision, vaginal infections, or poor wound healing. There is a stronger genetic contribution to the etiology of type 2 DM than type 1 DM. First-degree relatives of people with type 2 DM have a fourfold increased risk of type 2 DM than those in the general population (83). The prevalence of elevated basal insulin levels and impaired glucose homeostasis also has been found to be higher in nondiabetic relatives of people with type 2 DM than in the general population (13, 45).

Beck-Nielsen et al. have proposed a three-stage model for the pathophysiology of type 2 diabetes in which the first two stages are prediabetic states and the third stage is the fully expressed disease (3). During the first stage, insulin sensitivity is reduced and hyperinsulinemia is present, but the rate of liver glucose release is normal, and there is only a borderline elevation in fasting blood glucose levels and a normal or borderline glucose tolerance test response. At this stage, the main pathophysiological feature is postulated to be a genetically related defect in glycogen synthesis in skeletal muscle. If to this genetic defect are added obesity, a sedentary lifestyle, and aging, the second stage of the disease manifests itself by impaired glucose tolerance and relative insulin insufficiency. At this stage, hepatic glucose production and fasting blood glucose still remain normal, but postprandial plasma glucose levels are increased, which initially can be compensated for by hyperinsulinemia. In the third stage, DM is fully expressed with excess hepatic glucose release and fasting hyperglycemia. By then chronic vascular complications may already have started or in fact may be initial manifestations of the disease. This emphasizes not only the possibility and importance of early detection of the disease, but the value of primary prevention strategies, including exercise training.

Long-Term Complications

Prior to prescribing an exercise program, it is necessary to screen all individuals with DM for evidence of complications. Chronic complications in diabetic individuals are related to two types of vascular processes: microangiopathy and macroangiopathy. Microangiopathy refers to vascular alterations restricted to the blood capillaries (48), while macroangiopathy affects medium-sized and large arteries, and is a process characterized by premature atherosclerosis and increased risk of thrombosis. Pathophysiological macrovascular changes are why coronary heart disease, peripheral vascular disease, and stroke are much more common in diabetic than nondiabetic individuals (6). Epidemiological studies have demonstrated an exponential relationship between increased blood glucose values, hyperinsulinemia, and incidence of diabetic macrovascular and microvascular complications and premature mortality (18, 34, 78, 96).

Major atherosclerotic-thrombotic cardiovascular complications are the principal causes of morbidity and premature mortality in diabetic patients. Individuals with type 2 diabetes have a 27% greater chance of dying from CVD than matched nondiabetic people (6). Accelerated atherosclerosis in the presence of DM is due not only to endothelial cell injury by hyperglycemia, but also to the commonly associated dyslipidemias and elevated blood pressure levels. Accompanying coagulation defects also increase the risk of formation of a thrombus, causing obstruction of a coronary or cerebral artery and resulting in a myocardial infarct or stroke (28).

In addition, DM is responsible for about one-third of the cases of end-stage renal disease in the United States, requiring chronic dialysis and/or renal transplant. Microalbuminuria is the initial sign of diabetic nephropathy, and it is predictive of future development of overt proteinuria due to renal damage. The natural course of diabetic nephropathy is a progressive and relentless irreversible decline in renal function, refractory to treatment. The value of tight glycemic control in retarding the progression of diabetic nephropathy has been demonstrated (70).

Diabetic retinopathy is the most common cause of new cases of blindness among persons age 20-74 years in the United States (9). The earliest phase is called background diabetic retinopathy; the next phase is preproliferative diabetic retinopathy; and the last stage is proliferative retinopathy, in which neovascularization of the retina is the main feature. The fragile new blood vessels may rupture and bleed, producing vitreous hemorrhages and impaired vision (85). The resulting fibrous tissue deposition also can lead to retinal detachment (85). The presence of proliferative retinopathy is generally considered a relative or absolute contraindication for strenuous aerobic or resistance exercise, because of the fear that an associated excessive rise in blood pressure can promote vitreous hemorrhage and retinal detachment (4, 71).

DM patients commonly have less muscular strength than age-matched individuals (10). This may result from diabetic peripheral neuropathy, as well as from primary muscle damage and reduced vascular supply (1, 7, 8, 14). Muscle impairment limits the ability of diabetic individuals to exercise (79), contributing to further muscle atrophy and weakness. Muscle atrophy in turn adversely affects glucose control, making these individuals more susceptible to further disability from long-term complications. For that reason, designing proper exercise programs to help maintain muscle mass and function may permit the diabetic patient to perform activities of daily living more efficiently and thereby improve quality of life.

Treatment

The main goals in the treatment of DM are to achieve glycemic control, manage coexisting CVD risk factors, and prevent or reduce the progression of chronic complications. This is accomplished by the combination of diet, exercise, smoking cessation, and the use of insulin or oral hypoglycemic drugs to further improve glucose control, as well as pharmacological management of coexisting dyslipidemias and hypertension. Insulin is essential in the management of type 1 diabetes to prevent ketoacidosis. In type 2 DM patients, treatment with insulin generally is started only if blood glucose control cannot be achieved by the combined treatment of diet, exercise, and oral hypoglycemic agents. The currently recommended approach to achieve tight blood glucose control in type 1 DM is multiple subcutaneous injections of insulin with frequent self-monitoring of blood glucose levels. This ordinarily is accomplished by multiple doses of insulin. This includes administering 25% of the previous daily dose at bedtime as neutral protamine Hagedorn (NPH) or another long-acting type of insulin, and the remaining insulin requirements in divided doses 30 min before breakfast, lunch, and dinner on a sliding scale based on blood glucose levels (28).

The dietary plan for the patient with DM is individually prescribed based on nutritional assessments and treatment goals. The diet should provide an adequate intake of essential nutrients and provide proper energy intake for attaining or maintaining proper weight. This not only contributes to the management of hyperglycemia, but also can favorably affect associated dyslipidemias and elevated blood pressure. Generally, the recommended diet consists of 50-55% of energy obtained from carbohydrate, less than 30% of energy from fat, 15-20% of energy from protein, and reduction in saturated fat to less than 10% of total calories and cholesterol to less then 300 mg per day. For patients with type 2 DM, in the absence of severe hyperglycemia, management is commonly initiated with a diet and exercise program. Since the majority of patients with type 2 DM are obese and/or have excess body fat accumulated in central depots contributing to insulin resistance, weight reduction through diet and exercise is of primary importance for disease management. For type 2 DM patients, oral hypoglycemic agents are usually initiated when 3 months of exercise and dietary therapy fail to maintain plasma glucose within the goals of glycemic control. Optimal blood glucose targets to aim for are fasting levels less than 120 mg/dl, postprandial glucose levels less than 180 mg/dl, and a glycosylated hemoglobin level under 7%. Different types of oral hypoglycemic agents may be used alone or in combination. The mechanism of action of these drugs is either by improving insulin sensitivity, reducing hepatic glucose production, stimulating pancreatic insulin secretion, or by decreasing intestinal absorption of carbohydrates (23). The choice of which of these medications to use depends on the condition of the patient. Long-term type 2 DM patients often require multiple types of oral hypoglycemic agents and/or insulin to achieve glycemic control (93).

Exercise in the Prevention and Management of Type 2 DM

Cross-sectional (61) and long-term cohort epidemiological studies (35, 41, 59), as well as clinical trials (25, 66, 80) and experimental studies (26, 37, 51), provide data that strongly support the role of aerobic exercise in the prevention of type 2 DM, and as an adjunct therapy in the management of both types of DM. For example, in a cross-sectional study of 1600 men and women with variable glucose tolerance status, Mayer-Davis et al. assessed the association between insulin sensitivity and habitual physical activity (61). It was determined that insulin sensitivity was 59% and 77% higher in those who performed vigorous exercise 2-4 times a week and 5 times a week, respectively, as compared with those who performed no regular vigorous exercise over the previous year. Further, three longitudinal cohort studies observed a strong inverse relationship between levels of habitual physical activity and incidence of type 2 DM (35, 41, 59). One of these studies (41) involved about 6000 male college alumni, age 39 to 64, initially free of type 2 DM at entry, who were followed for 14 years. Data from this study revealed that for each increment of 500 kcal per week in energy expenditure during leisure-time physical activity, the age-adjusted risk of type 2 DM decreased 6% for those at increased risk for DM. These findings are similar to those of Lynch et al., who followed a population-based sample of 751 middle-age men for 4 years and determined that the risk of type 2 DM substantially decreased when individuals performed moderate to vigorous (≥5.5

METs[1]) leisure-time physical activity for at least 40 minutes per week (59). This observed association remained significant after adjusting for several risk factors for type 2 DM (59).

In a landmark randomized controlled clinical trial involving 577 men and women with impaired glucose tolerance (IGT), the effects of diet and aerobic exercise training alone or in combination on the incidence of type 2 diabetes were studied over a follow-up period of 6 years (66). The groups using diet alone, exercise alone, and a combined treatment experienced a 31%, 46%, and 42% reduction, respectively, in the risk of developing type 2 DM, as compared with a control group (66). In a population-based, long-term (12 years of follow-up) study, involving 423 men with IGT, participants were randomized to an intervention group that received dietary counseling plus an aerobic exercise program and a routine treatment control group that received only basic advice on lifestyle and diet. Mortality rates were compared with those of over 5000 healthy men with normal glucose tolerance. These investigators observed that the mortality rates in the active intervention group were not significantly different from rates in an inactive comparison group with normal glucose tolerance (21), and that both of these groups had significantly lower mortality rates than the routine treatment IGT control group. These results suggest that a combination of diet and exercise can reduce premature mortality in people at high risk for type 2 DM. In addition, in a clinical setting the inclusion of a supervised aerobic exercise program has been shown to reduce the requirements of insulin in type 1 DM patients (81). To date, there are no published epidemiological studies or clinical trials on the effects of resistance exercise in the prevention of type 2 diabetes or in glycemic management of type 1 or type 2 DM. More research is clearly needed in these areas.

The above epidemiological and clinical trial data demonstrating the benefits of aerobic exercise in improving glucose metabolism are supported by several experimental studies. It appears that improved insulin sensitivity and improved glycemic control with aerobic exercise in individuals with type 2 diabetes result both from short-term effects of single bouts of exercise (75) and from skeletal muscle adaptations to training (44, 49, 64, 69). The acute effect of aerobic exercise in both healthy individuals and those with type 2 DM results from an increased translocation of a glucose transporter protein labeled GLUT-4 in skeletal muscle to the cell surface (43, 51, 53). This effect was similar in older and younger subjects (15), may last up to 40 h after the last exercise bout (43, 52), and is independent of the training status of the subjects (43). This exercise-induced translocation of GLUT-4 and resulting

---

[1] MET = the energy expenditure at rest or an oxygen consumption of 3.5 ml · kg^{-1} · min^{-1}.

increased glucose uptake appears to be independent and additive to the effect of insulin on glucose uptake (37, 51).

The additional benefits of aerobic exercise training on glucose-insulin dynamics beyond that of a single exercise bout were recently reviewed by Ivy et al. (47). One or more of the following mechanisms are believed to play a role: a decrease in hepatic glucose output, a reduction in visceral adipose tissue, an increase in muscle mass, an increase in insulin-stimulated muscle blood flow, and/or an increase in intracellular muscle glucose oxidation and glycogen storage, due to increased activity of glycogen synthase (55) and hexokinase II enzymes (55, 65).

A significant percentage of individuals with DM have elevated blood pressure, high blood triglyceride levels, low blood high-density lipoprotein (HDL) cholesterol levels, and/or decreased fibrinolytic activity, which puts them at increased risk for CVD. Endurance exercise training favorably affects these risk factors for CVD in patients with both type 1 and type 2 DM (56, 57). Lehman et al. studied the effects of a 3-month regular aerobic exercise program in 16 well-controlled patients with type 2 DM (57). The authors reported a significant decrease in triglycerides and an increase in HDL cholesterol, as well as significant decreases in systolic and diastolic blood pressure in comparison to a control group (57). $\dot{V}O_2$max, which has consistently been shown to be decreased in patients with type 2 DM (74), also is improved with aerobic exercise in people with type 2 (82, 94) and also in type 1 DM patients (56). Additionally, after 6 weeks of a regular aerobic exercise program, fibrinolytic activity is reported to increase in type 2 DM patients (82). These findings strongly support the recommendation for including endurance exercise as an adjunct therapeutic strategy to decrease risk factors for atherogenesis and prevent CVD in patients with DM.

Resistance Exercise Training in DM Patients

Only limited direct evidence exists on the possible contribution of resistance exercise training in the management of DM. Tesch et al. demonstrated that muscle biopsy specimens from resistance-trained, nondiabetic men contained glycogen concentrations 50-100% higher than those of physically inactive men in the general population (90). Several exercise training studies have confirmed that as little as 4 weeks of resistance training increases muscle glycogen synthesis in elderly, previously sedentary, healthy subjects (62). Pascoe and Gladden concluded that the rate of glycogen synthesis with resistance training is increased considerably higher than after prolonged endurance exercise training (67). Recently, Tabata et al. determined that resistance training during 19 days of bed rest prevented the decline in GLUT-4 content in the vastus lateralis muscle in healthy young men in comparison to a control group that remained inactive during bed rest (89). However, it remains to be demonstrated whether resistance training also can stimulate muscle glycogen synthesis and GLUT-4 activity in individuals with diabetes in the presence of an absolute or relative insufficiency of insulin.

Another potential mechanism by which resistance training might help in the management of DM is by increasing skeletal muscle mass, since muscle is the principal source of glucose disposal (2, 17, 84). In cross-sectional studies comparing healthy male athletes with sedentary control subjects, a significant positive correlation ($r = 0.54$) was observed between muscle mass and insulin sensitivity (98). Resistance training clearly produces significant skeletal muscle hypertrophy even in elderly individuals (30, 33), with an associated increase in insulin sensitivity (99). Based on these observations, it is postulated that resistance training might be useful in the management of DM and perhaps also in the primary prevention of type 2 DM by reducing the development of or reversing some of the muscle atrophy associated with aging and physical inactivity.

However, absolute muscle mass clearly is not the only determinant of insulin sensitivity in the body. Obese individuals with an absolute muscle mass similar to that of weightlifters were reported to have significantly poorer glucose tolerance than the weightlifters. This is related to the fact that the body's fat mass is inversely related to insulin sensitivity (16, 36, 77), especially if fat has accumulated in the abdominal region (91, 92). Therefore, weight reduction also is important in the prevention and management of type 2 diabetes. However, weight reduction by dietary restriction is accompanied by a concomitant loss of muscle mass, though this loss can be significantly reduced by adding either regular aerobic or resistance exercise training. This is illustrated in a study by Rice et al., in which obese normoglycemic men were randomly assigned to one of the following three groups: a group on a weight-reduction diet plus aerobic exercise; a group receiving a similar diet plus resistance exercise; or a group on only a diet (76). These investigators reported an additive improvement in insulin sensitivity with a weight-reduction diet plus either aerobic or resistance training as compared with dieting alone (76). In another study involving men with hyperinsulinemia, the combination of resistance training and endurance exercise training was found to be more effective than endurance training alone in reducing fat mass, fasting insulin and glucose concentrations, and plasma triglycerides and systolic blood pressure levels, as well as in increasing HDL cholesterol levels (95). This latter study demonstrates the potential value of a combination of resistance exercise and aerobic training in the management, and possibly prevention, of type 2 DM and associated risk factors for CVD.

A limited number of studies, summarized in table 16.1, demonstrated the value of resistance training alone in improving glycemic control and glucose-insulin dynamics in type 1 and 2 DM. A single session of resistance exercise was reported to significantly improve insulin sensitivity in type 2 DM subjects as demonstrated by a reduced area under the insulin curve during an oral glucose tolerance test (OGTT) (31). The effects of resistance exercise training on insulin sensitivity and glycemic control in subjects with DM are summarized in table 16.1 and discussed in the following paragraphs. In these studies, glucose and insulin measurements were taken at least 48 h after the last exercise session to determine the true training adaptations.

Only two of these resistance training studies involved sedentary type 1 diabetic subjects (22, 63). In these studies, 10-12 weeks of resistance training, 3 times per week at 40-50% of one-repetition maximum (1-RM), was reported to significantly improve self-monitored blood glucose and Hb A_{1c} levels. Similarly, data on the effects of resistance exercise on

TABLE 16.1 Results From Studies on Effects of Resistance Exercise on Glucose Insulin Dynamics in Diabetics and Hyperinsulinemic Nondiabetic Subjects

Reference	Subjects	Frequency and duration	Intensity	Results
Durak et al. 1990 (22)	8 males with type 1 DM	3× week for 10 wks	Initially 50% BW on the bench press and 100% BW on the leg press	1.1% decrease in Hb A_{1c} and a reduction in self-monitored blood glucose levels
Mosher et al. 1998 (63)	10 previously sedentary men with uncomplicated type 1 DM	3× week for 12 wks	Initially 40% of 1-RM for upper body and 50% of 1-RM for lower body, with increases of 2.3 kg when more then 20 reps were accomplished	1% decrease in Hb A_{1c}
Wallace et al. 1997 (95)	16 sedentary, nondiabetic, but hyperinsulinemic men	3× week for 14 wks	75% of 1-RM; 4 sets of 8-10 reps	Significantly greater decrease in fasting insulin levels with endurance plus resistance exercise as compared with endurance training alone

Reference	Subjects	Frequency and duration	Intensity	Results
Smutok et al. 1993 (86)	40 sedentary men at high risk for CHD (half of whom had type 2 DM)	3× week for 20 wks	12-15 reps	Significant decrease in fasting insulin and in insulin area under the curve during an OGTT; no change in % body fat
Fluckey et al. 1994 (31)	17 sedentary men and 6 sedentary women with type 2 DM, and 7 healthy controls	Only one bout	75% 1-RM, 3 sets of 10 reps	Increase in insulin sensitivity 18 h after last exercise bout
Ishii et al. 1998 (46)	17 sedentary men with type 2 DM	5× week for 4-6 wks	2 sets, 10 reps upper body and 20 reps lower body	48% increase in insulin sensitivity during a hyperglycemic, euglycemic clamp technique; no change in $\dot{V}O_2max$
Eriksson et al. 1997 (24)	4 sedentary women and 4 sedentary men with moderate obesity and type 2 DM	2× week for 12 wks	Initially 50% of 1-RM, 1 set of 15-20 reps	Significant decrease in Hb A_{1c} and self-monitored blood glucose; no change in $\dot{V}O_2max$
Honkola et al. 1997 (42)	21 sedentary women and 17 sedentary men with obesity and type 2 DM	2× week for 20 wks	1-RM, 2 sets of 12-15 reps	Significant decrease in Hb A_{1c}
Dunstan et al. 1998 (21)	10 sedentary women and 17 sedentary men with obesity and type 2 DM	3× week for 8 wks	3 sets, 10-15 reps	Decrease in self-monitored blood glucose and increased insulin sensitivity

DM = Diabetes mellitus
BW = Body weight
1-RM = One-repetition maximum
CHD = Coronary heart disease
OGTT = Oral glucose tolerance test

glycemic control in individuals with type 2 DM are limited to only a few studies (24, 31, 42, 46, 86). In one of these studies, Ishii et al. had men with type 2 DM perform resistance exercise for the upper and lower body 5 times per week for 4-6 weeks (46). This training resulted in a 48% increase in insulin sensitivity over pretraining levels. In a study by Dunstan et al., involving 10 women and 17 men with type 2 DM, 3 sessions of resistance training per week for 8 weeks resulted in a significant decrease in self-monitored blood glucose levels and signifi-cant improvements in insulin sensitivity, as compared with a control group (21). In these studies, the beneficial effects of resistance training on glycemic control and insulin sensitivity in type 2 diabetic subjects were independent of both weight loss and the extent of improvement in $\dot{V}O_2$max (46). In addition, one resistance training study also demon-strated a concomitant improvement in the plasma lipid profile, with a reduction in plasma total and low-density lipoprotein (LDL) cholesterol and triglyceride levels in addition to improvements in glycemic control (42). However, in another study Eriksson et al. failed to find blood lipid changes following resistance training (24). Similar contradictory find-ings exist regarding the effects of aerobic exercise on the blood lipid profiles of nondiabetic individuals.

Although much additional research is required, these preliminary findings strongly suggest that resistance exercise is beneficial as an adjunct therapy in the management of diabetes, and perhaps in helping prevent type 2 DM in susceptible individuals. Postulated mechanisms by which resistance exercise training can improve blood glucose control include increased skeletal muscle mass, glucose uptake, and glycogen synthesis. It also appears from the above studies that the effects of resistance exercise in improving glucose tolerance can be achieved independent of weight loss or an increase in $\dot{V}O_2$max. Furthermore, when resistance exercise is combined with aerobic exercise and/or weight loss through diet, the effects on glycemic control and glucose tolerance would be expected to be significantly better than with any of the single-treatment modalities alone; however, this remains to be proven.

Safety of Resistance Exercise and Contraindications

Exercise in patients with DM occasionally results in adverse effects, ranging from slight soft tissue injuries to disabling and even life-threatening problems (12, 40). Therefore, before being prescribed an exercise program, the patient with DM should have a thorough medical evaluation to screen for the presence of predisposing factors for exercise-related complications and to rule out contraindications to exercise (see table 16.2). In addition, the patient needs to receive advice on proper

TABLE 16.2 Contraindications for Resistance Exercise for Patients With DM

1. Unstable angina
2. Uncontrolled hypertension; systolic blood pressure > 160 mmHg; diastolic blood pressure > 100 mmHg
3. Uncontrolled cardiac arrhythmias
4. Recent history of severe congestive heart failure
5. Aerobic capacity < 6 METs during symptom-limited exercise test
6. ST-segment depression before completion of stage 3 of the Bruce protocol
7. Left-ventricular ejection fraction < 45%
8. Active pericarditis or myocarditis
9. Thrombophlebitis
10. Third-degree AV block
11. Resting ECG ST-segment displacement > 3 mm
12. Severe proliferative retinopathy
13. Blood glucose values < 100 mg/dl or > 250 mg/dl

weightlifting techniques and about precautions that should be taken before engaging in an exercise program.

As previously indicated, DM is associated with increased risk of serious long-term complications, including diabetic retinopathy, chronic renal failure, peripheral neuropathy, and CVD. However, despite these potential complications, there are relatively few reported cases of serious adverse effects experienced by individuals with diabetes during resistance exercise. The relative safety of resistance training is illustrated by Powell et al., who in a recent observational study surveyed more than 5000 individuals in the general population for exercise participation and associated injuries (73). About 25% of this population engaged in weightlifting. Injuries related to weightlifting were reported in about 2% of those individuals, and in only 25% of those injured were the injuries serious enough to require medical attention or to miss half a day or more from work, housework, or school. In another study, from the Preventive Medicine Facility in the Cooper Clinic in Dallas, Texas, and the Center for Exercise Science at the University of Florida, not a single case of cardiovascular complications requiring medical intervention was observed during over 26,000 maximal strength assessments in almost 13,000 healthy people, some of whom had several risk factors for CVD (38). Despite these reassuring reports on the relative safety of resistance exercise, serious and potentially fatal complications during resistance exercise have been reported. For example, Haykowsky et al. reported three cases of subarachnoid hemorrhage in individuals during weight training sessions due to rupture of congenital cerebral artery aneurysms (40). In the relatively few resistance training studies previously referred to involving DM subjects, there were no reported serious complications during training (21, 22, 24, 31, 42, 46, 86). Therefore, in DM patients without major complications, well-supervised resistance exercise appears to be a safe mode of exercise for improving physical fitness and health status.

Since DM patients are at a higher risk of CVD than individuals without diabetes, the pre-exercise medical evaluation should include an exercise stress test for patients with type 1 DM over age 30 or for those who have had diabetes for over 15 years (58). Patients with type 2 DM should have a graded exercise test if they are over the age of 35 (58, 87). In addition, all patients with DM should be in reasonably good metabolic control before initiating an exercise program—that is, fasting blood glucose values should be between 100 and 250 mg/dl (58, 87).

Although to date no adverse effects of resistance training on preexisting diabetic retinopathy have been reported, severe proliferative retinopathy is generally considered a contraindication for strenuous aerobic or resistance exercise, because of concern about precipitating retinal hemorrhage (table 16.2). Duane coined the term Valsalva hemorrhagic retinopathy (VHR) to refer to development of retinal hemorrhage in response to a sudden rise in intrathoracic or intra-abdominal pressure (20). VHR has been observed during resistance exercise in healthy nondiabetic individuals (71) and was reported in a diabetic patient during an intense bout of emesis (50). To study the safety of exercise training in patients with proliferative diabetic retinopathy, Bernbaum et al. designed a 12-week aerobic exercise training program specifically for such patients (4). Forty-seven diabetic patients with moderate to severe retinopathy were exercised on a bicycle ergometer at increasing intensities until they achieved a systolic blood pressure 50 mmHg over baseline levels or a maximum of 200 mmHg. No new retinal hemorrhages were observed in any of the study participants. Based on these findings, it appears that diabetic patients with severe retinopathy can safely engage in exercise as long as they maintain systolic blood pressure levels below 200 mmHg; however, confirming evidence is needed.

Hypoglycemia is a common problem in diabetic individuals on insulin therapy. Hypoglycemic reactions are associated with blood glucose levels generally less than 60 mg/dl. Accompanying symptoms include hunger, anxiety, tachycardia, sweating, dizziness, and headache. One or more of these symptoms may provide the individual with DM with an early warning of the impending problem. Untreated severe hypoglycemia can lead to serious central nervous system problems, including mental confusion, abnormal behavior, loss of consciousness, and convulsions. Individuals with well-controlled DM are particularly prone to hypoglycemia, resulting either from a relative excess dose of insulin (or less commonly of an oral hypoglycemic agent), skipped meals, reduced food intake, or increased physical activity uncompensated for by extra food intake (60). Hypoglycemic episodes may occur before, during, and for up to 30 h after prolonged exercise. Exercising at the time of peak insulin activity, particularly if the insulin was administered into a limb participating in the activity, increases the likelihood of hypoglycemia. It is important for the individual with DM to self-monitor blood glucose levels before, during, and after exercise. If pre-exercise blood glucose levels are below 100 mg/dl, the individual with DM should delay initiating exercise until after consuming a snack containing 15-20 g of rapidly absorbed carbohydrates and monitoring the subsequent increase in blood glucose level. In addition, the diabetic exerciser should be trained to recognize early warning symptoms of hypoglycemia, and to promptly discontinue exercise and have a plan in place to manage the problem as outlined in table 16.3.

Resistance Exercise Prescription

Before starting a resistance exercise program, the exercise leader or health professional designing and supervising the exercise program should carefully demonstrate the proper weightlifting techniques and allow the patient to practice them, starting with very light weights or an unloaded bar. Each exercise session should be preceded by a warm-up period of 5-15 min, consisting of light aerobic exercises, calisthenics, and lifting light weights. Exercise sessions should be followed by a similar period of cool-down exercises. The patient also should be instructed not to excessively squeeze the bar handle, since this can cause an exaggerated rise in systolic blood pressure during the concentric phase of the contraction. Both concentric and eccentric contractions should be

TABLE 16.3 Recommendations in the Event of Hypoglycemia in a DM Patient, Before, During, or After a Bout of Exercise

1. If blood glucose is <100 mg/dl before starting an exercise session, consume 15-20 g of carbohydrates and wait 15-30 min; recheck blood glucose levels and only restart exercise if blood glucose is >100 mg/dl.
2. If symptoms appear during exercise, stop immediately and recheck blood glucose levels.
3. If blood glucose monitoring is not available at place of exercise, eat 15-30 g of fast-acting carbohydrates prior to prolonged exercise.
4. Also consume 15-30 g of carbohydrates as soon as possible if blood glucose following exercise is <60 mg/dl.

performed slowly for the whole range of motion. While performing the concentric contraction, the exerciser should exhale slowly in order to avoid the Valsalva maneuver and the subsequent rise in intra-arterial blood pressure. Every set of exercises should last between 45 and 180 s, with only about a minute between sets for optimal training effects (87).

General guidelines for prescribing resistance exercise for sedentary individuals with DM are outlined in table 16.4. The intensity of resistance exercise for each muscle group is determined after assessing the load that the individual can lift only one time (1-RM). This also establishes baseline values for subsequently assessing improvements in strength with training. To determine 1-RM, a weight estimated as approximately 50% of 1-RM is initially selected for the individual to perform a single lift. The load is then progressively increased in consecutive lifts until the actual 1-RM is achieved. Since individuals with DM are at increased risk for cardiovascular complications, and resistance exercise can abruptly increase systolic blood pressure, perhaps a safer approach is to determine the load that the individual can lift only 10 times (10-RM) instead of 1-RM (87). The initial weight for upper-body exercises should be 30-40% of 1-RM and 50-60% of 1-RM for lower body. Alternatively, intensity can be determined using Borg's rating of perceived exertion (RPE) scale (5). The starting weight for initiating a resistance training program should be perceived as light to somewhat hard (12-13 on the original Borg RPE scale). Reevaluations of an exercise program should initially be performed every 2-3 weeks in order to upgrade the exercise prescription. The intensity of resistance exercise should be gradually increased to a maximum of 70% of 1-RM or up to an RPE of 15-16 (29), based on the response and health of the patient. At this intensity level, systolic blood pressure generally will be maintained within clinically acceptable levels (below 200 mmHg) (72). When the recommended weights lifted are again perceived to be light to some-

TABLE 16.4 General Guidelines for Resistance Exercise Program for Type 2 DM Patients

1. Include 8-10 exercises involving all major muscle groups of the upper and lower body and the trunk.
2. Frequency: 2-3 times per week.
3. Intensity should start at 40-50% of 1-RM and be gradually increased every 2-3 weeks up to 70% of 1-RM, depending on health status of the patient.
4. 1-2 sets of 12-15 repetitions, with not more than 60 s between sets.
5. Follow proper weightlifting techniques and precautions.
6. First exercise large muscle groups, then small muscle groups.

what hard (RPE 12-13), or if the exerciser is able to perform more repetitions than initially recommended, the amount of weight lifted should be increased by about 5% increments. However, if an individual is not able to lift a weight more than 8 times, the weight should be lowered to reduce risk of injuries (72).

An optimal resistance exercise training program should include sets of at least 8-9 different exercises that involve large and small muscle groups of the upper and lower body, back, chest, and abdominal muscles. Ten to 15 repetitions each of a set of these exercises should be performed in about 30-45 min. A recent review by Feigenbaum and Pollock on resistance exercise training concluded that a single set of repetitions per muscle group was as effective as 3 sets in improving muscular strength (29), but this requires further confirmation. In the studies previously mentioned, 1 or 2 sets of 12 or 15 repetitions, 2-3 times per week for up to 5 months, were reported to significantly improve glucose tolerance in type 2 DM and decrease Hb A_{1c} and blood glucose levels in diabetic patients (20, 21, 23, 30, 41, 45, 81).

For an ideal resistance exercise program, the following types of exercises are advised: leg presses, leg extensors, leg curls, torso extension, bench press, lateral pull-down, shoulder press, biceps curl, triceps extension, abdominal crunch, and back extension. For elderly patients, machine exercises provide a safer option than free weights, especially if balance is a problem. However, lifting free weights more closely resembles activities of daily living, such as carrying bags or lifting objects; therefore the principle of specificity should be applied, depending on the needs and condition of the patient.

Despite a strong effort from public health advocates to increase the level of habitual physical activity in the general population, the percentage of people who engage in the recommended minimal amount of physical activity (at least 30 min on most, preferably all, days of the week) is very low (32, 68, 88). Data from the National Health Interview Survey showed that people with diabetes were less likely to report exercising regularly than people without the disease (32). Furthermore, individuals with diabetes engage less frequently in jogging, aerobics, dancing, calisthenics, bicycling, weightlifting, several ball sports, and skiing than people without the disease (32). In addition, only 50% of those who initiate an exercise program continue the program after 24 weeks (19). Therefore, special efforts must be made by the health care team to encourage diabetic patients to start and continue on a regular exercise program. Some of the behavior modification methods utilized to increase adherence to an exercise program are summarized in table 16.5. These include helping the participant identify times and places to exercise, making the exercise enjoyable, exercising in groups, and having spouse or friends participate and support exercise activities.

TABLE 16.5   Guidelines for Improving Exercise Adherence

1. Make the exercise enjoyable. Be creative.
2. Tailor the intensity, duration, and frequency of the exercise to patient needs and capabilities. Don't overtrain or undertrain.
3. Promote exercising with a group for social support.
4. Set goals and reinforce success.
5. Help locate a convenient place to exercise.
6. Use music while exercising. Don't lose the rhythm.
7. Explain the beneficial effects of exercise in helping control diabetes and preventing complications, especially CVD.

Adapted from Weinberg and Gould 1995 (97).

An exercise prescription should be tailored to the individual's needs and preferences. Regular aerobic and resistance exercise generally is recommended to patients with DM to improve glucose control, increase cardiovascular fitness, lose excess weight, reduce risk factors for CVD, and improve quality of life. Resistance exercise also may be prescribed to improve athletic performance in young type 1 DM individuals participating in competitive sports as well as for diabetic master athletes. The goal should be to design an individualized exercise program that properly balances the potential benefits and risks of exercise.

Summary and Conclusions

Diabetes mellitus is a major and growing public health problem in the United States and other economically developed Western countries. It is associated with excess morbidity and mortality related to microvascular and macrovascular complications resulting in loss of vision, renal failure, neurological damage, and coronary heart disease, stroke, and peripheral vascular disease. The value of regular endurance exercise as an adjunct therapy for improving glycemic control alone or in combination with diet, insulin, or hypoglycemic drugs has long been recognized. More recently, epidemiological cohort studies and clinical trials have demonstrated that regular endurance exercise is of value in the primary prevention of type 2 diabetes. Multiple mechanisms appear to contribute to the apparent beneficial effects of aerobic exercise in the management of this disease. These include enhanced glucose uptake, oxidation, and storage as glycogen independent of and additive to the effects of insulin. In addition, exercise also increases muscle blood flow and mitochondrial oxidative capacity, and reduces body fat, particularly from central and visceral fat depots. Endurance exercise training can also decrease mean blood pressure and triglyceride levels and increase blood levels of HDL, thereby decreasing important risk factors for CVD.

Recently a limited number of small-scale studies also have demonstrated the potential value and relative safety of resistance training as an adjunct therapy in the management of diabetes. The principal apparent biological mechanism involved is skeletal muscle hypertrophy, with an associated increased glucose uptake and insulin sensitivity.

Medical screening of diabetic individuals prior to initiating an exercise program is recommended, and exercise prescription guidelines for a progressive resistance exercise training program for type 2 DM patients are presented in table 16.4. Individuals with DM who follow these guidelines should be able to safely improve muscular strength and endurance, which can not only improve diabetic control, but also substantially improve capacity for independent living and enhanced quality of life in older individuals with diabetes.

Acknowledgment

The authors wish to thanks Dr. Judith Regensteiner for her thorough review and critique of this manuscript and her helpful comments.

References

1. Andersen, H., P.C. Gadeberg, and J. Jakobsen. 1997. Muscular atrophy in diabetic neuropathy: A sterological magnetic resonance imaging study. *Diabetologia* 40: 1062-1069.
2. Baron, A.D., G. Brechtel, P. Wallace, and S.V. Edelman. 1988. Rates and tissue sites of non-insulin- and insulin-mediated glucose uptake in humans. *American Journal of Physiology* 255: E769-E774.
3. Beck-Nielsen, H., J.E. Henriksen, A. Vaag, and O. Hother-Nielsen. 1995. Pathophysiology of non-insulin-dependent diabetes mellitus (NIDDM). *Diabetes Research and Clinical Practice* 28: S13-S25.
4. Bernbaum, M., S.G. Albert, J.D. Cohen, and A. Drimmer. 1989. Cardiovascular conditioning in individuals with diabetic retinopathy. *Diabetes Care* 12: 740-742.
5. Borg, G.A. 1982. Psychophysical bases of perceived exertion. *Medicine and Science in Sports and Exercise* 14: 377-381.
6. Bruno, G., F. Merletti, P. Boffetta, P. Cavallo-Perin, G. Bargero, G. Gallone, and G. Pagano. 1999. Impact of glycaemic control, hypertension and insulin treatment on general and cause-specific mortality: An Italian population-based cohort of type II (non-insulin-dependent) diabetes mellitus. *Diabetologia* 42: 297-301.
7. Cameron, N.E., M.A. Cotter, and S. Robertson. 1990. Changes in skeletal muscle contractile properties in streptozocin-induced diabetic rats and role of polyol pathway and hypoinsulinemia. *Diabetes* 39: 460-465.
8. Cameron, N.E., M.A. Cotter, and S. Robertson. 1992. Angiotensin converting enzyme inhibition prevents development of muscle and nerve dysfunction and stimulates angiogenesis in streptozotocin-diabetic rats. *Diabetologia* 35: 12-18.
9. Centers for Disease Control and Prevention. 1996. Blindness caused by diabetes—Massachusetts, 1987-1994. *Morbidity and Mortality Weekly Report* 45: 937-941.

10. Centers for Disease Control and Prevention. *Diabetes surveillance, 1997.* **http://www.cdc.gov/diabetes/statistics/surv197/pdf/**

11. Centers for Disease Control and Prevention. 1999. Self-reported prevalence of diabetes among Hispanics—United States, 1994-1997. *Morbidity and Mortality Weekly Report* 48: 8-12.

12. Compton, D., P.M. Hill, and J.D. Sinclair. 1973. Weight-lifters' blackout. *Lancet* 2: 1234-1237.

13. Costa, A., M. Rios, R. Casamitjana, R. Gomis, and I. Conget. 1998. High prevalence of abnormal glucose tolerance and metabolic disturbances in first degree relatives of NIDDM patients. A study in Catalonia, a Mediterranean community. *Diabetes Research and Clinical Practice* 41: 191-196.

14. Cotter, M., N. Cameron, S. Robertson, and I. Ewing. 1993. Polyol pathway-related skeletal muscle contractile and morphological abnormalities in diabetic rats. *Experimental Physiology* 78: 139-155.

15. Cox, J.H., R.N. Cortright, G.L. Dohm, and J.A. Houmard. 1999. Effect of aging on response to exercise training in humans: Skeletal muscle GLUT-4 and insulin sensitivity. *Journal of Applied Physiology* 86: 2019-2025.

16. Craig, B.W., J. Everhart, and R. Brown. 1989. The influence of high-resistance training on glucose tolerance in young and elderly subjects. *Mechanisms of Ageing and Development* 49: 147-157.

17. DeFronzo, R.A., E. Jacot, E. Jequier, E. Maeder, J. Wahren, and J.P. Felber. 1981. The effect of insulin on the disposal of intravenous glucose. Results from indirect calorimetry and hepatic and femoral venous catheterization. *Diabetes* 30: 1000-1007.

18. Diabetes Control and Complications Trial Research Group. 1993. The effect of intensive treatment of diabetes on the development and progression of long-term complications in insulin-dependent diabetes mellitus. *New England Journal of Medicine* 329: 977-986.

19. Dishman, R.K. 1988. *Exercise adherence: Its impact on public health.* Champaign, IL: Human Kinetics.

20. Duane, T.D. 1973. Valsalva hemorrhagic retinopathy. *American Journal of Ophthalmology* 75: 637-642.

21. Dunstan, D.W., I.B. Puddey, L.J. Beilin, V. Burke, A.R. Morton, and K.G. Stanton. 1998. Effects of a short-term circuit weight training program on glycaemic control in NIDDM. *Diabetes Research and Clinical Practice* 40: 53-61.

22. Durak, E.P., L. Jovanovic-Peterson, and C.M. Peterson. 1990. Randomized crossover study of effect of resistance training on glycemic control, muscular strength, and cholesterol in type I diabetic men. *Diabetes Care* 13: 1039-1043.

23. Edelman, S.V. 1998. Type II diabetes mellitus. *Advances in Internal Medicine* 43: 449-500.

24. Eriksson, J., S. Taimela, K. Eriksson, S. Parviainen, J. Peltonen, and U. Kujala. 1997. Resistance training in the treatment of non-insulin-dependent diabetes mellitus. *International Journal of Sports Medicine* 18: 242-246.

25. Eriksson, K.F., and F. Lindgarde. 1998. No excess 12-year mortality in men with impaired glucose tolerance who participated in the Malmo Preventive Trial with diet and exercise. *Diabetologia* 41: 1010-1016.

26. Etgen, G.J., J. Jensen, C.M. Wilson, D.G. Hunt, S.W. Cushman, and J.L. Ivy. 1997. Exercise training reverses insulin resistance in muscle by enhanced recruitment of GLUT-4 to the cell surface. *American Journal of Physiology* 272: E864-E869.

27. Expert Committee on the Diagnosis and Classification of Diabetes Mellitus. 1997. Report of Expert Committee on the diagnosis and classification of diabetes mellitus. *Diabetes Care* 20: 1183-1197.

28. Fauci, A.S., E. Braunwald, K.J. Isselbacher, J.D. Wilson, J.B. Martin, D.L. Kasper. 1997. *Harrison's principles of internal medicine.* 14th ed. New York: McGraw-Hill.

29. Feigenbaum, M.S., and M.L. Pollock. 1999. Prescription of resistance training for health and disease. *Medicine and Science in Sports and Exercise* 31: 38-45.

30. Fiatarone, M.A., E.C. Marks, N.D. Ryan, C.N. Meredith, L.A. Lipsitz, and W.J. Evans. 1990. High-intensity strength training in nonagenarians. Effects on skeletal muscle. *Journal of the American Medical Association* 263: 3029-3034.

31. Fluckey, J.D., M.S. Hickey, J.K. Brambrink, K.K. Hart, K. Alexander, and B.W. Craig. 1994. Effects of resistance exercise on glucose tolerance in normal and glucose-intolerant subjects. *Journal of Applied Physiology* 77: 1087-1092.

32. Ford, E.S., and W.H. Herman. 1995. Leisure-time physical activity patterns in the U.S. diabetic population. Findings from the 1990 National Health Interview Survey—Health Promotion and Disease Prevention Supplement. *Diabetes Care* 18: 27-33.

33. Frontera, W.R., C.N. Meredith, K.P. O'Reilly, H.G. Knuttgen, and W.J. Evans. 1988. Strength conditioning in older men: Skeletal muscle hypertrophy and improved function. *Journal of Applied Physiology* 64: 1038-1044.

34. Gaster, B., and I.B. Hirsch. 1998. The effects of improved glycemic control on complications in type 2 diabetes. *Archives of Internal Medicine* 158: 134-140.

35. Godsland, I.F., F. Leyva, C. Walton, M. Worthington, and J.C. Stevenson. 1998. Associations of smoking, alcohol and physical activity with risk factors for coronary heart disease and diabetes in the first follow-up cohort of the Heart Disease and Diabetes Risk Indicators in a Screened Cohort study (HDDRISC-1). *Journal of Internal Medicine* 244: 33-41.

36. Goodpaster, B.H., F.L. Thaete, J.A. Simoneau, and D.E. Kelley. 1997. Subcutaneous abdominal fat and thigh muscle composition predict insulin sensitivity independently of visceral fat. *Diabetes* 46: 1579-1585.

37. Goodyear, L.J., and B.B. Kahn. 1998. Exercise, glucose transport, and insulin sensitivity. *Annual Review of Medicine* 49: 235-261.

38. Gordon, N.F., H.W. Kohl III, M.L. Pollock, H. Vaandrager, L.W. Gibbons, and S.N. Blair. 1995. Cardiovascular safety of maximal strength testing in healthy adults. *American Journal of Cardiology* 76: 851-853.

39. Harris, M.I., K.M. Flegal, C.C. Cowie, et al. 1998. Prevalence of diabetes, impaired fasting glucose, and impaired glucose tolerance in U.S. adults. The Third National Health and Nutrition Examination Survey, 1988-1994. *Diabetes Care* 21: 518-524.

40. Haykowsky, M.J., J.M. Findlay, and A.P. Ignaszewski. 1996. Aneurysmal subarachnoid hemorrhage associated with weight training: Three case reports. *Clinical Journal of Sports Medicine* 6: 52-55.

41. Helmrich, S.P., D.R. Ragland, R.W. Leung, and R.S. Paffenbarger Jr. 1991. Physical activity and reduced occurrence of non-insulin-dependent diabetes mellitus. *New England Journal of Medicine* 325: 147-152.

42. Honkola, A., T. Forsen, and J. Eriksson. 1997. Resistance training improves the metabolic profile in individuals with type 2 diabetes. *Acta Diabetologica* 34: 245-248.

43. Host, H.H., P.A. Hansen, L.A. Nolte, M.M. Chen, and J.O. Holloszy. 1998. Rapid reversal of adaptive increases in muscle GLUT-4 and glucose transport capacity after training cessation. *Journal of Applied Physiology* 84: 798-802.

44. Hughes, V.A., M.A. Fiatarone, R.A. Fielding, C.M. Ferrara, D. Elahi, and W.J. Evans. 1995. Long-term effects of a high-carbohydrate diet and exercise on insulin action in older subjects with impaired glucose tolerance. *American Journal of Clinical Nutrition* 62: 426-433.

45. Humphriss, D.B., M.W. Stewart, T.S. Berrish, L.A. Barriocanal, L.R. Trajano, L.A. Ashworth, M.D. Brown, M. Miller, P.J. Avery, K.G. Alberti, and M. Walker. 1997. Multiple metabolic abnormalities in normal glucose tolerant relatives of NIDDM families. *Diabetologia* 40: 1185-1190.

46. Ishii, T., T. Yamakita, T. Sato, S. Tanaka, and S. Fujii. 1998. Resistance training improves insulin sensitivity in NIDDM subjects without altering maximal oxygen uptake. *Diabetes Care* 21: 1353-1355.

47. Ivy, J.L., T.W. Zderic, and D.L. Fogt. 1999. Prevention and treatment of non-insulin dependent diabetes mellitus. In *Exercise and sport sciences reviews*, vol. 27, 1-35, edited by J.O. Holloszy. Philadelphia: Lipincott Williams & Wilkins.

48. Jaap, A.J., and J.E. Tooke. 1995. Pathophysiology of microvascular disease in non-insulin-dependent diabetes [editorial]. *Clinical Science* 89: 3-12.

49. Kang, J., R. Robertson, J.M. Hagberg, D.E. Kelley, F.L. Goss, S.G. DaSilva, R.R. Suminski, and A.C. Utter. 1996. Effect of exercise intensity on glucose and insulin metabolism in obese individuals and obese NIDDM patients. *Diabetes Care* 19: 341-349.

50. Kassoff, A., R.A. Catalano, and M. Mehu. 1988. Vitreous hemorrhage and the Valsalva maneuver in proliferative diabetic retinopathy. *Retina* 8: 174-176.

51. Kawanaka, K., M. Higuchi, H. Ohmori, S. Shimegi, O. Ezaki, and S. Katsuta. 1995. Muscle contractile activity modulates GLUT-4 protein content in the absence of insulin. *Hormone and Metabolic Research* 28: 75-80.

52. Kawanaka, K., I. Tabata, S. Katsuta, and M. Higuchi. 1997. Changes in insulin-stimulated glucose transport and GLUT-4 protein in rat skeletal muscle after training. *Journal of Applied Physiology* 83: 2043-2047.

53. Kennedy, J.W., M.F. Hirshman, E.V. Gervino, J.V. Ocel, R.A. Forse, S.J. Hoenig, D. Aronson, L.J. Goodyear, and E.S. Horton. 1999. Acute exercise induces GLUT4 translocation in skeletal muscle of normal human subjects and subjects with type 2 diabetes. *Diabetes* 48: 1192-1197.

54. King, H., R.E. Aubert, and W.H. Herman. 1998. Global burden of diabetes, 1995-2025: Prevalence, numerical estimates, and projections. *Diabetes Care* 21: 1414-1431.

55. Koval, J.A., R.A. DeFronzo, R.M O'Doherty, et al. 1998. Regulation of hexokinase II activity and expression in human muscle by moderate exercise. *American Journal of Physiology* 274: E304-308.

56. Lehmann, R., V. Kaplan, R. Bingisser, K.E. Bloch, and G.A. Spinas. 1997. Impact of physical activity on cardiovascular risk factors in IDDM. *Diabetes Care* 20: 1603-1611.

57. Lehmann, R., A. Vokac, K. Niedermann, K. Agosti, and G.A. Spinas. 1995. Loss of abdominal fat and improvement of the cardiovascular risk profile by regular moderate exercise training in patients with NIDDM. *Diabetologia* 38: 1313-1319.

58. Leon, A.S. 1989. Patients with diabetes mellitus. In *Exercise in modern medicine*, 118-145, edited by B.A. Franklin, S. Gordon, and G.C. Timmis. Baltimore: Williams & Wilkins.

59. Lynch, J., S.P. Helmrich, T.A. Lakka, G.A. Kaplan, R.D. Cohen, R. Salonen, and J.T. Salonen. 1996. Moderately intense physical activities and high levels of cardiorespiratory fitness reduce the risk of non-insulin-dependent diabetes mellitus in middle-aged men. *Archives of Internal Medicine* 156: 1307-1314.

60. MacDonald, M.J. 1987. Postexercise late-onset hypoglycemia in insulin-dependent diabetic patients. *Diabetes Care* 10: 584-588.

61. Mayer-Davis, E.J., R. D'Agostino, A.J. Karter, S.M. Haffner, M.J. Rewers, M. Saad, and R.N. Bergman. 1998. Intensity and amount of physical activity in relation to insulin sensitivity (The Insulin Resistance Atherosclerosis Study). *Journal of the American Medical Association* 279: 669-674.

62. Miller, J.P., R.E. Pratley, A.P. Goldberg, P. Gordon, M.A. Rubin, M.S. Treuth, A.S. Ryan, and B.F. Hurley. 1994. Strength training increases insulin action in healthy 50- to 65-yr-old men. *Journal of Applied Physiology* 77: 1122-1127.

63. Mosher, P.E., M.S. Nash, A.C. Perry, A.R. LaPerriere, and R.B. Goldberg. 1998. Aerobic circuit exercise training: Effect on adolescents with well-controlled insulin-dependent diabetes mellitus. *Archives of Physical Medicine and Rehabilitation* 79: 652-657.

64. Mourier, A., J.-F. Gautier, E. De Kerviler, A.X. Bigard, J.-M. Villette, J.-P. Garnier, A. Duvallet, C.Y. Guezennec, and G. Cathelineau. 1997. Mobilization of visceral adipose tissue related to the improvement in insulin sensitivity in response to physical training in NIDDM. *Diabetes Care* 20: 385-391.

65. Nakatani, A., D.H. Han, P.A. Hansen, L.A. Nolte, H.H. Host, R.C. Hickner, and J.O. Holloszy. 1997. Effect of endurance exercise training on muscle glycogen supercompensation in rats. *Journal of Applied Physiology* 82: 711-715.

66. Pan, X.R., G.W. Li, Y.H. Hu, A. Zuoxin, W. Jixing, P.H. Bennett, and B.V. Howard. 1997. Effects of diet and exercise in preventing NIDDM in people with impaired glucose tolerance. The Da Qing IGT and Diabetes Study. *Diabetes Care* 20: 537-544.

67. Pascoe, D.D., and L.B. Gladden. 1996. Muscle glycogen resynthesis after short term, high intensity exercise and resistance exercise. *Sports Medicine* 21: 98-118.

68. Pate, R.R., M. Pratt, S.N. Blair, W.L. Haskell, C.A. Macera, C. Bouchard, D. Buchner, C.J. Caspersen, W. Ettinger, G.W. Heath, A.C. King, A.M. Kriska, A.S. Leon, B.H. Marcus, J. Morris, R. Paffenbarger, K. Patrick, M. Pollock, J.M. Rippe, J. Sallis, and J.H. Wilmore. 1995. Physical activity and public health. A recommendation from the Centers for Disease Control and Prevention and the American College of Sports Medicine. *Journal of the American Medical Association* 273: 402-407.

69. Perseghin, G., T. Price, K. Falk Petersen, M. Roden, G.W. Cline, K. Gerow, D.L. Rothman, and G.I. Shulman. 1996. Increased glucose transport-phosphorylation and muscle glycogen synthesis after exercise training in insulin-resistant subjects. *New England Journal of Medicine* 335: 1335-1357.

70. Pirson, Y. 1998. Physiopathology of diabetic nephropathy: What we learn from transplantation (in French). *Nephrologie* 19: 105-109.

71. Pitta, C.G., R.F. Steinert, E.S. Gragoudas, and C.D. Regan. 1980. Small unilateral foveal hemorrhages in young adults. *American Journal of Ophthalmology* 89: 96-102.

72. Pollock, M.L., B.A. Franklin, G.J. Balady, B.L. Chaitman, J.L. Fleg, B. Fletcher, M. Limacher, I.L. Piña, R.A. Stein, M. Williams, and T. Bazzarre. 2000. Resistance exercise in individuals with and without cardiovascular disease: Benefits, rationale, safety and prescription. *Circulation* 101 (7): 828-833.

73. Powell, K.E., G.W. Heath, M.J. Kresnow, J.J. Sacks, and C.M. Branche. 1998. Injury rates from walking, gardening, weightlifting, outdoor bicycling, and aerobics. *Medicine and Science in Sports and Exercise* 30: 1246-1249.

74. Regensteiner, J.G., J. Sippel, E.T. McFarling, E.E. Wolfel, and W.R. Hiatt. 1995. Effects of non-insulin-dependent diabetes on oxygen consumption during treadmill exercise. *Medicine and Science in Sports and Exercise* 27: 875-881.

75. Ren, J.-M., C.F. Semenkovich, E.A. Gulve, J. Gao, and J.O. Holloszy. 1994. Exercise induces rapid increases in GLUT-4 expression, glucose transport capacity and insulin-stimulated glycogen storage in muscle. *Journal of Biological Chemistry* 269: 14396-14401.

76. Rice, B., I. Janssen, R. Hudson, and R. Ross. 1999. Effects of aerobic or resistance exercise and/or diet on glucose tolerance and plasma insulin levels in obese men. *Diabetes Care* 22: 684-691.

77. Ryan, A.S., R.E. Pratley, A.P. Goldberg, and D. Elahi. 1996. Resistive training increases insulin action in postmenopausal women. *Journal of Gerontology. Series A, Biological Sciences and Medical Sciences* 51: M199-M205.

78. Salomaa, V., W. Riley, J.D. Kark, C. Nardo, and A.R. Folsom. 1995. Non-insulin-dependent diabetes mellitus and fasting glucose and insulin concentrations are associated with arterial stiffness indexes. The ARIC Study. Atherosclerosis Risk in Communities Study. *Circulation* 91: 1432-1443.

79. Salsich, G.B., and M.J. Mueller. 1997. Relationships between measures of function, strength and walking speed in patients with diabetes and transmetatarsal amputations. *Clinical Rehabilitation* 11: 60-67.

80. Schneider, S.H., and H. Kanj. 1986. Clinical aspects of exercise and diabetes mellitus. *Current Concepts in Nutrition* 15: 145-182.

81. Schneider, S.H., A.K. Khachadurian, L.F. Amorosa, L. Clemow, and N.B. Ruderman. 1992. Ten-year experience with an exercise-based outpatient life-style modification program in the treatment of diabetes mellitus. *Diabetes Care* 15: 1800-1810.

82. Schneider, S.H., H.C. Kim, A.K. Khachadurian, and N.B. Ruderman. 1988. Impaired fibrinolytic response to exercise in type II diabetes: Effects of exercise and physical training. *Metabolism: Clinical and Experimental* 37: 924-929.

83. Shaw, J.T., D.M. Purdie, H.A. Neil, J.C. Levy, and R.C. Turner. 1999. The relative risks of hyperglycaemia, obesity and dyslipidaemia in the relatives of patients with Type II diabetes mellitus. *Diabetologia* 42: 24-27.

84. Shulman, R.G., G. Bloch, and D.L. Rothman. 1995. In vivo regulation of muscle glycogen synthase and the control of glycogen synthesis. *Proceedings of the National Academy of Sciences of the United States of America* 92: 8535-8542.

85. Singer, D.E., D.M. Nathan, H.A. Fogel, and A.P. Schachat. 1992. Screening for diabetic retinopathy. *Annals of Internal Medicine* 116: 660-671.

86. Smutok, M.A., C. Reece, P.F. Kokkinos, C. Farmer, P. Dawson, J. Shulman, J. De Vane-Bell, J. Patterson, C. Charabogos, A.P. Goldberg, and B.F. Hurley. 1993. Aerobic versus strength training for risk factor intervention in middle-aged men at high risk for coronary heart disease. *Metabolism: Clinical and Experimental* 42: 177-184.

87. Soukup, J.T., T.S. Maynard, and J.E. Kovaleski. 1994. Resistance training guidelines for individuals with diabetes mellitus. *Diabetes Educator* 20: 129-137.

88. Surgeon general's report on physical activity and health. From the Centers for Disease Control and Prevention. 1996. *Journal of the American Medical Association* 276: 522.

89. Tabata, I., Y. Suzuki, T. Fukunaga, T. Yokozeki, H. Akima, and K. Funato. 1999. Resistance training affects GLUT-4 content in skeletal muscle of humans after 19 days of head-down bed rest. *Journal of Applied Physiology* 86: 909-914.

90. Tesch, P.A., E.B. Colliander, and P. Kaiser. 1986. Muscle metabolism during intense, heavy-resistance exercise. *European Journal of Applied Physiology and Occupational Physiology* 55: 362-366.

91. Treuth, M.S., G.R. Hunter, R. Figueroa-Colon, and M.I. Goran. 1998. Effects of strength training on intra-abdominal adipose tissue in obese prepubertal girls. *Medicine and Science in Sports and Exercise* 30: 1738-1743.

92. Treuth, M.S., G.R. Hunter, T. Kekes-Szabo, R.L. Weinsier, M.I. Goran, and L. Berland. 1995. Reduction in intra-abdominal adipose tissue after strength training in older women. *Journal of Applied Physiology* 78: 1425-1431.

93. Turner, R.C., C.A. Cull, V. Frighi, and R.R. Holman. 1999. Glycemic control with diet, sulfonylurea, metformin, or insulin in patients with type 2 diabetes mellitus: Progressive requirement for multiple therapies (UKPDS 49). UK Prospective Diabetes Study (UKPDS) Group. *Journal of the American Medical Association* 281: 2005-2012.

94. Verity, L.S., and A.H. Ismail. 1989. Effects of exercise on cardiovascular disease risk in women with NIDDM. *Diabetes Research and Clinical Practice* 6: 27-35.

95. Wallace, M.B., B.D. Mills, and C.L. Browning. 1997. Effects of cross-training on markers of insulin resistance/hyperinsulinemia. *Medicine and Science in Sports and Exercise* 29: 1170-1175.

96. Wang, P.H., J. Lau, and T.C. Chalmers. 1993. Meta-analysis of effects of intensive blood-glucose control on late complications of type I diabetes. *Lancet* 341: 1306-1309.

97. Weinberg, R.S., and D. Gould. 1995. *Foundations of sport and exercise psychology.* Champaign, IL: Human Kinetics.

98. Yki-Jarvinen, H., V.A. Koivisto, M.R. Taskinen, and E. Nikkila. 1984. Glucose tolerance, plasma lipoproteins and tissue lipoprotein lipase activities in body builders. *European Journal of Applied Physiology and Occupational Physiology* 53: 253-259.

99. Zachwieja, J.J., G. Toffolo, C. Cobelli, D.M. Bier, and K.E. Yarasheski. 1996. Resistance exercise and growth hormone administration in older men: Effects on insulin sensitivity and secretion during a stable-label intravenous glucose tolerance test. *Metabolism: Clinical and Experimental* 45: 254-260.

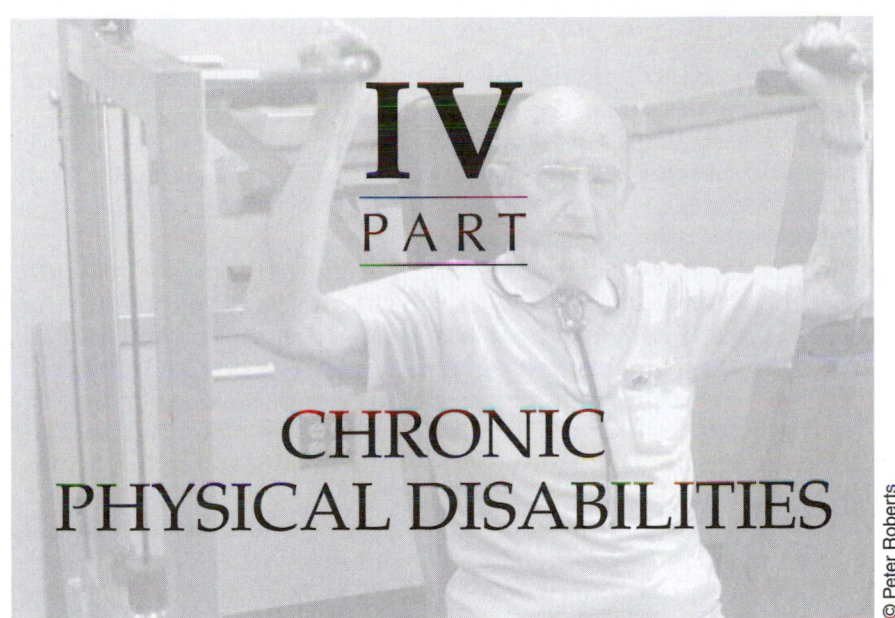

© Peter Roberts

IV PART

CHRONIC PHYSICAL DISABILITIES

Disability is defined as an impairment that limits one or more activities of daily living. This constellation of medical conditions, which affect nearly 49 million Americans, has a profound impact on the U.S. healthcare system. Recently, increased attention has been directed toward the role of exercise for improving the health and fitness of the general population. There is also significant knowledge about the detrimental physiological effects of inactivity on both physical functioning and health. Less is known, however, about designing aerobic and resistance training programs for persons with disabilities. Yet, optimizing physical conditioning programs for people with disabilities may be even more important to their general welfare.

Common medical disabilities such as spinal cord injury, multiple sclerosis, postpolio syndrome, cerebral palsy, and stroke can lead to debilitating sequelae, including muscle paralysis, paresis, and spasticity. These commonly cause a cycle of deconditioning in which physical functioning deteriorates, leading to secondary complications such as reduced aerobic fitness, muscle atrophy, osteoporosis, impaired circulation to the lower extremities, and in some cases, thrombus formation or decubitus ulcers. In addition, a diminished self-efficacy, greater dependence on others for daily living, and reduced ability for normal societal interactions can have a deleterious psychological impact.

Properly designed and implemented physical activity programs for persons with physical disabilities should include developing and maintaining cardiovascular endurance, flexibility, and muscular strength. Nevertheless, exercise training programs for this patient population must be tailored to a myriad of associated considerations, including localized weakness or paralysis; progressive disorders; spasticity / contracture; flaccid (loose) or hypotonic muscle tone; damage to sensory nerves; and muscle groups that may be functional, partially functional, or nonfunctional.

Arthritis and related musculoskeletal disorders are the leading cause of physical disability in the United States. Although exercise appears to be beneficial for most people with arthritis, the physical conditioning program should be tailored to the individual, depending on the type and severity of arthritis, the patient's age and physical function, and comorbid conditions. Resistance training has been shown to increase muscle strength, reduce pain and disability, and improve other measures of psychosocial well-being and health-related quality of life in persons affected by arthritis.

Low back pain is one of the most common and costly medical problems in our society, especially among persons under 45 years of age. While the specific cause of this anomaly is often unknown, it has increasingly been associated with poor physical fitness and our hypokinetic lifestyle. Muscular strength training through properly prescribed resistance exercise is increasingly promulgated to help overcome structural weaknesses that may serve as the precursor to low back pain.

Finally, a decrease in bone mineral density, or bone loss, is inevitable as people age. Until about age 20, bone growth outpaces bone breakdown (resorption). But as people age, this process reverses, which causes bone loss, or osteoporosis ("porous bone"). This condition is defined by the National Osteoporosis Foundation as "a disease characterized by low bone mass and structural deterioration of bone tissue, leading to bone fragility and an increased susceptibility to fractures of the hip, spine, and wrist."

Type I osteoporosis is the accelerated loss of bone density that occurs when women reach menopause. Type II osteoporosis occurs in both men and women after about age 70. One-third to one-half of all postmenopausal women and nearly half of all persons over age 75 will be affected by one of these types of bone loss. Women are affected at a much higher rate than men; moreover, osteoporosis is responsible for about 1.5 million bone fractures in the United States annually.

It is well documented that weight-bearing exercise such as walking, jogging, or aerobic dance helps maintain bone density. Fortunately, resistance training is a potent prevention and treatment strategy for osteoporosis and may be optimally effective when combined with an adequate intake of calcium and vitamin D, increased lifestyle activity, and appropriate medications.

Resistance Training for Persons With Physical Disabilities

James H. Rimmer, PhD
University of Illinois at Chicago

Federal officials and members of the public health community are growing concerned that as persons with disabilities age, they will have increasing difficulty performing self-care activities of daily living (ADL) (e.g., dressing, showering) and related instrumental activities of daily living (IADL) (e.g., ambulation, doing laundry, and grocery shopping) at a much earlier rate than the general population (9, 33). Persons with physical disabilities are often confronted with many physical challenges as a result of their functional limitations (e.g., inability to walk) and associated health conditions (e.g., spasticity, weakness, fatigue). When combined with the natural aging process, these difficulties and challenges substantially increase the likelihood of becoming physically dependent on others for assistance with ADL and IADL (5). Some experts believe that the high incidence of inactivity and poor health practices seen in persons with disabilities (13, 28), combined with the natural aging process and the potential loss of function from the disability itself, creates a destructive combination for those people living at or close to the "threshold" of physical dependence.

Maintaining a high level of fitness among persons with physical disabilities has even greater importance than in the general population, because a loss in strength can diminish a person's ability to care for himself or herself, to work, and to recreate or engage in community events (e.g., attend worship services, socialize with friends). Persons with physical disabilities would benefit greatly from participation in resistance training programs and would be more likely to maintain their physical function and independence (7, 8, 18).

As persons with physical disabilities age, the interaction between the natural aging process and the disability creates a demanding physical environment. Tasks that could be accomplished in younger adulthood become major barriers in middle and later adulthood. Climbing stairs, walking with a cane or walker, carrying packages, transferring from a wheelchair to a bed, commode, chair, or car, pushing a wheelchair up a ramp or over a curb, and standing for long periods of time become difficult or impossible tasks. As illustrated in figure 17.1, when a person's strength level drops below the "physical dependence" threshold, the individual is no longer capable of performing certain ADL and IADL and will need personal assistance to complete these tasks. Figure 17.1 also illustrates that if persons with physical disabilities achieve an optimum level of strength during their younger years, and attempt to maintain or improve these levels as they grow older, they are more likely to maintain physical independence in later life. Likewise, when strength decreases below a certain threshold, certain tasks require a greater percentage of maximum strength, which increases the likelihood of overuse injuries and fatigue, a common problem in persons with physical disabilities (14).

Many persons with physical disabilities are deconditioned and lack adequate muscular strength and endurance (27, 31). Fitness professionals can play an important role in improving the health of persons with physical disabilities by developing resistance training programs that will help them maintain adequate levels of muscular strength and endurance (29). The physical challenges that many people with disabilities face on a daily basis are exacerbated by poor strength levels. If persons with physical disabilities are unable to transfer from their wheelchair to their car, or walk from their home to the bus stop or train station, they will have difficulty working and participating in social and community events. This will impose a substantial physical and psychological hardship and will reduce the person's overall quality of life (29).

Improving strength levels in persons with physical disabilities is, in some ways, even more important than improving strength levels in the general population. A comprehensive strength training program can help persons with physical disabilities achieve greater confidence in

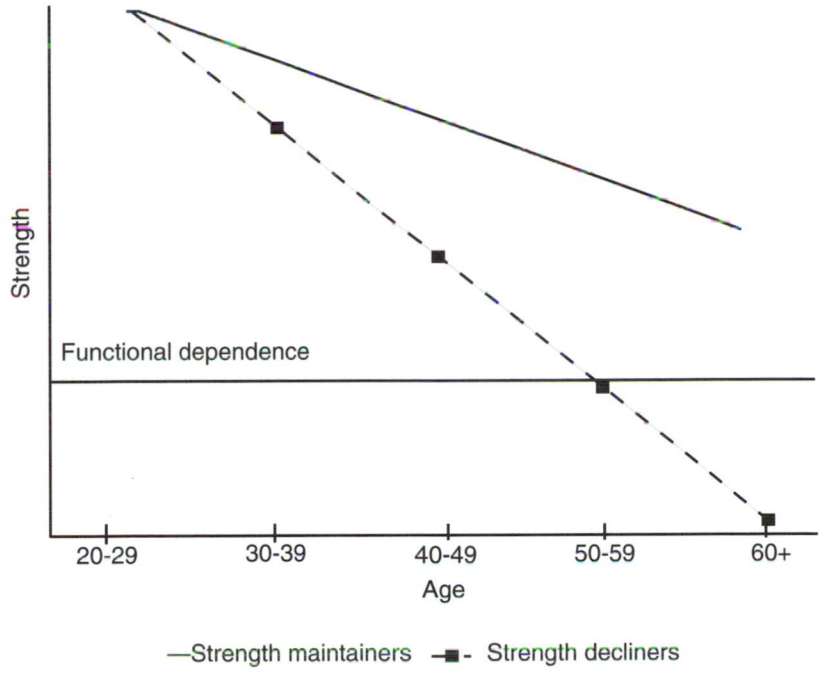

Figure 17.1 The relationship between strength and physical function among persons with disabilities.

accomplishing more physically demanding tasks, and greatly improve their ability to overcome physical barriers in their environment. Strength improvements will ultimately result in greater freedom and physical independence.

This chapter will discuss resistance training guidelines for persons with physical disabilities. The first section will focus on associated conditions and general resistance training guidelines. The last section will discuss guidelines for specific disability groups. Although the emphasis of this chapter is on five disabilities—spinal cord injury, multiple sclerosis, postpolio syndrome, cerebral palsy, and stroke—the general guidelines section will be useful for other types of physical disabilities that produce similar movement limitations (e.g., spina bifida, amputations, brain injury).

Conditions Associated With Physical Disabilities

Because of the extensive medical nature of many physical disabilities, it is important for the exercise professional to understand the associated conditions that accompany the disability. Because many persons with physical disabilities often have a localized weakness or paralysis, it is important to understand the terminology used to refer to movement limitations. A few of these terms are defined in table 17.1.

Progressive Versus Nonprogressive Disabilities

Some physical disabilities are classified as *progressive* in nature. This means that the condition will worsen over time. Some forms of multiple sclerosis and postpolio syndrome are considered progressive disorders, while other conditions such as cerebral palsy and spinal cord injury are considered *nonprogressive*. Progressive disorders will require more careful monitoring to ensure that the resistance training program is not causing the condition to worsen, which is referred to as an *exacerbation*.

Asymmetrical Weakness

Persons with physical disabilities often exhibit asymmetrical weakness. Many individuals with cerebral palsy or stroke have *hemiplegia* (weakness or paralysis on the right or left side of the body), which results in significant differences in strength between the stronger side and weaker side of the body. It is important to improve the affected side as much as

TABLE 17.1   Glossary of Common Terms Related to Limitations in Movement in Persons With Disabilities

Hemiplegia—involvement of both limbs on one side of the body

Paraplegia—involvement of both legs

Quadriplegia (also referred to as tetraplegia)—involvement of all four limbs

Diplegia—involvement of all four limbs, with more involvement in the lower limbs than the upper

Paresis—partial weakness in one or more limbs

Spasticity—an involuntary increase in muscle tone

Muscle tone—amount of tension in a muscle group

High tone (spasticity or hypertonicity)—excessive amount of tone in a muscle group

Low tone (hypotonia or flaccidity)—decreased amount of tone in a muscle group

Functional muscle mass—muscle mass that still has nerve innervation and can be improved in a resistance training program

Contracture—shortening of a muscle group and tendon usually seen in persons with spasticity

Progressive disorder—condition that gets worse over time

Exacerbation—a flare-up in which symptoms deteriorate in a particular condition

Remission—symptoms stabilize or slightly improve

possible without neglecting the nonaffected side. There may be circumstances in which the nerves controlling the affected side have been partially or completely damaged. When this occurs, the magnitude of improvement in the affected muscle groups will be greatly reduced. However, if there is still some nerve innervation on the weakened side, a resistance training program should result in measurable improvements in strength. Having hemiplegia may require active-assistive resistance exercise on the affected side while using standard exercises on the nonaffected side.

Spasticity

Spasticity is a general term used to describe various types of rigid or hypertonic muscle tone. It results in an exaggerated contractile response to stretch. It is often seen in persons who have damage to their central nervous system, such as individuals with cerebral palsy, stroke, multiple sclerosis, and spinal cord injury. The condition occurs in one of three ways:

1. loss of control from the damaged portion of the brain or spinal cord;
2. hypersensitivity of nerve receptors that are no longer being supplied with control after the injury; or
3. growth of new nerve pathways (17).

The amount of spasticity that a person has can be mild, moderate, or severe.

Spastic muscles are very rigid and are often accompanied by a "clasped-knife" position, which refers to the arm or leg maintaining a flexed position. Some individuals will have severe spasticity, which often makes it difficult or impossible to extend the limb. Severe spasticity usually results from the muscle groups being placed in a fixed position for a significant period of time, resulting in a *contracture*. Contractures can often be stretched, except in severe cases where the muscle group is permanently shortened.

Since many individuals with physical disabilities will have some degree of spasticity (tightness), flexibility training should always be combined with resistance training. It is important for the instructor to identify the "spastic" muscle groups and develop a long-term plan to increase range of motion. If the joint has been in a "fixed" position for many years, or if the spasticity is severe, it may not be possible to fully extend the joint. The instructor should consult with a physical therapist, physician, or appropriate medical professional to determine how to stretch a spastic muscle without causing injury. As with resistance training, use active-assistive stretching for certain muscle groups that are too weak (paresis) or tight (spasticity) to be moved independently.

Additional guidelines for working with spasticity are noted in table 17.2.

Contractures and Hypertonicity

Some individuals with physical disabilities develop *contractures,* which are shortened muscle groups and connective tissues surrounding the joint. The muscle tone is very high, which is referred to as *hypertonicity.* A contracture occurs when a body part (arm or leg) is placed in a flexed position over an extended period (weeks or months), usually resulting from spasticity. Sometimes this cannot be avoided due to the neurological involvement, while at other times it can be prevented by constantly stretching the muscle group. Contractures may be permanent or temporary depending on the severity of spasticity and the length of time that the joint has been placed in a "fixed" position. Some muscle groups with contractures may be able to obtain minimal improvements in strength, while others will be unable to benefit from a resistance training program. The exercise professional should consult with a physical therapist or qualified health professional to determine if contractures can be strengthened. Flexibility training should always be integrated in the exercise prescription for persons who have contractures, since the primary

TABLE 17.2   Resistance Training Guidelines for Persons With Spasticity

1. Involved limbs may experience a temporary increase in tone after resistance training on the affected (spastic) or nonaffected side. This should dissipate soon after the exercise session is completed.

2. Occasionally, the person may experience muscle spasms. These are often transient and should not present a problem in resistance training routines unless they occur often. They can often be stopped by placing the limb (arm or leg) in an extended position.

3. Avoid quick movements that may increase spasticity or cause a muscle spasm. Slow, controlled movements are often best in avoiding increases in spasticity or muscle spasms.

4. Most experts recommend that high-intensity training be avoided in spastic muscle groups.

5. When training spastic muscle groups, emphasize slow and fluid movements within the person's capability. It may be impossible for some clients to move the limb in a completely smooth fashion due to high levels of spasticity.

6. To improve or maintain muscle balance between flexors and extensors, strengthen muscle groups that oppose the spastic muscle. For example, if the biceps have a high level of spasticity, work on strengthening the triceps.

7. Remember: tight muscle groups (spastic) are not necessarily strong and also need to be strengthened.

problem is shortening of muscle fibers and connective tissues surrounding the joint.

Hypotonia

On the other end of the spectrum are persons who have *hypotonia,* or flaccid (loose) muscle tone. This condition is often seen in persons with postpolio syndrome and some persons with spinal cord injury and cerebral palsy. Persons with hypotonic muscle tone may or may not have enough nerve innervation to obtain improvements in strength. If there is some nerve innervation, the hypotonic muscle groups will be very weak and will require considerable physical therapy.

Progressive Weakness

Some individuals with neurological conditions (e.g., multiple sclerosis, postpolio syndrome) get progressively weaker as they age. This may be related to the condition or may be associated with an inactive lifestyle compounded by the aging process. Consult with the client's physician if you are concerned about a noticeable decline in strength.

Exacerbation

At certain times in the person's life, it may be necessary to temporarily stop the training program because of an exacerbation. Exacerbations occur most often in persons with multiple sclerosis. These can occur frequently or infrequently depending on the amount of involvement. After an exacerbation, it will often be necessary to start out at a much lower resistance because of complications from the exacerbation. When the person is ready to resume activity, the exercise professional should contact the client's physician to determine the appropriate training progression. Although the person may be unable to reach the level of strength he or she had before the exacerbation, it is important that the exercise professional reassure the client that strength levels can be improved. Persons who have had exacerbations should understand that they begin with a "new slate" and that the goal is to always attain the highest strength level possible.

Pressure Sores

Damage to sensory nerves occurs with many types of physical disabilities. It results in an inability to detect pressure against the skin, which, if left untreated, could result in a pressure sore (3). A pressure sore is an area of damage to the skin and underlying tissues resulting from unrelieved pressure and inadequate circulation (5). Because many people with physical disabilities who wear braces or use wheelchairs have a high risk of incurring a pressure sore, it is extremely important that they frequently check all parts of their body for skin irritations that may result from a new resistive exercise or piece of equipment. These injuries often start with a small area of redness (about the size of a quarter) and then gradually get larger if untreated.

Muscle and Joint Functionality

Depending on the disability, muscle groups may be functional, partially functional (paresis), or nonfunctional (paralysis). The exercise professional will need to obtain information on which muscle groups fall into each category. There may also be some joint irregularity to consider in the exercise prescription. For example, individuals with cerebral palsy often have hip dislocations due to the strong pull of the adductor muscles. If there has been a history of hip displacement, the instructor should check with the client's physician to determine if modifications need to be made to the resistance training program.

Loss of Muscle Strength in Progressive Disorders

Progressive disorders will often result in a gradual loss of muscle mass and strength. When muscle soreness occurs in persons who have a progressive condition, it may be an indication that the overload or intensity was excessive. Although it has not been well established in the research literature, it is generally assumed that this could lead to a permanent loss of strength (17). Until more research is conducted, it is important to be extremely cautious when working with individuals who have progressive disorders. Get approval and recommendations from the client's physician for the optimal training volume and specific resistance exercises that may prevent injury to the client.

Depression

Individuals who have physical disabilities must overcome the physical and psychological challenges of living with a disability. This often results in bouts of depression, which is a commonly associated condition in persons with physical disabilities. The exercise professional must be aware of any signs of depression and contact the client's physician or health care provider if it becomes evident that the client is struggling with this condition. Occasionally, the person may drop out of the program because of the severity of the depression.

It is important to keep detailed records on each client. Because there are often several associated conditions that accompany a physical disability (e.g., spasticity, hypertension, joint pain, exacerbations, pressure sores), the exercise professional should maintain current records and note any new medical conditions that develop during the training program.

Resistance Exercise Guidelines for Persons With Physical Disabilities

There are several factors to consider when prescribing resistance exercise to persons with physical disabilities. Most importantly, the resistance training program will depend on the severity of the disability and its associated conditions. Some clients will be able to train at very high intensity levels, while others will be able to perform at only minimal levels of resistance (e.g., lifting a body part against gravity). The training load (number of sets and repetitions, frequency, rest interval between sets) will also vary in persons with similar and different types of physical disabilities. For example, two individuals with multiple sclerosis may require a completely different training regimen because of the type of multiple sclerosis, the length of time they have had the condition, and their age. On the other hand, two individuals with stroke and cerebral palsy may have a similar program, because they exhibit the same associated conditions (e.g., nonprogressive hemiplegia, spasticity) and are at the same baseline level of strength.

A major determinant of training volume is the amount of muscle mass that is still functional. Persons with paralysis, hemiplegia, impaired motor control, or limited joint mobility have less *functional muscle mass* and will therefore require a lower training volume. For those who cannot lift the minimal weight on certain resistance machines, resistance bands or cuff weights are recommended. If bands and cuff weights are too difficult, use the person's own body weight as the initial resistance. For example, lifting an arm or leg for 5-10 seconds may be the initial starting point for clients with very low levels of strength.

The training load will also depend on the type of disability. In general, individuals who do not have a progressive disorder (e.g., spinal cord injury, cerebral palsy) will be able to work at higher intensity levels than persons with progressive disorders (e.g., multiple sclerosis, postpolio).

Training volume will also depend on the person's health status. For example, a person with stroke and hypertension should not perform high-intensity exercise. Individuals who are prone to seizures or fatigue require a reduction in training volume. Many individuals with physical disabilities who have been inactive for much of their lives need only a small amount of resistance exercise during the initial stage of the program to obtain a training effect. How quickly a person is able to progress during the conditioning stage will depend on the person's health status. For individuals who start out at very low levels of strength, significant improvements can be made with very light resistance.

Modes of resistance exercise come in three general categories: free weights, portable equipment (e.g., elastic bands, tubing), and machines.

Any of these modalities is acceptable for improving strength levels except in cases where the individual is at risk for injury. For example, persons with multiple sclerosis and cerebral palsy often have impaired motor control and may have a higher risk of dropping a free weight or having an elastic band snap back too quickly. When it appears that the resistance mode presents a danger to the client, the exercise routine should be either adapted (e.g., securing the weight to the hand, changing the movement) or substituted with a safer piece of equipment.

Some experts argue that free-weight exercises have greater value for persons with physical disabilities because the resistance can be tailored to resemble a functional daily activity (16). Free weights also require the action of stabilizing muscles around the torso and joints while lifting and lowering the resistance, and these are muscle groups that persons with physical disabilities need to strengthen to be able to perform ADL and IADL. However, free-weight exercises require good trunk stability and may be difficult to perform by individuals who have severe limitations in motor control and coordination.

Gravity-resistance exercise may be all that persons with very low strength levels are capable of performing. Performing 8-12 repetitions of a certain movement, such as abducting an arm or extending a leg, may be a good entry point. These exercises can be used with extremely weak musculature, while other modes of resistance exercise can be used with stronger muscle groups. Once an individual is able to complete 8-12 repetitions of a gravity-resistance exercise, he or she can progress to free weights, bands, or machines. If a client is unable to move a limb against gravity because of extreme weakness (often seen in the late stages of multiple sclerosis or in persons with high-level quadriplegia), one can place the limb in a certain position (e.g., shoulder abduction) and have the client hold the position isometrically for a few seconds or longer.

Active-assistive exercise may be required for certain individuals who do not have enough strength to overcome the force of gravity. The exercise professional can assist the client in performing the movement by providing as much physical assistance as necessary to complete the repetition. At various points in the concentric phase (against gravity), one may have to help the client maintain the resistance. During the eccentric phase (with gravity), the instructor controls the movement so that the weight is not lowered too quickly. In many instances, active-assistive exercise can be used with severely weak musculature while active-resistance exercise (performed without assistance) is used with stronger muscle groups.

The exercise professional should make every effort to help individuals with physical disabilities avoid fatigue and delayed-onset muscle soreness. Although this is a common side effect of any new resistance training program, it could present a problem for clients if the soreness prevents them from conducting their normal ADL. Even if a client with a physical disability aspires to make rapid gains in strength and can train at a moderate to high intensity level, the instructor should be cautious in not overworking the muscle groups, particularly in clients with progressive disorders. Use light resistance for at least the first month of the program (30-50% of 1-RM) and proceed to higher training loads only if muscle soreness and fatigue are not present.

If soreness in certain muscle groups prevents the person from performing routine daily activities, the exercise should be stopped until the pain subsides. If it continues after the program resumes, the exercise professional may need to reduce the training volume or avoid certain exercises that evoke pain or fatigue. If there are prolonged bouts of pain or soreness 24-48 h after exercise, the client should consult with his or her physician to determine the cause.

Developing the greatest amount of strength in the affected muscle groups may result in a "reservoir" of strength that can help decrease the severity of an exacerbation. Theoretically, the more muscle strength one has before an exacerbation, the more likely one will be able to maintain a high enough level of strength to stay above the "physical dependence" threshold. Progressive disorders (e.g., multiple sclerosis) make it very difficult to determine the success of the resistance training program. However, the general feeling among rehabilitation professionals is that improvements in strength may help delay the progression of muscle weakness and permanent disability. If an individual achieves a gain of 30-40% in strength before an exacerbation, a loss of strength may still keep the individual at a high enough level to be able to perform ADL and IADL.

Many physical disabilities result in hand dysfunction. This may make it difficult to grasp barbells or handles on different strength machines. There are several versions of specially designed gloves, available commercially, that will allow the person's hand to maintain contact with the resistance equipment. Gloves will also protect the hand from injury while the person performs resistance training routines. Participants who do not have good grip strength can use wrist cuffs or leather mitts with Velcro and buckles to secure their hands to dumbbells or weight equipment.

Many individuals with physical disabilities will exhibit asymmetrical weakness or will have disproportionately weaker flexor or extensor muscle groups. This will depend on where the injury site is in the brain or spinal cord and whether or not the condition is progressive in nature. It is important to evaluate individual muscle groups on both sides of the body, as well as anteriorly and posteriorly, to isolate the degree of weakness to key muscle groups.

Individuals with asymmetrical weakness will often "hike" their body toward the weaker side in order to compensate for this weakness while lifting the resistance. This could impose mild or moderate muscle strain. Make sure that the client is lifting the weight with proper form. If there is a tendency to "hike" the body, lower the resistance and emphasize good form.

Blood pressure should be monitored frequently during the early stages of the program. In some individuals with physical disabilities (e.g., from stroke, spinal cord injury), hypertension or hypotension is a common problem. It is recommended that blood pressure be measured before exercise and before and after each set. Once the client adjusts to the program and there are no wide fluctuations in blood pressure, it can be measured before and after each training session.

Guidelines for Wheelchair Users

Wheelchair users encompass a large proportion of the disabled population. Manual wheelchair users engage in a significant amount of arm and shoulder activity and are prone to repetitive motion musculoskeletal problems. Maintaining a sitting posture for extended periods of time also has adverse effects on many manual wheelchair users.

Anterior Shoulder Muscles

Persons in wheelchairs often have overdeveloped anterior shoulder muscles (pectoralis major and minor, anterior deltoid) from pushing their chair (16). This is usually accompanied by overstretched back musculature from chronic sitting. The exercise professional should develop strength in the shoulder abductors, adductors, refractors, elevators, and depressors to ensure greater "balance" between the anterior and posterior musculature. Because overloading the anterior muscle groups from wheeling the chair can result in an overuse injury, it is important to not overwork these muscle groups unless they are low in strength. Pain or soreness 24-48 h after activity is an indication that the joint and muscle group may have been excessively loaded.

Overuse of certain muscle groups can also cause stress fractures or cumulative trauma disorders. Manual wheelchair users are particularly prone to rotator cuff tears, lateral epicondylitis, and carpal tunnel syndrome, which result from repetitive motions to small muscle groups as a result of propelling the wheelchair (6).

Triceps and Biceps Brachii

Transfers and seated push-ups (used to prevent pressure sores) are essential movements to be performed several times a day, and the exercise professional should make them a primary goal of the resistance training program. Two important muscle groups needed to perform these tasks are the triceps and biceps brachii. Improved strength in these muscle groups is also very important for getting up from the floor. Persons with balance impairments such as cerebral palsy and multiple sclerosis have a higher incidence of falls and will occasionally have to lift themselves up from the floor.

Trunk Musculature

Many individuals who use wheelchairs have poor trunk musculature (27). This often requires the person to wear some type of strap or harness to prevent falling out of the chair. The exercise professional should evaluate upper-trunk stability by having the person flex their spine while sitting in the chair and then returning to the straight-up position. Someone who has difficulty performing this task may need to wear a chest strap that attaches to the back of the wheelchair in order to maintain good trunk stability. These straps or belts can be purchased in most medical supply stores.

Sitting Posture

Persons who use wheelchairs will often exhibit poor sitting posture. It is important to remind the client not to slump in his or her chair. Emphasize good sitting posture while performing the resistance training program. Mirrors will often facilitate good body awareness and might help the client become more aware of his or her sitting posture. If the person is unable to maintain good posture, it may be necessary to work with a physical therapist or physician to devise ways to improve posture. Sometimes it is necessary to facilitate improved sitting posture by having a rehabilitation engineer or assistive technology specialist design a seat cushion that supports the weak side of the body.

Range of Motion

Establishing and maintaining optimal range of motion in the affected limbs are paramount. Wheelchair users often have limited range of motion from sitting in the chair for long periods and will therefore need a complementary flexibility program. It is important to understand the limitations in range of motion at certain joints that result from wheelchair use (e.g., spasticity). Muscle groups that are severely shortened (contractures) may need to be strengthened through isometric exercise.

Breathing

Some persons with severe physical disabilities have difficulty performing the correct breathing pattern during the resistance training program (exhaling while raising the weight and inhaling while lowering it). With certain progressive disorders such as multiple sclerosis and postpolio syndrome, breathing may worsen at certain stages in life. During the initial training phase, teach the client the appropriate breathing technique with little or no resistance until he or she becomes accustomed to performing it correctly. Because resistance training requires a substantial increase in breathing rate and volume, diaphragmatic and pursed lip breathing is recommended for clients who have difficulty maintaining a normal breathing pattern during the exercise regimen.

Wheelchair Transfers

The exercise professional may have to transfer individuals who are in wheelchairs to machines or the floor in order for them to use certain pieces of equipment. Although one-person transfers are done routinely by rehabilitation professionals, they are difficult to perform and present a high risk of injury to both the instructor and client. Whenever possible, perform a two-person wheelchair transfer. Guidelines on how to transfer clients can be found in Baxter and Lockette (3) or Rimmer (27). General information on wheelchair safety is listed in table 17.3.

TABLE 17.3 General Safety Guidelines for Wheelchair Users

1. Reduce the distance between the transfer surface and the wheelchair. Removing armrests and detachable footrests will permit closer positioning to the transfer surface.
2. Always secure wheelchair locks (one on each side of chair). The major cause of injury to wheelchair users is being transferred to or from a wheelchair that has one or both brakes unlocked.
3. Provide surfaces of equal height if possible. It is much more difficult lifting someone onto a surface of greater height than the wheelchair.
4. Keep a wide base of support and use legs and not back musculature to lift the person.
5. Make sure the person knows when you are ready to transfer them.
6. When you are going to push a client in a wheelchair, make sure the person is prepared to move.
7. If you ever have to tip the wheelchair to get over an obstacle such as a curb or door threshold, never tip the wheelchair forward. This could cause the person to fall out of the chair. Always tip the chair backward onto the larger, posterior wheels. Remind the client to sit back in the chair.
8. A transfer of a client from the chair to the floor or a machine should be performed by two people. One-person transfers are very difficult and can result in a higher risk of injury to the client or instructor.

Resistance Training Guidelines for Specific Disability Groups

Although most individuals with disability can benefit from resistance training, all have unique characteristics that influence the exercise prescription. In this section we consider the guidelines for prescribing resistance training to persons with spinal cord injury, multiple sclerosis, postpolio syndrome, cerebral palsy, and stroke.

Spinal Cord Injury

There are approximately 250,000-400,000 people living in the United States with a spinal cord injury (SCI). Eighty-two percent of these injuries occur in young males age 16-30 years. The most common cause of SCI is motor vehicle accidents (44%), followed by acts of violence (24%) and falls (22%) (24). Persons who have sustained an SCI will lose nerve innervation to various musculature depending on where the spinal cord has been damaged. For example, if a person's injury occurs between the fifth (T5) and sixth (T6) thoracic vertebrae and is a complete lesion (some injuries result in an incomplete lesion, which allows some muscle innervation), loss of function will occur from the point of injury to all nerve innervation below it. In complete lesions, the musculature has no innervation, and a resistance training program will not be effective for the involved muscle groups. Instead, the emphasis should be placed on maintaining good range of motion while focusing on strengthening the muscle groups that are still functional. Table 17.4 provides a brief listing of the functional level at each injury site.

The following items are resistance training guidelines for persons with spinal cord injury.

1. Many persons who have sustained a spinal cord injury will require a significant increase in upper-body strength in order to manage transfers, push a wheelchair, and perform activities of daily living (e.g., bathing and dressing). Pushing a wheelchair up a ramp or curb cut can be a significant physical challenge to persons with SCI who are deconditioned. The exercise professional should have a good understanding of what muscle groups are still functional and should help the person develop adequate amounts of strength in those muscle groups, since they will be used more often to assist with transfers and performing ADL and IADL.

2. Individuals with a complete SCI will use a manual or power wheelchair to ambulate. High cervical injuries usually require a power wheelchair, while lower-level injuries leave enough muscle innervation in the hands to allow use of a manual wheelchair. However, some individuals who have the necessary muscle and nerve innervation to

TABLE 17.4   Spinal Cord Injury Location and Function of Major Muscle Groups*

Cervical 4—Retain function of only the scapular elevators (trapezius) and the diaphragm. Unable to use arms, trunk, or lower extremities. Individual needs a power wheelchair to ambulate and will use a mouthstick to operate the wheelchair.

Cervical 5—Functional muscle groups include the deltoids, part of the biceps, and part of the scapular adductors (rhomboids). The innervation of these muscles allows the arm to be used for some activities. There is no control at the wrist or hand.

Cervical 6—Functional muscle groups include biceps, brachioradialis, wrist extensors, and partial use of the latissimus dorsi and pectoralis muscles. There is no control at the hand.

Cervical 7-8—Use of triceps, some finger extensors, and long finger flexors. May still have some dexterity problems with the hands and fingers.

Thoracic 1-8—Has complete use of the hands. Poor trunk control because of affected abdominal muscles.

Thoracic 9-12—Good trunk control because of full use of abdominals.

Lumbar 1-3—Use of hip flexors and hip adductors.

Lumbar 4-Sacral 2—Use of hamstrings. Some ankle and foot musculature may be present.

*All muscle groups above the lesion location will also be functional.

use a manual wheelchair prefer to use a power wheelchair to preserve energy.

3. Persons with SCI must do everything possible to avoid pressure sores (also known as decubitis ulcers or pressure ulcers). If left untreated, pressure sores can cause tissue necrosis, which often has to be removed surgically. One way to avoid pressure sores is to perform wheelchair push-ups every 15-20 minutes. This requires the person to lift his or her body out of the chair by grabbing the armrests and pressing up with the arms. The position should be held for 5-15 seconds to allow blood flow to the tissues that make contact with the chair (primarily the gluteals and hamstrings). Clients with injuries C6 or higher will not be able to perform this exercise independently because of damage done to the nerves controlling triceps innervation. Some clients may be able to pull one side of the body off the chair by using the biceps to grab a bar or other object located on the side of the wheelchair at approximately shoulder height. The exercise professional should develop biceps and forearm strength to help facilitate this important movement.

4. Many persons with SCI have a condition known as autonomic dysreflexia (AD). Individuals with SCI at the T6 level or higher have the greatest risk (24). This condition results in an excessive rise in blood

pressure that could be extremely dangerous if not treated immediately (25). AD often occurs when an individual has a distended (full) bladder. Symptoms include headache, facial flush, perspiration, and a stuffy nose. It is important to make sure that the client has voided his or her bladder before starting the program. It is also important to measure the individual's blood pressure and monitor how the person feels before each exercise session to assure that AD is not present.

Multiple Sclerosis

Multiple sclerosis is a progressive disorder that results in a deterioration of the myelin sheath around the spinal nerves. As the disease progresses, secondary conditions may include impaired gait, genitourinary dysfunction (incontinence), and loss of movement in some or all limbs (12). The disease affects more women than men and is often diagnosed in the person's 20s and 30s (20).

Persons with multiple sclerosis may exhibit several symptoms. These include fatigue, occasionally severe enough that activities of daily living cannot be performed independently, and weakness in one or more extremities. The hands are often affected in the later stages of the disease, which makes it difficult to grasp objects.

Multiple sclerosis is characterized by periods of exacerbation and remission. An exacerbation results in the condition worsening. The individual may incur additional weakness or complete loss of function in several different muscle groups. Some individuals with multiple sclerosis have few exacerbations and little disability, while others get progressively worse. Because multiple sclerosis affects each person differently, it is difficult to make generalizations about the progression of the disease and the amount of disability that may result from it.

The following are resistance training guidelines for persons with multiple sclerosis:

1. Persons with multiple sclerosis have an attenuated or absent sweating response (19). Performing resistance exercise in warm environments could result in early-onset fatigue and should therefore always be performed in cool environments. If the room is warm, use fans to improve air circulation. Make sure the client drinks water before, during, and after the activity, since dehydration can also result in higher core temperatures. Persons with multiple sclerosis would also benefit from resistance training exercises performed in a cool swimming pool (77-80°F). The water will help maintain or lower the person's core temperature and can simultaneously serve as a resistance mode. Certain commercial resistance devices are also available to help develop strength in the water.

2. Balance is often impaired in persons with multiple sclerosis, particularly as the condition progresses (19). Make sure that balance is

assessed on a regular basis, so that if it does decline to where standing exercises are difficult or dangerous, the instructor can switch to routines from a chair or provide support for standing exercise (e.g., parallel bars, holding on to a railing, leaning against a wall).

3. Tremor and incoordination may prevent the performance of smooth movements, causing the movement to look somewhat "choppy." Provide assistance as necessary to help the client move the resistance through the full range of motion as smoothly as possible, but don't overemphasize this, because the client may be incapable of it because of the neurological involvement.

4. Blurred vision and double vision are commonly associated conditions in persons with multiple sclerosis (26). Make sure that equipment is marked clearly. Use bright colors (yellow tape on a black weight plate) or magnets to identify where to place the pin on weight machines. Small weights and objects should not be left in the middle of the floor where a person could trip over them.

5. Persons with multiple sclerosis may need to urinate frequently during the resistance training program, particularly if there is pressure displaced on the urinary bladder. Because of neurological involvement, the person may be unable to sense the need to void their bladder. Make sure that the bladder is voided before exercise and intermittently during the training program, particularly if the client is drinking fluids to prevent dehydration and overheating.

Postpolio Syndrome

Polio, which is sometimes referred to as poliomyelitis, is caused by an acute virus that attacks the anterior horn cells of lower motor neurons (4). These motor neurons are located in the front part of the spinal cord and are essential for muscle activity. The extent of motor neuron damage and the progression of the disease vary considerably in individuals with postpolio syndrome, depending on which muscle groups were affected and how much damage was sustained during the acute stages of the disease (23).

Postpolio syndrome occurs several decades after the onset of polio. Approximately 25% of individuals who contracted the polio virus during the 1940s and 1950s report late-onset symptoms in their 40s and 50s (24). Although polio became quite rare in this country after the discovery of the Salk vaccine, persons with this condition who were born in the 1940s and 1950s and are now in their 50s and 60s are starting to experience significant mobility limitations. Common symptoms associated with postpolio syndrome include

1. fatigue, generally described as a feeling of extreme exhaustion after minimal activities;

2. decreased endurance, which is manifested by the inability to sustain general activity;

3. new joint and muscle pain;

4. progressive weakness in muscles due to the polio and also new muscle weakness;

5. respiratory insufficiency, which often requires ventilatory support; and

6. cold intolerance that contributes to muscle weakness (15).

There is some debate about whether or not persons with postpolio syndrome should perform resistance training exercise (4). Because progressive weakness is a hallmark of postpolio syndrome in the later years, the theory is that excessive exercise can cause an accelerated loss in function. In a recent study on resistance training in persons with postpolio syndrome, Agre, Rodriquez, and Franke examined the effects of a combined program of dynamic and isometric muscle-strengthening exercises in seven individuals with postpolio syndrome and concluded that muscle strength can be significantly increased without adversely affecting neurological function (1). Although there are few well-controlled studies on resistance training in persons with postpolio syndrome (4), most experts agree that not performing muscle-strengthening exercises will result in a loss in function with age.

The following are resistance training guidelines for persons with postpolio syndrome:

1. Many polio survivors complain of new musculoskeletal pain as they grow older (4). The most common complaints are difficulty in walking and stair climbing. This may be related to a progressive loss of muscle strength (1). The exercise professional must understand that postpolio is a progressive disorder that may result in weakness as the person ages. To determine if a resistance training program should be maintained, reduced, or eliminated, it is important to communicate with the client's physician or other qualified health professional. The medical advisor should be able to determine if the program should be modified or stopped in a person who is complaining of pain or fatigue. High-intensity resistance exercise is not recommended for persons with postpolio syndrome, since it is not known if this type of exercise can cause permanent loss of function (4).

2. Although resistance training should be part of an exercise program for persons with postpolio syndrome, it is extremely important to keep muscle fatigue to a minimum. Overworking affected muscle groups could result in fatigue and decreased muscle function. The development of strength in persons with postpolio syndrome must be carefully monitored to ensure that the program is not compromising the person's health. The exercise professional should monitor the

client closely for any signs of pain, discomfort, or fatigue resulting from the program.

3. Begin with minimal resistance and progress slowly. Stay within the client's comfort level. The more deconditioned the client is, the more important it is to prevent fatigue by starting with very light resistance. If pain or fatigue is present, switch to cardiovascular and flexibility training until they subside.

4. Because postpolio syndrome often results in asymmetrical muscle weakness, the fitness instructor should evaluate each limb separately. The instructor should document the training protocol and determine if any new muscle weakness is associated with other aging-related changes or the resistance training program. If there is a sudden loss of function or enhanced pain or fatigue resulting from the activity, contact the client's physician or health provider to determine if the exercise program should be modified or discontinued.

Cerebral Palsy

Cerebral palsy is a nonprogressive disorder that results in physical impairment and causes postural and balance problems. It affects approximately 25,000 children each year (32). The disorder is caused by an injury to the brain before, during, or after birth. To be diagnosed with cerebral palsy, the person must have a nonprogressive lesion to the brain that causes motor dysfunction usually before the age of 3 (32). The damage is not to the muscles or nerves in the spinal cord, but rather to the motor center of the brain that controls muscle function. The more severe the injury to the brain, the greater the limitation in movement and function (10).

The following are resistance training guidelines for persons with cerebral palsy:

1. The strong pull of the hip adductors seen in many persons with cerebral palsy will require a resistance training program that emphasizes strengthening the hip abductors. This does not necessarily mean that the hip adductors do not need to be strengthened. While the adductor muscles are often very tight due to spasticity, they may also be very weak. Therefore, both sets of muscle groups must be strengthened even though the abductors might need a greater amount of work. Before working these muscle groups in a client, make sure the client has not had a hip dislocation. If he or she has had a hip dislocation, consult with the primary care physician or health provider to determine if hip exercises can be conducted safely.

2. Flexibility training is an important part of the exercise prescription for persons with cerebral palsy because of the high level of spasticity. Resistance training programs should include nearly the same amount of

attention to enhancing and/or maintaining good range of motion in the affected limbs.

3. A common type of cerebral palsy that results in weakness or paralysis to the right or left side of the body is spastic hemiplegia. (A similar condition occurs in persons with stroke.) This condition will often require greater attention to developing strength on the weaker side of the body. The amount of improvement that can be made to the hemiplegic side will depend on the amount of damage that was sustained to that part of the central nervous system. If the person has complete paralysis to one side of the body, resistance training should be substituted with flexibility training.

4. Because balance is often impaired in ambulatory persons with cerebral palsy, it is important to protect clients from injury by developing safe resistance training programs that do not expose them to a high risk of injury. Some clients will be able to work on strength exercises in a standing position with physical assistance from the therapist, while others will have to perform the exercise routines from a chair. The exercise professional should measure the client's static and dynamic balance before developing the resistance training program to determine if standing exercises are safe.

5. In individuals who have spastic cerebral palsy, the antagonistic muscles, which directly oppose the action of the prime mover, are not inhibited. This is the result of a hyperactive stretch reflex that responds to the change in length of the muscle fibers by overreacting with a forceful contraction (17). For example, during elbow flexion, the triceps are supposed to serve as the antagonists, directly opposing the biceps and brachialis. When reciprocal innervation is absent, both muscles contract simultaneously, causing significant movement dysfunction and jerky actions. The therapist should try to work with the client to ensure the smoothest movement possible but should not be alarmed if there is some jerkiness during the movement phase. This is normal for persons with this condition.

6. Certain individuals with cerebral palsy have a condition known as athetosis. This condition results in involuntary movements in one or more of the person's limbs. The movements are uncontrollable and are often referred to as slow and "writhing." Facial muscles are also involved, which make the person appear to be laughing or crying. Since the movement of muscle groups is involuntary, use of free weights may not be possible because the hand may open reflexively during the weight routine. Elastic bands may be inappropriate since the resistance may be difficult to control and result in the band snapping back too quickly. Cuff weights and machines are the preferred modalities. Active-assistive exercise may be needed to perform the motion smoothly.

Stroke

Stroke is the third leading cause of death in the United States and affects 731,000 people annually, of whom 570,000 survive (22). There are currently 4 million stroke survivors living in the United States (11). The newer term for stroke is *brain attack*, which has been adopted by the American Heart Association to indicate that the same level of urgency applies in seeking emergency medical care as with a heart attack. Stroke is also referred to as a cerebrovascular accident, or CVA.

Strokes occur when the blood supply to the brain is interrupted. There are generally two types of stroke. One is called an *ischemic* stroke, which results from a blood clot. The second type is called a *hemorrhagic* stroke, which results from a ruptured blood vessel in the brain. Either of these conditions will result in a disruption to the motor and sensory pathways that are involved in voluntary movement (32). Approximately 83% of all strokes are of the ischemic type (22).

Aside from the emotional setback resulting from stroke, there is often complete or partial loss of muscle function on either the right side (right hemiplegia) or left side (left hemiplegia) of the body, depending on where the injury occurs in the brain (the right brain controls the left side of the body and vice versa). The severity of stroke can vary from person to person. Some individuals who have had a mild stroke, or what is commonly referred to as a trans-ischemic attack (TIA), will maintain full function after the injury, while others who have suffered a severe stroke often lose significant physical function on the right, left, or both sides of the body.

The following are resistance training guidelines for persons who have suffered a stroke:

1. Blood pressure must be monitored very closely in persons with stroke. Since a common associated condition is hypertension, follow the resistance training guidelines for persons with hypertension as noted in chapter 13. It is especially important to make sure that the person's hypertension is under control before initiating the resistance training program. If blood pressure fluctuates during the first few weeks of the training program, contact the client's physician to determine how to proceed with a safe program. Under no circumstances should a person who has had a stroke and continues to have difficulty maintaining a stable blood pressure be permitted to exercise.

2. A recent paper noted that persons with stroke and hypertension can safely participate in rehabilitation therapy provided blood pressure does not fluctuate widely. The investigators recommended that mean arterial pressure (MAP = diastolic pressure + 1/3 [systolic pressure − diastolic pressure]) not go above 130 mmHg until blood pressure is under better control (4). During the early stages of the program, blood

pressure should be monitored before, during, and at the end of the exercise to ensure that wide variations are not occurring. Once the client adjusts to the program and there are no complications, blood pressure can be taken before and after each set (30).

3. How much recovery will occur after a stroke is a question many stroke survivors and family members ask (2). Most persons with stroke go through a significant recovery period during the first six months after having a stroke, while others can see significant recovery for up to a year or longer (17). The goal of resistance training is to maximize recovery. Because most stroke survivors will return home shortly after their injury, the exercise professional should work closely with the client's physician or physical therapist in developing a safe and effective program.

Conclusion

Persons with physical disabilities are often limited in their mobility and therefore face secondary health problems associated with a sedentary lifestyle. Resistance training can improve functional capacity and attenuate the detrimental health consequences of immobility. Recent research clearly documents the benefits of participation in resistance training by individuals with spinal cord injury, multiple sclerosis, postpolio syndrome, cerebral palsy, and stroke. Further research is required, however, to identify the most appropriate resistance exercises in different physically disabled populations. A summary of resistance training guidelines for persons with physical disabilities is given in table 17.5.

TABLE 17.5 Summary of Resistance Training Guidelines for Persons With Physical Disabilities

1. Know and understand the pathology of each condition and how it may interact with a resistance training program (e.g., progressive disorders often result in increased weakness and high levels of fatigue).

2. Determine which muscle groups are still functional (neurological innervation) and which muscle groups are weak (paresis) or paralyzed (paralysis).

3. Determine the progression of resistance exercise through consultation with the client's physician, physical therapist, or qualified health provider. With certain individuals, the progression may vary regularly because of exacerbations that occur throughout the person's lifetime. Periods of exacerbation may require the instructor to return to baseline or below baseline levels of strength.

4. Focus on muscle groups that are essential for performing ADL (e.g., shoulder abductors for combing hair and dressing) and IADL (e.g., triceps and forearm and shoulder stabilizers for wheelchair transfers).

(continued)

TABLE 17.5 *(continued)*

5. Make sure that blood pressure and heart rate responses remain in a safe zone.

6. Make sure that associated conditions (e.g., autonomic dysreflexia, hypertension) are dealt with properly.

7. Make sure that exercise facility is accessible for wheelchair users. Guidelines can be obtained from the Americans With Disabilities Act.

8. For more information on physical activity and disability, contact the National Center on Physical Activity and Disability at **http:// www.ncpad.org**. Information on exercise guidelines for all disabilities can be obtained here.

References

1. Agre, J.C., A.A. Rodriquez, and A. Franke. 1997. Strength, endurance, and work capacity after muscle strengthening exercise in postpolio subjects. *Archives of Physical Medicine and Rehabilitation* 78: 681-686.

2. American Heart Association. 1994. *Family guide to stroke. Treatment, recovery, prevention.* Dallas, TX: Author.

3. Baxter, K.F., and K.F. Lockette. 1995. Resistance training with stretch bands: Modifying for disability. In *Fitness programming and physical disability*, edited by P.D. Miller, 91-100. Champaign, IL: Human Kinetics.

4. Birk, T.J. 1997. Polio and post-polio syndrome. In *ACSM's exercise management for persons with chronic diseases and disabilities*, edited by J.L. Durstine, 194-199. Champaign, IL: Human Kinetics.

5. Brandt E, and A. Pope, eds. 1997. *Enabling America: Assessing the role of rehabilitation science and engineering.* Institute of Medicine. Washington, DC: National Academy Press.

6. Cooper, R.A., L.A. Quatrano, P.W. Axelson, W. Harlan, M. Stineman, and B. Franklin. 1999. Research on physical activity and health among people with disabilities: A consensus statement. *Journal of Rehabilitation Research and Development* 36: 142-154.

7. Cress, M.E., D.M. Buchner, K.A. Questad, P.C. Esselman, B.J. deLateur, and R.S. Schwartz. 1999. Exercise: Effects on physical functional performance in independent older adults. *Journal of Gerontological Medicine and Science* 54A: M242-M248.

8. Ferketich, A.K., T.E. Kirby, and S.E. Always. 1998. Cardiovascular and muscular adaptations to combined endurance and strength training in elderly women. *Acta Physiologica Scandinavica* 164: 259-267.

9. Freedman, V.A., and L.G. Martin. 1999. Understanding trends in functional limitations among older Americans. *American Journal of Public Health* 88: 1457-1462.

10. Gersh, E.S. 1991. What is cerebral palsy? In *Children with cerebral palsy*, edited by E. Geralis, 57-89. Washington, DC: Woodbine House.

11. Gorelick, P.B., R.L. Sacco, D.B. Smith, M. Alberts, L. Mustone-Alexander, D. Rader, J. Ross, E. Raps, M. Ozer, L. Brass, M. Malone, S. Goldberg, J. Booss, D. Hanley, J. Toole, N. Greengold, and D. Rhew. 1999. Prevention of a first stroke. A review of guidelines and a multidisciplinary consensus statement from the National Stroke Association. *Journal of the American Medical Association* 281: 1112-1120.

12. Greenspun, B., M. Stineman, and R. Agri. 1987. Multiple sclerosis and rehabilitation outcome. *Archives of Physical Medicine and Rehabilitation* 68: 434-437.

13. Heath, G.W., and P.H. Fentem. 1997. Physical activity among persons with disabilities—A public health perspective. In *Exercise and sport sciences reviews*, edited by J.O. Holloszy, 195-234. Baltimore: Williams & Wilkins.

14. Janssen, T.W.J., C. Van Oers, L. Van Der Woude, and A.P. Hollander. 1994. Physical strain in daily life of wheelchair users with spinal cord injuries. *Medicine and Science in Sports and Exercise* 26: 661-670.

15. Jones, D.R., J. Speier, K. Canine, R. Owen, and G.A Stull. 1989. Cardiorespiratory responses to aerobic training by patients with postpoliomyelitis sequelae. *Journal of the American Medical Association* 261: 3255-3258.

16. Lockette, K.F. 1995. Resistance training: Program design. In *Fitness programming and physical disability,* edited by P.D. Miller, 79-90. Champaign, IL: Human Kinetics.

17. Lockette, K.F., and A.M. Keys. 1994. *Conditioning with physical disabilities.* Champaign, IL: Human Kinetics.

18. Morey, M.C., C.F. Pieper, and J. Cornoni-Huntley. 1998. Physical fitness and functional limitations in community-dwelling older adults. *Medicine and Science in Sports and Exercise* 30: 715-723.

19. Mulcare, J.A. 1997. Multiple sclerosis. In *ACSM's exercise management for persons with chronic diseases and disabilities,* edited by J.L. Durstine, 189-193. Champaign, IL: Human Kinetics.

20. National Multiple Sclerosis Society. MS information. **http://www.nmss.org/**

21. National Spinal Cord Injury Association. 1999. Spinal cord injury statistics. **http://www.spinalcord.org/**

22. National Stroke Association. 1999. Brain attack statistics. **http://www.stroke.org/brain_stat.cfm**

23. Nollet, F., and A. Beelen. 1999. Strength assessment in postpolio syndrome: Validity of a hand-held dynamometer in detecting change. *Archives of Physical Medicine and Rehabilitation* 80: 1316-1323.

24. Pauls, J.A., and K.L. Reed. 1996. *Quick reference to physical therapy.* Gaithersburg, MD: Aspen.

25. Phillips, W.T., B.J. Kiratli, M. Sarkarati, G. Weraarchakul, J. Myers, B.A. Franklin, I Parkash, and V. Froelicher. 1998. Effect of spinal cord injury on the heart and cardiovascular fitness. *Current Problems in Cardiology* 23 (11): 641-720.

26. Poser, C.M., and M. Ronthal. 1991. Exercise and Alzheimer's disease, Parkinson's disease, and multiple sclerosis. *Physician and Sportsmedicine* 19: 85-92.

27. Rimmer, J.H. 1994. *Fitness and rehabilitation programs for special populations.* Dubuque, IA: WCB McGraw-Hill.

28. Rimmer, J.H. 1999. Health promotion for people with disabilities: The emerging paradigm shift from disability prevention to prevention of secondary conditions. *Physical Therapy* 79: 495-502.

29. Rimmer, J.H., D. Braddock, and K.H. Pitetti. 1996. Research in physical activity and disability: An emerging national priority. *Medicine and Science in Sports and Exercise* 28: 1366-1372.

30. Rimmer, J.H., and G. Hedman. 1998. A health promotion program for stroke survivors. *Topics in Stroke Rehabilitation* 5 (2): 30-44.

31. Rimmer, J.H., S.S. Rubin, D. Braddock, and G. Hedman. 1999. Physical activity patterns of African-American women with physical disabilities. *Medicine and Science in Sports and Exercise* 31: 613-618.

32. Schwartz, L., J.M. Engle, and M.P. Jensen. 1999. Pain in persons with cerebral palsy. *Archives of Physical Medicine and Rehabilitation* 78: 1243-1246.

33. Sherwood, A.M. 1999. Aging in America. *Journal of Rehabilitation Research and Development* 36: vii-viii.

Arthritis and Related Musculoskeletal Disorders

Walter H. Ettinger, MD
Virtua Health, Inc.

Introduction

Arthritis in its various forms affects 50 million Americans of all ages. Moreover, arthritis and related musculoskeletal disorders are the leading cause of physical disability in the United States. Although the cause of disability from arthritis is complex, poor muscular and aerobic conditioning are important contributors to loss of function (figure 18.1) (6, 8, 18, 19). Thus, physical activity and in particular structured exercise has an important therapeutic role for people affected by arthritis.

Over the past decade extensive research has shown that people with arthritis are able to undertake therapeutic exercise safely and that they accrue benefit from regular physical activity (7, 9-12, 16, 17, 20, 24, 25, 27, 30-34). However, in prescribing exercise the clinician must appreciate that arthritis is not one disease, but rather multiple conditions that affect health and function in different ways. Exercise appears to be beneficial for nearly all types of people with arthritis but must be tailored to the individual depending on the type of arthritis, the severity of the arthritis, the person's age and physical function, and coexistent conditions.

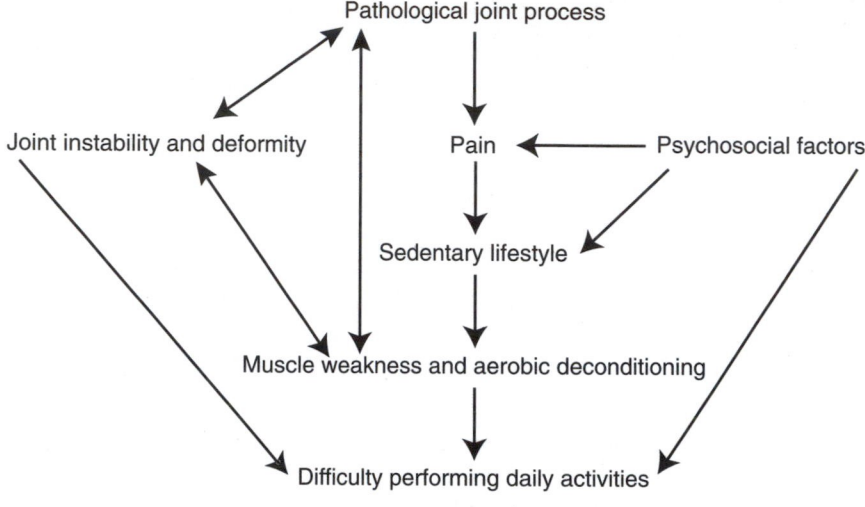

Figure 18.1   Mechanism of physical disability from arthritis.

This chapter reviews the major types of arthritis and the risks and benefits of resistance exercise for persons with arthritis, and provides guidelines for the prescription of resistance training for such individuals.

Types of Arthritis

There are over one hundred types of arthritis. For the purpose of prescribing resistance training, arthritis can be divided into three broad categories: osteoarthritis, systemic inflammatory arthritides, and soft tissue rheumatism.

Osteoarthritis is the most common type of arthritis. It is characterized by degeneration of the hyaline cartilage of diarthrodial joints with concomitant bony hypertrophy of subchondral bone. Clinically, patients with osteoarthritis experience pain, especially while using the affected joints, and stiffness after prolonged periods of immobility. People with osteoarthritis do not experience systemic symptoms such as fatigue and fever, and other organ systems are not involved.

The joints that are affected by osteoarthritis include any or all of the small joints of the fingers (distal and proximal interphalangeal joints), the base of the thumb, the spine, hips, knees, and small joints of the feet. The affected joints may be tender, swollen, or deformed, but these findings are usually mild. Clinically, osteoarthritis of the knees and hips is the most debilitating because pain and stiffness of these joints lead to problems with mobility and therefore adversely affect a person's quality of life and ability to function independently.

The major risk factor for the development of osteoarthritis is age. Most people with symptomatic osteoarthritis are over the age of 60. Other risk factors for osteoarthritis include obesity (13), injury, and periarticular muscle weakness (2, 21, 26, 28). The latter is thought to cause instability of the joint, which can lead to structural damage. Thus, resistance training may have a preventive as well as a therapeutic role in osteoarthritis.

The second group of arthritides is the systemic inflammatory disorders. The most common type of inflammatory polyarthritis is rheumatoid arthritis. Affecting mostly middle-aged and older adults, rheumatoid arthritis is a chronic, serious disease that causes marked inflammation of the small joints of the hands, wrists, elbows, shoulders, temporomandibular joints, spine, hips, knees, ankles, and feet. Generally, all joints are affected in a symmetrical fashion. Swelling, redness, and tenderness are prominent. Over time, the underlying joint structures are damaged or destroyed, and marked deformities can occur. In 20% of cases, other organ systems, such as the heart and lungs, are involved. Other common types of inflammatory arthritis include systemic lupus erythematosis and the spondyloarthropathies.

Systemic lupus erythematosis (SLE) is an inflammatory disease that causes mild arthritis, primarily of the small joints of the hands and feet, although other joints can be affected. The distinguishing feature of SLE is involvement of other organ systems, including the skin, bone marrow, lungs, heart, kidneys, and nervous system.

The spondyloarthropathies, including ankylosing spondylitis, Reiter's disease, enteropathic arthritis, and, in some cases, psoriatic arthritis, are characterized by inflammation of the sacroiliac joints and axial spine. In more advanced cases the spine fuses, restricting rotation, flexion, and extension.

People with rheumatoid arthritis and other inflammatory diseases may take certain medications that must be considered when prescribing resistance training. Many patients use prednisone or other corticosteroids. These drugs can cause a myopathy that results in weakness and loss of muscle mass. Additionally, the immunosuppressive drugs that are prescribed for these disorders may lead to infection, fatigue, and weakness due to bone marrow suppression.

The third category of musculoskeletal disorders is classified as nonarticular, or soft tissue, rheumatism. The most common is fibromyalgia. Muscle pain and tenderness at trigger points along the trunk and limbs characterize this disorder of unknown etiology. The joints and muscles do not show pathological changes, and laboratory tests are normal. Fibromyalgia is chronic but usually not progressive in nature. Two other types of nonarticular rheumatism are bursitis and tendinitis. These disorders are local and lead to pain and limitation of motion of the affected areas.

Evidence for Resistance Training as Therapy for Arthritis

Resistance training may improve health outcomes in people with arthritis in two different ways. First, it may attenuate the clinical consequences of the underlying condition. Patients with arthritis have weaker musculature than age- and gender-matched controls (2, 3, 8, 14). The muscle weakness is due to disuse (the pain of arthritis causes people to be sedentary) and to the joint pain and inflammation that leads to periarticular muscle atrophy (28, 29). The muscle weakness that accompanies arthritis contributes to difficulty with ambulating, transferring, and lifting and carrying objects (10, 21). In addition, weak quadriceps and ankle musculature is associated with poor balance and may increase the risk of falls (18, 19).

Recently, a hypothesis has been put forth that muscle weakness may lead to or hasten the progression of osteoarthritis by causing instability of the joint (2). Such instability is thought to alter the biomechanics of the joint, resulting in destruction of cartilage. Indeed, recent data suggests that persons who developed osteoarthritis of the knee had weaker quadriceps muscles than age-matched control subjects (26, 28, 29). Thus, resistance training has the potential to improve clinical outcomes in patients with arthritis.

Over the past decade numerous studies have been undertaken to examine the effects of resistance training on muscle strength, pain, physical function, and health-related quality of life in patients with arthritis (7-12, 16, 17, 25, 31). The data are consistent and compelling that resistance training improves muscle strength, balance, and function, thereby reducing dependency and disability. In addition, patients with arthritis and other musculoskeletal diseases who undertake regular resistance training report improvement in pain, mood, and well-being compared with inactive controls. The positive effects of resistance training on pain, function, and well-being are modest, but clinically significant.

The mechanisms responsible for the clinical improvements associated with resistance training are not fully understood. In some studies there were concomitant improvements in strength, pain levels, and physical function. However, in other studies, improvements in well-being, pain, and disability were independent of changes in muscular strength. Part of the benefit of combined resistance training and aerobic exercise appears to be due to improvements in self-efficacy and sense of control (23).

A legitimate question is whether exercise, both aerobic and resistance training, will exacerbate the underlying pathological process in the joint by producing biomechanical stress on joint structures (1, 14, 15). Currently, the weight of the scientific evidence suggests that regular exercise is safe for people with arthritis (6, 14).

In all reported research to date involving resistance training and aerobic training, patients have reported improvement in symptoms, and both types of training have been well tolerated. The risks of exercise are limited to injury from dropping weights and from falls due to increased ambulation. In general, such untoward events are rare. In one study of resistance training in older adults, there was no increase in joint pain in those who exercised compared with sedentary controls (5).

In animals, repetitive or high-impact loading has been shown to damage cartilage and subchondral bone, sequelae that may lead to osteoarthritis (1, 15). Human studies suggest that competitive weightlifters and other athletes who put repetitive mechanical stress on their joints are at greater risk for osteoarthritis (8, 14). These studies are limited, however, as they are not population-based samples and do not control for injuries that increase the risk of osteoarthritis. Two epidemiological studies have shown that older patients that are physically active are more likely to develop radiographic evidence of osteoarthritis, while another study showed no increase in radiographic arthritis with activity. The relevance of these data to the question of whether resistance training can accelerate damage to joint structures is unclear, but at the very least suggests that excessive resistance should be avoided during training.

The second category of health benefits that accrue from resistance training includes reducing risk factors for heart disease, preventing diabetes, treating obesity, and attenuating the potential for osteoporosis.

Persons with both osteoarthritis and the inflammatory arthritides often have unfavorable risk factor profiles for heart disease (22). Individuals with lower-extremity osteoarthritis tend to be more obese, less fit, and hypertensive, with higher fasting glucose levels and lower high-density lipoprotein levels than age-matched controls. Similarly, those affected by inflammatory disorders are less aerobically fit and more commonly have dyslipidemia. Much of this can be attributed to the low level of activity of persons with arthritis (4). Because of pain and stiffness, patients may severely limit their activity, resulting in obesity, insulin resistance, or both. In addition, the systemic inflammation that characterizes these disorders may adversely affect lipid and lipoprotein levels, particularly by lowering high-density lipoprotein cholesterol. Anti-rheumatic medications may also adversely affect a person's coronary risk factor profile.

Corticosteroids cause insulin resistance and diabetes, hypertension, and dyslipidemia, and the nonsteroidal anti-inflammatory agents that are frequently used for symptom relief may elevate blood pressure.

In addition, people with inflammatory arthritis are at risk for developing osteoporosis, both as a result of the underlying disease process and as an adverse effect of medication, especially corticosteroids (12).

Collectively, these data suggest that patients afflicted with arthritis are at higher risk for heart disease, diabetes, hypertension, and osteoporosis, and that they would benefit from resistance training. Moreover, there is no a priori reason to believe that patients affected with arthritis would not gain the same benefits as their counterparts who do not have musculoskeletal disorders. However, data that resistance training unequivocally improves the general health of arthritis patients are lacking because, with a few exceptions, studies examining the benefits of resistance training in arthritis have not focused on cardiovascular and metabolic outcomes. Nonetheless, this author believes that such benefits would likely occur.

Exercise Prescription

The American College of Sports Medicine guidelines for screening and resistance exercise prescription should be used to develop resistance programs for persons with arthritis and related musculoskeletal disorders. However, modifications need to be made based on the individual's type and severity of arthritis, age, medication use, and comorbid conditions to increase safety and enhance the effectiveness of training.

In all cases, careful consideration must be given to the issue of where resistance training is conducted and to what extent expert supervision is necessary to prevent injury and foster long-term compliance. Although home-based exercise can be efficacious, it is this author's recommendation to begin all resistance training programs for persons with arthritis under the supervision of an exercise professional who has training in working with such individuals. There are several reasons to support this rationale. First, persons with arthritis are likely to be deconditioned and will need to have their exercise prescription tailored carefully to avoid injury and/or excessive muscular soreness that could lead to discontinuation of training and dropping out of the program.

Second, the exercise program should be viewed as an integral part of a comprehensive intervention that teaches patients self-help skills and provides necessary physical and occupational therapy for restoration of ambulation and activities of daily living. Moreover, the exercise prescription should include activities to improve aerobic function since cardiorespiratory fitness may be a limiting factor in the performance of daily activities.

Third, clinicians prescribing exercise for patients with arthritis must be cognizant of the individual's type of arthritis and the associated prescriptions (see table 18.1). In patients with systemic inflammatory arthritis, exercise should be stopped or curtailed during flare-ups that result in fever or extreme fatigue. Similarly, if patients report excessive fatigue, the exercise therapist should consider the possibility of underlying conditions such as anemia, gastrointestinal bleeding, or bone marrow suppression from medication.

Rarely, patients with inflammatory arthritides develop myositis or inflammation of the muscles. If patients report the onset of muscle weakness or pain after the initial muscle soreness that comes from initiating resistance training, exercise should be stopped until the cause of the symptoms is clarified.

TABLE 18.1 Resistance Training in Various Types of Arthritis

Type of arthritis	Evidence for efficacy of resistance training	Prescription caveats
Osteoarthritis	++++	Avoid excessive resistance when joint is unstable.
Inflammatory polyarthritides		Systematic symptoms preclude exercise training; medications and potential side effects must be known; avoid excessive resistance when joint is unstable.
Rheumatoid arthritis	++++	Avoid hyperextension of cervical spine; hand deformities may preclude use of handheld weights or equipment.
Systemic lupus erythematosis and related disorders	+	Subjects may have other organ system involvement that will alter exercise prescription and risk.
Spondyloarthropathies	++	Avoid excessive spine rotation, extension, or flexion against resistance.
Other (microcrystalline disease, vasculitis, etc.)	None	Subjects may have other organ system involvement that will alter exercise prescription and risk.
Soft tissue rheumatism		
Tendinitis and bursitis	None	To avoid rupture, use light resistance or adapt prescription if tendon is painful.
Fibromyalgia	+++	

+ = little, ++ = moderate, +++ = moderate to strong, ++++ = strong.

Biomechanical abnormalities or deformities can make resistance training challenging or even dangerous if the physical conditioning program is not appropriately modified by the exercise professional. Persons whose hands are inflamed or deformed from arthritis may have difficulty gripping handheld weights or using exercise equipment. In such cases, strap-on weights can be used, or custom devices or braces can be fashioned by an occupational therapist for use during resistance training. Similarly, instability of the shoulder or knee joint can make use of standard equipment tenuous at best. The exercise professional should consult with the patient's physician or physical or occupational therapist if there is concern over whether it is safe to put a resistance load across a deformed or unstable joint.

Three important caveats are to be understood at all times. First, patients with rheumatoid arthritis should not do exercises that result in extension of the neck. If the disease affects a patient's cervical spine and there is instability of the C1-C2 joint, hyperextension can result in spinal cord injury. Second, patients with ankylosing spondylitis should not perform exercises that forcibly rotate, flex, or extend the back. Fusion of the spinal column may have occurred, and fractures can result from excessive force. Finally, persons with tendinitis, especially of the shoulder and wrist joints, should have their exercise prescription modified to avoid excessive strain on the affected tendon in order to avoid rupture. The latter may lead to long-term loss of function.

Summary

Arthritis and related musculoskeletal disorders are common and result in significant physical disability. Resistance training has been shown to increase muscle strength, reduce pain and disability, and improve other measures of health-related quality of life in all cohorts of persons with arthritis. The clinician who is prescribing exercise for a person with arthritis must have an understanding of the individual's type and severity of arthritis, and modify the prescription accordingly. Long-term adherence to an exercise program will likely be enhanced by incorporating the prescription into a multidisciplinary, multimodal treatment plan (13).

References

1. Armstrong S.J., R.A. Read, P. Ghosh, and D. Wilson. 1993. Moderate exercise exacerbates the osteoarthritic lesions produced in cartilage by meniscectomy: A morphological study. *Osteoarthritis and Cartilage* 1: 89-96.
2. Brandt K.D. 1997. Putting muscle into osteoarthritis. *Annals of International Medicine* 127: 154-155.
3. Carter R., P. Riantawan, S.W. Banham, R.D. Sturrock. 1999. An investigation of factors limiting aerobic capacity in patients with ankylosing spondylitis. *Respiratory Medicine* 93:700-708.

4. Centers for Disease Control and Prevention. 1997. Prevalence of leisure-time physical activity among persons with arthritis and other rheumatic conditions—United States, 1990-1991. *Morbidity and Mortality Weekly Report* 46: 389-393.

5. Coleman E.A., D.M. Buchner, M.E. Cress, B.K. Chan, and B.J. de Lateur. 1996. The relationship of joint symptoms with exercise performance in older adults. *Journal of the American Geriatrics Society* 44: 14-21.

6. Ettinger W.H., and R.D. Afable. 1994. Physical disability from knee osteoarthritis: The role of exercise as an intervention. *Medicine and Science in Sports and Exercise* 26: 1435-1440.

7. Ettinger W.H., R. Burns, S.P. Messier, W. Applegate, W.J. Rejeski, T. Morgan, S. Shumaker, M.J. Berry, M. O'Toole, J. Monu, and T. Craven. 1997. A randomized trial comparing aerobic exercise and resistance exercise with a health education program in older adults with knee osteoarthritis. The Fitness Arthritis and Seniors Trial (FAST). *Journal of the American Medical Association* 277: 25-31.

8. Ettinger W.H. 1998. Physical activity, arthritis, and disability in older people. *Clinics in Geriatric Medicine* 14: 633-639.

9. Fisher N.M., and D.R. Pendergast. 1994. Effects of a muscle exercise program on exercise capacity in subjects with osteoarthritis. *Archives of Physical Medicine and Rehabilitation* 75: 792-797.

10. Fisher N.M., S.C. White, H.J. Yack, R.J. Sholinski, and D.R. Pendergast. 1997. Muscle function and gait in patients with knee osteoarthritis before and after muscle rehabilitation. *Disability Rehabilitation* 19: 47-55.

11. Gowans S.E., A. deHueck, S. Voss, and M. Richardson. 1999. A randomized, controlled trial of exercise and education for individuals with fibromyalgia. *Arthritis Care Research* 12: 120-128.

12. Hakkinen A., T. Sokka, A. Kotaniemi, H. Kautiainen, I. Jappinen, L. Laitinen, et al. 1999. Dynamic strength training in patients with early rheumatoid arthritis increases muscle strength but not bone mineral density. *Journal of Rheumatology* 26: 1257-1263.

13. Jakicic J.M., R.R. Wing, B.A. Butler, and R.J. Robertson. 1995. Prescribing exercise in multiple short bouts versus one continuous bout: Effects on adherence, cardiorespiratory fitness, and weight loss in overweight women. *International Journal of Obesity* 19: 893-901.

14. Lane N.E., and J.A. Buckwalter. 1999. Exercise and osteoarthritis. *Current Opinions in Rheumatology* 11: 413-416.

15. Little C.B., P. Ghosh, and R. Rose. 1997. The effect of strenuous versus moderate exercise on the metabolism of proteoglycans in articular cartilage from different weight-bearing regions of the equine third carpal bone. *Osteoarthritis and Cartilage* 5: 161-172.

16. Maurer B.T., A.G. Stem, B. Kinossian, K.D. Cook, and H.R. Schumacher Jr. 1999. Osteoarthritis of the knee: Isokinetic quadriceps exercise versus an educational intervention. *Archives of Physical Medicine and Rehabilitation* 80: 1293-1299.

17. McMeeken J., B. Stillman, I. Story, P. Kent, and J. Smith. 1999. The effects of knee extensor and flexor muscle training on the timed-up-and-go test in individuals with rheumatoid arthritis. *Physiotherapy Research International* 4: 55-67.

18. Messier S.P., R.F. Loeser, J.L. Hoover, et al. 1992. Osteoarthritis of the knee: Effects on gait, strength and flexibility. *Archives of Physical Medicine and Rehabilitation* 73: 20-36.

19. Messier, S.P., T.D. Royer, T.E. Craven, M.L. O'Toole, R. Burns, and W.H. Ettinger. 2000. Long-term exercise and its effect on balance in older, osteoarthritic adults: Results from the Fitness, Arthritis, and Seniors Trial (FAST). *Journal of the American Geriatrics Society* 48 (2): 131-138.

20. Minor M.A., and N.E. Lane. 1996. Recreational exercise in arthritis. *Rheumatic Diseases Clinics of North America* 22: 563-577.

21. O'Reilly S.C., A. Jones, K.R. Muir, M. Doherty. 1998. Quadriceps weakness in knee osteoarthritis: The effect on pain and disability. *Annals of the Rheumatic Diseases* 57: 588-594.

22. Philbin E.F., M.D. Ries, G.D. Groff, K.A. Sheesley, T.S. French, and T.A. Pearson. 1996. Osteoarthritis as determinant of an adverse coronary heart disease risk profile. *Journal of Cardiovascular Risk* 3: 529-533.

23. Rejeski W.J., W.H. Ettinger, K. Martin, and T. Morgan. 1998. Treating disability in knee osteoarthritis with exercise therapy: A central role for self-efficacy and pain. *Arthritis Care Research* 11: 94-101.

24. Rossy L.A., S.P. Buckelew, N. Dorr, K.J. Hagglund, J.F. Thayer, M.J. McIntosh, J.E. Hewett, and J.C. Johnson. 1999. A meta-analysis of fibromyalgia treatment interventions. *Annals of Behavioral Medicine* 21: 180-191.

25. Scholten C., T. Brodowicz, W. Graninger, I. Gardavsky, K. Pils, B. Pesau, E. Eggl-Thyl, A. Wanivenhaus, and C. Zielinski. 1999. Persistent functional and social benefit 5 years after a multidisciplinary arthritis training program. *Archives of Physical Medicine and Rehabilitation* 80: 1282-1287.

26. Slemenda C., D.K. Heilman, K.D. Brandt, B.P. Katz, S.A. Mazzuca, E.M. Braunstein, and D. Byrd. 1998. Reduced quadriceps strength relative to body weight: A risk factor for knee osteoarthritis in women. *Arthritis and Rheumatism* 41: 1951-1959.

27. Stenstrom C.H., B. Arge, and A. Sundbom. 1997. Home exercise and compliance in inflammatory rheumatic diseases—A prospective clinical trial. *Journal of Rheumatology* 24: 470-476.

28. Suter E., and W. Herzog. 2000. Does muscle inhibition after knee injury increase the risk of osteoarthritis? *Exercise and Sport Sciences Reviews* 28: 15-18.

29. Suter E., W. Herzog, K. Desouza, and R.C. Bray. 1998. Inhibition of the quadriceps muscles in patients with anterior knee pain. *Journal of Applied Biomechanics* 14: 360-373.

30. Tan J., N. Balci, V. Sepici, and F.A. Gener. 1995. Isokinetic and isometric strength in osteoarthrosis of the knee. A comparative study with healthy women. *American Journal of Physical Medicine and Rehabilitation* 74: 364-369.

31. Van Baar M.E., W.J. Assendelft, J. Dekker, R.A. Oostendorp, and J.W. Bijlsma. 1999. Effectiveness of exercise therapy in patients with osteoarthritis of the hip or knee: A systematic review of randomized clinical trials. *Arthritis and Rheumatism* 42 (7): 1361-1369.

32. Van den Ende C.H., T.P. Vliet Vlieland, M. Munneke, and J.M. Hazes. 1998. Dynamic exercise therapy in rheumatoid arthritis: A systematic review. *British Journal of Rheumatology* 37: 677-687.

33. Viitanen J.V., K. Lehtinen, J. Suni, and H. Kautiainen. 1995. Fifteen months' follow-up of intensive inpatient physiotherapy and exercise in ankylosing spondylitis. *Clinical Rheumatology* 14: 413-419.

34. Yocum D.E., W.L. Castro, and M. Cornett. 2000. Exercise, education, and behavioral modification as alternative therapy for pain and stress in rheumatic disease. *Rheumatic Diseases Clinics of North America* 26: 145-159.

19

CHAPTER

Resistance Training for Low Back Pain and Dysfunction

James E. Graves, PhD
John Mayer, DC, PhD
Syracuse University

Ted Dreisinger, PhD
Progressive Spine Care and Rehabilitation

Vert Mooney, MD
U.S. Spine and Sport

Epidemiology and the Theoretical Considerations

Low back pain (LBP) is one of the most common and costly medical problems in modern societies. Although it is not as serious a condition as heart disease or cancer in terms of mortality, LBP is the most common cause of disability in the United States for persons under 45 years of age (22), and it has an estimated annual cost (medical cost and disability payments) of between \$20 and \$50 billion (85). One of the problems in the prevention and treatment of LBP is that the etiology is diverse, and the specific cause is often unknown (24). Many cases of LBP, however, have been associated with poor physical conditioning (14, 86, 116). For this reason, LBP is considered one of the major hypokinetic diseases (13).

Although the exact role of physical activity in the prevention and rehabilitation of LBP is not clear (10), active exercise has long been recognized as an effective approach for both prevention and rehabilitation (23, 36). Indeed, the major emphasis in LBP rehabilitation has recently shifted from pain management to the restoration of functional capacity (42). Muscular strength training through properly prescribed progressive resistance exercise, in particular, is thought to help overcome structural weakness that may predispose one to LBP (96). This chapter will discuss restorative lumbar exercise training for health, prevention, and rehabilitation, outline strength testing for spinal function, review the physiological considerations for exercising the low back musculature, and make recommendations for the prescription of progressive resistance exercise for the prevention and rehabilitation of LBP.

The Cost of Back Pain to Society and Industry

Low back pain has become the most expensive health care problem in the United States in people 25 to 50 years of age. Whether this impact is measured in terms of frequency of doctor visits, industrial injury claims, or disability pensions, back pain complaints remain the most costly musculoskeletal problem in developed countries (126). The total compensation for low back pain was estimated at $6,000 per patient in 1990 and has greatly increased since (5). The expense of back pain to society consists not only of the costs related to therapy, but also the cost of time lost from work due to permanent or partial disability. It is generally agreed that medical costs account for about one-third of the total of back pain costs. Disability payments account for the remaining two-thirds. The direct and indirect costs have been carefully analyzed and in 1990 were thought to exceed $24 billion (29). With a decade of inflation and increasing medical costs, an estimated total annual expense exceeding $50 billion is not unreasonable.

Although greater biomechanical knowledge has resulted in improved ergonomic conditions in the workplace, and automated devices have made jobs less strenuous, the financial impact of back pain continues to grow. With increased subsidization of medical care in industrialized societies, public perception of back pain has shifted from unpleasant fact of life to treatable medical problem (4). This shift in perception has led to greater expectation for resolution. The perception that back pain often results from industrial injury has also brought about a host of problems related to workplace liability and society's responsibility for disability.

Those who do the heaviest work are at the greatest risk. Nurse's aides, for example, are more likely than supervising nurses to have back pain (125). It has also been demonstrated that people in good physical shape have a lower incidence of back pain than those who are less well conditioned (14). Such studies might lead us to believe that screening for weakness will help prevent the occurrence of back pain in the work place. Yet only one study in the literature suggests that industrial back pain is more likely to occur if the back is considered weak during pre-employment evaluation (18). Other studies have not found a relationship between back pain complaints and pre-employment tests of functional capacity (56, 79). In a prospective longitudinal study of more than 3000 manufacturing workers in the United States, data on more than 50 commonly suspected risk factors explained less than 10% of the variation in predicting who would file a complaint of low back pain (8). Thus, susceptibility to an initial episode of low back pain is difficult to identify.

On the other hand, diminished lumbar extensor strength can be a significant predictor of low back pain in previously injured workers (80). In a prospective study by Mooney et al., 80% of the workers who volunteered for a once-a-week lumbar strength training program had a history of back pain (80). These workers were weaker than the 20% without a history of back pain, even though they had no pain at the time of testing. This strength deficit was correctable. Following the strengthening program, both groups of workers improved their functional capacity to the same level. The incidence of back injury following training was reduced relative to untrained controls during a one-year follow-up.

The Role of Strength in Back Pain Prevention

Although social and cultural factors influence back pain, there is also an inherent structural change that develops secondary to injury of the soft tissues. This structural alteration explains the frequency of back pain complaints even when there are no economic factors involved, and structural weakness is often implicated in the literature as a predisposing risk factor for low back pain.

Although exercise is known to improve muscular strength and functional capacity (26), the role of exercise for the prevention of low back pain is equivocal. The most recent summary of pertinent literature has been published by the Agency for Health Care Policy and Research (9). Although the summary encourages an active exercise program, no specific guidelines or rationale are provided for the prevention of low back pain.

There is, however, good theoretical support for the role of exercise in the prevention of low back pain. The human lumbar spine functions in a unique posture. Other primates stand and walk in a forward flexed position without lordosis (curvature of the lumbar spine). Lordosis is prevalent in quadrupeds, but in these animals the spine does not function under high axial loads, as it does in erect humans. The muscle group most responsible for maintaining a lordotic posture in humans is the multifidus. The multifidus has five separate bands, each consisting of sections that stem from the spinous process and lamina of the lumbar vertebrae and covering from one to four segments (64). The deepest sections are shorter than the more superficial transverse segments. Some of the deepest multifidus fibers attach to the capsules of the zygapophyseal (facet) joints. This attachment to the joint capsules keeps the capsule taut and free from impingement between the articular cartilage (64). Because the majority of torso weight is anterior to the spine, these muscles have the most direct control in maintaining the lordotic position. Muscle activity is a defense against sudden overload of connective tissue. The normal events of daily life present many opportunities for an "unguarded moment." A sudden change of position, or arrival of an unsuspected force, can place an unusual load on the vulnerable connective tissues of the spine and intervertebral discs when the spine is flexed and rotated.

Another unique biomechanical function of the human spine is to provide support for a great array of precise and powerful arm and hand functions. Torso stability serves as the foundation for many upper-limb movements. The transverse abdominis in humans is a unique muscle due to its extensive attachment to the thoracical lumbar fascia through multiple layers (117). The thoraco-lumbar fascia has attachments not only to the lumbar vertebrae by way of the transverse processes and the ligaments, but also to the erector spinae muscle fascia.

The importance of the transverse abdominis is highlighted in studies that demonstrate its constant role in upper-extremity manual activity and spinal stability (19). Using fine wire electrodes placed during real-time ultrasound, it is possible to isolate abdominal muscle activity (20). In all movements of the trunk, the transverse abdominis is activated slightly sooner (200 ms) than the other abdominal muscles, and in coordination with the multifidus. Transverse abdominis activity also occurs sooner than arm muscle activity when sudden unguarded movements occur (21). Under all conditions studied, when the transversalis is activated in normals, the multifidus is activated (21). Transverse abdominis activity also occurs without regard to lateralization, that is, left arm movement versus right arm movement, flexion versus extension, or lateral bending (45).

The importance of these muscles becomes apparent when they are studied in patients. When a subject with low back pain flexes, abducts, or extends the spine, there is a delay in transverse abdominis firing with shoulder motion (44). Likewise, multifidus activation is delayed. The anticipatory function of the transversalis and the multifidus is also observed during leg movement in normals but not in patients with back pain (43). The inhibition of the transverse abdominis leaves the trunk more vulnerable to physical stress during the unguarded moment.

Multifidus function is deficient in chronic low back pain patients (2, 93, 102, 109). The multifidus has been identified as the most at risk lumbar musculature during lifting because it is the first to fatigue (103). Fatigue is greater in patients with chronic low back pain compared to normal subjects. Fatty infiltration of the lumbar extensors in patients with chronic low back pain (93) has also been observed (2). Myoelectric activation of the lumbar extensors is also considerably less than expected in low back pain patients (102). The flexors often function normally in patients with low back pain, while the extensors do not (27). In normal subjects, there is no difference in size of the extensor muscles between the right and left side. In patients with low back pain, however, the symptomatic side can be over 40% smaller. This size differential in low back pain patients occurs within 2 weeks of symptoms and persists for 10 weeks despite symptomatic relief. When subjects participate in a progressive resistance training program to strengthen the multifidus and transversalis muscles, only 30% of those subjects who train have a recurrence of back pain at long-term follow-up. Patients who do not train have an 80% recurrence rate (41).

There is a relationship between back extensor strength and back pain. Biering-Sorensen (7) completed an extensive physical examination of lumbar strength and range of motion. One year later, back injuries were evaluated by questionnaire. There was a direct correlation between the incidence of back pain and isometric back extensor weakness. A subsequent study showed that individuals with poor performance on the Biering-Sorenson muscular endurance test were three times more likely to have back pain than those who had good performance (61).

Another recent study clearly demonstrates postinjury inhibition, as well as the trainability of lumbar extensor muscles (78). In this study, surface EMG of the lumbar musculature was measured before and after an 8-week low back training program. MRIs were also taken before and after the training program to assess the cross-sectional area of the multifidus muscles. The patients averaged about 40% less lumbar extensor strength at the beginning of the training program than asymptomatic controls. At the conclusion of training, the patients were able to lift 100% more weight than when they started. When the amplitude of the lumbar extensors' EMG activity was evaluated after training, it had decreased by one-third compared to amplitude at the start. Thus, neural efficiency greatly increased. There was only a 10% increase in strength in the normals. The size of the multifidus muscles in the normals did not change. Cross-sectional images of the patients' multifidus showed significant hypertrophy. These data demonstrate that physical training that focuses on specific activation of the back extensors can increase size and improve functional capacity in muscles that tend to be inhibited in patients with back pain.

A one-year follow-up study of 400 patients from two separate clinical centers using a standardized protocol for lumbar extensor strength testing and training (58) evaluated patients with chronic recurrent back pain who were treated in a standardized progressive exercise program for approximately 8 weeks (training twice per week). Over 80% of the patients reported attenuated levels of pain and discomfort after the training program. Interestingly, all patients had previous physical therapy and chiropractic manipulation, and 12% had previous surgical care. In both centers, the particular medical diagnosis was not a predictor of efficacy, as all conditions improved about the same. At one-year follow-up, there was an 11% reutilization of medical care due to back pain. By comparison, Carey et al. reported a 73% utilization of the health care system in a group that had not had strength training (15).

In summary, there is convincing scientific evidence to support a specific exercise program for the development of lumbar extensor muscular strength to restore lumbar muscle function and prevent future episodes of low back pain. The deficit in lumbar extensor function seen in patients with low back pain is reversible and can be corrected by an active strength training program.

Strength Testing of the Spine: A Historical Perspective

Soft-tissue weakness is often considered a primary risk factor for LBP (96). As a result, the lumbar extensor musculature is considered by some to be the weak link in the kinetic chain that makes many individuals susceptible to LBP. Quantitative assessment of lumbar muscle function dates back to the 1940s when investigators postulated the need for strong trunk muscles to prevent back injury and dysfunction (53, 73). These ideas were based on biomechanical and clinical principles rather than empirical evidence, since there were no devices to accurately measure strength of the lumbar musculature at the time. There were several difficulties facing early investigators attempting to evaluate the relationship between clinical low back pain and strength. They would need patients willing to have their painful backs tested and tools that could provide valid and reliable measurements from which to make clinical judgments.

In 1969, Nachemson and Lindh studied 160 subjects, including 63 patients with low back pain, 80 subjects without history of low back pain who served as controls, and 17 women who had worn a corset for support for at least 6 months (86). Trunk extension strength was measured in both the standing and prone positions. Abdominal strength was measured while subjects lay supine with knees bent. In all three measures, the body was restrained to minimize the influence of other musculature. A spring dynamometer was used to measure extensor and flexor strength through three trials. Test values were unaffected by age, body height, or weight. There was little difference in strength between patients and those without back pain. The researchers concluded there was no evidence to suggest that back pain could be related to weakness of trunk muscles and that spinal and abdominal strength were not important for the prevention of low back syndrome (86).

In 1980, Hasue, Fujiwara, and Kikuchi (37) used a modified isokinetic knee extension device to measure dynamic and static strength of the lumbar extensors and trunk flexors. One hundred normals and 26 patients with chronic low back pain were studied. Extensor strength was measured in the prone position with the force arm of the dynamometer placed across the lower pole of the scapula. The feet were held to reduce motion artifact. Flexion strength was measured with subjects in the supine position with the force arm of the dynamometer placed across the xiphoid process. Knees were bent and the feet held, once again to reduce motion artifact. Measurements were taken dynamically at 360°/ s (extensors) and 720°/s (flexors). Single-position isometric measures were also taken for flexion and extension. The results indicated that the extensor muscles were stronger than the flexors, and age was inversely related to strength. Flexor muscles fatigued more easily than extensors, and isometric testing was more fatiguing than dynamic testing. In contrast to Nachemson's data (86), strength of trunk muscles was reduced in patients with low back pain. This difference was probably due to the level of sophistication of the testing apparatus that had evolved by the 1980s. Although the pelvis was not well restrained to isolate the trunk musculature, the data were better quantified.

In 1980, Smidt and others recognized that gravity would affect trunk strength measures taken in the supine or prone positions (112). The weight of the trunk alone would cause the "measured strength" of the dynamometer to inaccurately reflect torque output of the subject. They developed a device called the "Iowa table" whereby subjects lay on their side with a dynamometer attached to their trunks (112). The pelvis was stabilized in the front and the back with pads. Torque was measured in four positions (–20°, 0°, 20°, and 40°). Zero degrees was considered the neutral position, –20° was considered full extension, and 40° was considered full flexion. The observed torque measures indicated that extensor strength was greater than flexion strength at all angles. The data also demonstrated that eccentric strength was much greater than concentric strength. These investigators realized two important concepts relative to spinal testing methodology: that gravity would affect the observed results, and that not all trunk positions generate the same amount of torque. This was the first published observation that single-position isometric testing of the lumbar spine did not provide a clear picture of the strength of the trunk (flexors or extensors) through the full range of motion.

In 1983, Smidt et al. developed a seated dynamometer using a modified isokinetic knee machine (111). This device provided pelvic stability using knee and thigh restraints. This was the first study to focus on the important issue of stabilizing the pelvis to restrict pelvic rotation when measuring back extensor strength. Pelvic restraint limited the patients' range of motion more than that of the controls, and the rate of torque development in the patients was slower.

In 1983, Suzuki and Endo (115) reproduced the study by Hasue et al. (37) on a larger group of patients with back pain. Ninety men with low back pain and 50 asymptomatic controls participated. The subjects were tested in the supine and prone positions to assess flexion and extension strength. The controls were stronger during flexion only when the knees were straight, but always stronger during extension. As previously demonstrated, fatigue was greater in flexors than extensors. Length of time from injury was unrelated to the ability to generate torque.

In 1984, Langrana et al. (55), using a similar but less restraining device than that of Smidt (111), showed that patients with low back pain had lower peak torque and less range of motion than controls with no back pain. The researchers suggested that these differences were due to the restrictions of low back pain.

In 1985, Smith et al. gathered strength data using two standing isokinetic dynamometers that had been designed specifically for testing flexion, extension, and rotation of the spine (113). The study was designed to examine dynamic and isometric torque output of the subjects and assess the reliability of the data collection. As previously shown, men were stronger than women. Test reliability was good, suggesting that standardized protocols could be developed and reproduced. However, during several tests, dynamic torque measures exceeded those of isometric torque. This was surprising since the force velocity curve indicates that concentric dynamic torques should always be less than static measures. The elevated torque measures in flexion and rotation were probably due to the artifact of impact forces (torque overshoot) during directional change rather than representing true torque values (113).

In 1995, Petersen et al. continued to explore the importance of pelvic stabilization during trunk strength testing (95). Ten subjects (5 men and 5 women) were tested while seated with a strain gauge attached to their trunk and fixed to a restraining device. Torque measures were taken during four different constraint configurations: pelvic pad fixation with no leg restraint, pelvic pad fixation with leg restraint, pelvic belt fixation with no leg restraint, and pelvic belt fixation with leg restraint. The investigators found that pelvic motion was unaffected by leg stabilization, but that pelvic stabilization increased torque values, suggesting that stabilization is important for accurate torque measurements. An important implication of this study is that by stabilizing the pelvis, torque measures more accurately reflect forces generated by the lumbar spine. Methods of testing without pelvic stabilization (as previously described) were likely measuring compound trunk extension. Trunk extension during most lifting activity occurs as a result of combined contraction of the hamstring and gluteal muscles (the hip extensors) as well as the lumbar extensors. Without appropriate stabilization during back testing, it is virtually impossible to determine what specific muscle groups are contributing to the generation of torque.

In 1988, Seeds et al. introduced a so-called isoinertial testing device (106). Unlike the isokinetic machines that are "constant velocity," the isoinertial machine is a constant mass device. In other words, speed is allowed to vary in the dynamometer, but the mass against which the forces are applied remains constant. This device recorded torque measures in all three planes. The study compared healthy controls (normals) and a patient population. The normals showed greater ranges of motion in flexion, extension, and lateral flexion/extension. The flexion/extension data were similar to those of Smidt et al. (111), suggesting that individuals without back pain had greater range of motion than individuals with back pain. It was also found that normals had greater torque production in all planes. Parnianpour et al. used a similar device on healthy populations and found that when exercising to fatigue, torque values decreased and muscle substitution occurred (94). This finding suggests that in a person who is at high risk for low back pain, muscle substitution due to fatigue might further increase the risk by creating unfavorable postural changes or reducing the ability of the spine to protect against an "unguarded" movement.

In 1989, Battie et al. used a modified "platform dynamometer" to measure "back strength" in a large industrial population (6). There was no restraint system in this particular device. The subject stood in a flexed position, held a gripping device in their hands that was anchored to a static dynamometer, and extended with an isometric contraction of the back. The device was not a back dynamometer, per se; it was simply designed to measure gross strength. The investigators concluded that height, weight, gender, and age were not predictors of strength. Moreover, there appeared to be a higher incidence of back problems in subjects who were stronger, but the results of strength testing were not predictive of back problems. These data contrasted with findings of

Chaffin et al. (using a similar system) who in 1978 showed that back strength was a risk factor for injury in industry (17). The discrepancy is likely due to the nature of the industrial setting to which the test was applied.

The historical review of spinal strength testing to this point highlights several issues and concerns. Patients with low back pain do not perform as well as persons with healthy backs. The ability to generate torque is reduced with age. Pelvic restraint is important for the accurate measurement of lumbar extension torque output. Single-position isometric tests do not provide a valid assessment of back strength through a full range of motion. Pelvic stabilization during multiposition isometric testing has emerged as an effective strategy for the accurate measurement of functional capacity of the spine. In addition, comparisons among studies are difficult because the measurement devices used have been dissimilar. They vary from recumbent-position strain gauges and isokinetic dynamometers to seated/standing isokinetic dynamometers and standing isoinertial dynamometers. The absence of standardized protocols as well as a lack of established reliability and validity for the devices themselves have also been important limitations (25).

In 1989, Pollock et al. published validity/reliability and training data with a new lumbar extension dynamometer (97). This machine provided several new and unique characteristics. Testing was done in the seated position. Gravity was compensated for via a trunk counterweight, pelvic stabilization was used to minimize the contribution of the hip extensor muscle groups, and multipositional isometric torque measurements were taken to quantify functional capacity (torque output) of the spine through its full range of motion. Dynamic strength training was prescribed based on the multipositional isometric test. Graves et al. followed this pilot training study with a thorough analysis of the reliability of the testing protocol (32), and several training studies were subsequently performed to design the most appropriate testing and training protocols (34, 35).

Russell et al. treated 91 patients with low back pain (63 men and 28 women) with varying diagnoses (e.g., lumbar strain, herniated lumbar disc, degenerated lumbar disc) with this new dynamometer (104). The treatment protocol involved 8 weeks of progressive resistance exercise preceded and followed by isolated isometric testing. Stabilization of the pelvis to isolate the lumbar extensors has the added clinical value of requiring movement by the lumbar spine, which typically moves little in the patients with low back pain. Significant gains in strength and range of motion were seen in all groups. Perceived pain also decreased following training. Although there were some differences among groups prior to training, there were no significant differences between diagnostic groups following the training program. The investigators concluded that this approach was safe for these patients and that trainability (improvement in functional capacity) was unrelated to initial diagnosis.

In 1993, Newton and Waddell published a review of the scientific literature to date on the clinical efficacy of isodynamic dynamometers (89). They concluded that there was "inadequate scientific evidence to support the use of iso-machines in preemployment screening, routine clinical assessment, or medico-legal evaluation" (89, p. 801). The paper emphasized that poor reliability, cross-equipment comparisons, inadequate normative data, and lack of standard protocols have made interpretation of the data tenuous at best.

Research using isometric measurement with pelvic stabilization, however, has had the advantage of standardized protocols across clinics in order to provide a more consistent clinical picture of patient strength deficits. Normative data, standard protocols, and emerging industrial, clinical, and outcomes data permit valid and reliable comparisons among clinical sites. Indeed, the clinical efficacy for testing and treating patients with low back pain has been established in several recent studies (80, 88, 99).

In summary, lumbar spine testing has a history dating back to the 1940s. Since that time, investigators have been intrigued by the relationship between functional capacity and low back pain. Studies suggest that reduced strength and range of motion are common among individuals with low back pain. Strength training can counteract this association. Patients who increase low back strength have demonstrated reductions in pain (99, 104), less reutilization of health care (88), and reduced workers' compensation costs (80).

Difficulties in interpreting the published research are largely attributed to a lack of standardization among testing devices, inadequate normative data, and varying protocols, as noted by Newton and Waddell in their review of dynamic back-testing machines (89). Fortunately, new technology and standardized protocols have provided normative data and a better ability to study lumbar muscle function and its relationship to low back pain. The strong clinical and industrial data now emerging from this approach are proving that strength training of the isolated lumbar spine can have favorable medical and fiscal implications. Most recent data indicate that isolation of the lumbar musculature via pelvic restraint allows for the accurate evaluation of lumbar muscle function and effective progressive resistance exercise training.

Physiological Considerations for the Prescription of Resistance Training for the Prevention and Rehabilitation of Low Back Pain

The lumbar extensor musculature consists of two muscle groups: the erector spinae and the multifidus (12). The erector spinae group, which lies lateral to the multifidus, is divided into the iliocostalis lumborum and longissimus thoracis muscles (11). These muscles are separated from each other by the lumbar intramuscular aponeurosis, with the longissimus lying medially (63). The longissimus and iliocostalis are composed of several multisegmental fascicles (62), which allow for sagittal rotation (extension) and posterior translation when the muscles are contracted bilaterally. The fascicular arrangement of the multifidus muscle suggests that the multifidus acts primarily as a sagittal rotator (extension without posterior translation). Lateral flexion and axial rotation are possible for both the multifidus and erector spinae musculature during unilateral contraction (12, 52). Because of these anatomical and biomechanical properties, it has been suggested that the lumbar extensor musculature is particularly adapted to maintain posture (49) and stabilize the spine and trunk (49, 91).

Functional Capacity

The functional capacity of skeletal muscle is usually quantified by measures of muscular strength and endurance. Muscular strength refers to the ability to generate force during a single muscle action. Muscular endurance is the ability to resist fatigue during repeated muscle actions.

The relationship between morphological and physiological characteristics of the lumbar musculature and low back extension strength has been explored extensively using isometric strength testing procedures. The mean fiber size of the erector spinae muscles is positively correlated ($r = 0.60, p \leq 0.05$) with isometric trunk extension strength (31, 48). It has been estimated that the absolute strength of the erector spinae is approximately 48 N (Newtons)/cm^2, based on cross-sectional area and morphological analyses (98). Mean values for isometric trunk extension strength while standing have been reported between 675 N and 1034 N for males and between 410 N and 823 N for females (48). Furthermore, males are stronger than females even after total body mass and lean body mass are taken into consideration (48). This is consistent with gender comparisons of the relative strength of other muscle groups located in the upper body and is likely due to the fact that men have a greater proportion of lean mass in the upper body than women do. Patients with LBP have been shown to have lower trunk extension strength values than healthy individuals (16, 74, 75, 77, 78, 99). However, the force generated during maximum voluntary contraction (MVC) of the trunk extensors has failed to be a predictive factor for future LBP (6).

Morphological and histochemical characteristics of the lumbar extensor musculature are also related to isometric trunk extension endurance (resistance to fatigue). The relative area of the erector spinae muscle occupied by type I fibers has a significant positive correlation to static endurance (isometric holding) time ($p \leq 0.05$) (67). The lumbar extensor muscles also have higher endurance times at various levels of submaximal forces than other skeletal muscles (48). Additionally, women have approximately 33% greater endurance times during a prone isometric test than men (7, 50, 61, 67). Lower endurance values for patients with LBP have been reported (7, 46, 61), and, unlike MVC, endurance values have been predictive of future LBP (7, 61). Therefore, the prescription of resistance exercise for the prevention and rehabilitation of LBP should probably focus on the development of muscular endurance (lower load, higher repetitions) as opposed to muscular strength (higher load, lower repetitions).

Exercise Training

A common belief within the exercise and rehabilitation communities is that conditioning the trunk flexors (abdominal musculature) should be the highest priority for exercise training protocols designed to relieve back pain. This belief arises from the theory that strengthening the abdominal muscles will increase intra-abdominal pressure and also maintain a favorable balance between the strength of the abdominal muscles and the back extensors. Increasing intra-abdominal pressure diminishes compressive forces on the spine and reduces the load on the intervertebral discs and posterior spinal structures (83). However, studies have shown that intra-abdominal pressure is not increased during contraction of the abdominals (38). Furthermore, it is not increased following an abdominal strength training program (38). Thus, the anterior trunk muscles are at best only of secondary importance in the pathogenesis and management of spinal disorders.

Current evidence suggests that it is weakness in the lumbar musculature (possibly resulting from disuse) that is closely linked to LBP, rather than weak abdominals. Weak and highly fatigable trunk extensor muscles have been consistently reported in populations with low back pain (23, 52, 60, 63, 68, 77, 91). Those who suffer from low back pain also have a decreased trunk extensor to trunk flexor strength ratio compared with asymptomatic individuals (54, 107). In addition, morphological changes, such as atrophy of the lumbar multifidus and erector spinae muscles, have been reported in patients with acute and chronic low back pain (40). Morphological changes to the lumbar extensors often persist long after the remission of symptoms from the first episode of back pain, leaving the individual at risk for future pathology (39). In vitro studies, for example, have shown that multifidus dysfunction results in intersegmental instability and excessive vertebral rotation (91) and may lead to facet capsulitis, arthrosis of the facet joint, annular tears, disc herniation, and spondylosis (52).

For these reasons, spinal rehabilitation programs often attempt to incorporate back extensor muscle conditioning exercises. Progressive resistance training regimens involving the low back extensor muscles have been largely successful, with increased cross-sectional area of the lumbar extensors (39, 101), decreased fatty infiltration of the lumbar extensors (78), increased strength (58, 74, 80, 88, 99, 101), increased endurance (66), decreased pain (65, 66, 74, 99), improved psychosocial function (99), decreased rates of future spinal surgery (87), and reduction in lost work time (80, 88, 99) reported following training in patients with chronic low back pain. Recently, the U.S Agency for Health Care Policy and Research (AHCPR) concluded that back extensor muscle conditioning exercises are helpful in the management of low back pain (9).

While the lumbar extensors appear to be the weak link in the development of LBP (as opposed to the trunk flexors), it is our firm belief that conditioning of all of the major muscle groups is important for the development of overall functional capacity and the health benefits associated with physical activity. Therefore, although the lumbar extensors should be targeted for the prevention and rehabilitation of LBP, a well-rounded exercise program that incorporates a variety of progressive resistance exercises should be promulgated.

Progressive resistance exercise training with pelvic stabilization on a lumbar dynamometer effectively increases functional capacity in both healthy and LBP patient populations. Pollock et al. found that 10 weeks of dynamic progressive resistance training was capable of eliciting 42-102% increases in isometric lumbar extension strength (97). Surprisingly, the subjects in Pollock's study trained at a relatively low frequency and with a low training volume (1 set, 1/week, 8-12 repetitions to volitional exhaustion). A follow-up study indicated that a training frequency of 1 session per week was as effective as training 2 times and 3 times per week in developing isometric lumbar extension strength (33). Furthermore, after subjects achieve strength gains from this relatively low training frequency, reduced training frequencies as low as 1 session every 4 weeks allow maintenance of the lumbar extension strength gains (122).

The lumbar extensor muscles exhibit morphological changes (hypertrophy) that exceed those found in other muscle groups following a low volume of training. A 5-8% increase in cross-sectional area of the erector spinae musculature has been observed after a 12-week resistance training program of 1 exercise session per week (28, 59), while a 15% increase in cross-sectional area has been noted following training at a frequency of 3 times per week (59). The greater increase in cross-sectional area associated with more frequent training raises interesting and important questions about the prescription of lumbar extension exercise for the prevention of LBP. Low-volume (1 set), low-frequency (1/week) training is likely associated with significant neural (learning) adaptations

(59). If improving the structural integrity of the vulnerable area through morphological adaptation is important, more frequent training may be advantageous even though functional measures (isometric strength) are identical in low-frequency and more frequent training.

The relatively large strength gains (compared to gains reported following training with other skeletal muscle groups [26]) associated with a low volume of exercise have been attributed to a low initial trained state of the low back extensor muscles (97). Because there is little pelvic stabilization during normal activities of daily living, the lumbar muscles rarely experience an overload stimulus sufficient to elicit strength gains (33). Thus, the powerful gluteus and hamstring muscles, instead of the smaller lumbar paraspinals, may be responsible for the majority of torque generation during compound trunk extension. The postulation of a low initial trained state of the lumbar extensors is supported by histochemical data that have revealed a smaller type II fiber size of the lumbar extensor muscles than what is typically observed in other skeletal muscles (67, 69, 70, 90).

It has been suggested that isolating the lumbar area through pelvic stabilization eliminates the contribution of the gluteal and hamstring muscle groups during exercise training, thereby allowing the lumbar extensor muscles to receive the stimulus necessary for strength gains (97). To test this hypothesis, the effect of pelvic stabilization during resistance training on lumbar extension strength has been studied by several investigators. In a 12-week training study by Graves et al. (34), exercise training with pelvic stabilization (PSTAB) on a lumbar extension dynamometer (MedX) was compared with exercise training without pelvic stabilization (NOSTAB) on other machines (Cybex or Nautilus). All training groups exhibited significant increases in dynamic exercise load, but only PSTAB showed an increase in isometric lumbar extension strength. It was concluded that pelvic stabilization is required during training to strengthen the lumbar extensor muscles. However, there may have been issues of specificity of testing and training related to the testing machine employed, since the PSTAB group exercised on the lumbar extension dynamometer used to obtain criterion measures, while the NOSTAB groups did not (34).

To minimize these exercise specificity issues, Mayer et al. completed a study that allowed both the PSTAB and NOSTAB groups to train on the same lumbar extension dynamometer that was utilized for the isometric strength tests (71). In this study, isometric strength tests were performed by 33 healthy subjects with and without the pelvis stabilized on the dynamometer prior to training. Interestingly, lumbar extension torque values were similar for the stabilized and unstabilized tests at five of the seven angles of lumbar flexion tested. The unstabilized test produced higher torque values than the stabilized test only at the two most extended angles in the range of motion (0° and 12°). Following 12 weeks of progressive resistance exercise, both the PSTAB and NOSTAB groups increased lumbar extension isometric torque output during the test with the pelvis stabilized. However, only the NOSTAB group increased torque output in the unstabilized test. The investigators concluded that pelvic stabilization during testing of lumbar muscle function may not be as important as once thought. Additionally, they emphasized that training with pelvic stabilization on the dynamometer is not necessary to increase lumbar extension strength and that training without pelvic stabilization on the dynamometer is more versatile. Training without stabilization may be more closely correlated with performance of normal activities (unstabilized).

In support of the Mayer et al. (71) study, Parkkola et al. (92) reported that training on a low back machine (Nautilus) that makes little to no attempt to stabilize the pelvis was successful in increasing back extension strength and the cross-sectional area of the lumbar extensor muscles. In addition, Lee reported that exercise on a Roman chair (an exercise device that allows lumbar extension from a prone position) or lumbar dynamometer was successful in increasing back extension static endurance times on the Roman chair and isometric torque values on the dynamometer following 4 weeks of training by healthy, sedentary subjects and female volleyball players (57).

Fujita et al. compared 12 weeks of exercise training on a dynamometer with straight-legged dead lifts and Roman chair exercise (30). Outcomes were assessed using all exercise techniques and included a seven-angle isometric lumbar extension torque test on a dynamometer, a five-repetition maximum (5-RM) test on a Roman chair, and a dead lift. Following training, all groups showed significant improvement in the 5-RM test on the Roman chair and the dead lift ($p \leq 0.05$). The dynamometer group improved significantly at all angles of lumbar flexion during the seven-angle isometric torque test ($p \leq 0.05$). The dead-lift group increased at 0°, 12°, 60°, and 72° of lumbar flexion. The Roman chair group did not increase their isometric torque output at any angle of lumbar flexion measured on the dynamometer ($p > 0.05$). The investigators concluded that the Roman chair is not effective for increasing lumbar extension strength when testing is performed on a dynamometer. Mayer et al. also reported no gain in isometric torque production on a dynamometer following 12 weeks of training with a Roman chair (71). The findings of these studies contradict the finding by Lee that Roman chair training can develop lumbar extension torque output on the dynamometer (57). The lack of improvement with Roman chair training in two of the three studies discussed above suggests that there may be significant specificity of testing and training effects associated with measures of functional capacity obtained using a lumbar dynamometer.

The above studies indicate that the need for pelvic stabilization during lumbar extension testing and training is inconclusive and perhaps not as important as once thought. Intuitively, stabilization is essential for the isolation of specific muscle groups during progressive resistance exercise training. It is important to recognize, however, that individual muscles rarely work in isolation in the real world. The trade-off between the need to isolate a muscle to achieve maximum strength benefit versus training the ability of a muscle to work in concert with other muscle groups to produce patterned movements will continue to be debated.

The feasibility of widespread clinical or home use of lumbar extension dynamometers has been limited by the expense and lack of portability of these machines, despite their clinical efficacy (72). Furthermore, the high cost of dynamometric methods (1, 47, 100, 105) and the unusual posture often required for testing has put into question the true benefits of the various sophisticated dynamometric devices. In addition, the seated upright posture, which is necessary for the performance of lumbar extension exercise on some dynamometers, is associated with increased compressive forces on the spine and lumbar discs (84) and may be detrimental for some patients with low back pain. However, at present, there are no known low-cost, low-tech alternatives to safely and effectively measure the functional capacity of the lumbar extensor musculature.

Stationary Roman chair machines, such as 45° and 90° benches, are unable to provide a level of resistance that is appropriate for clinical back pain populations. The lightest load for resistance on a Roman chair depends on upper-body mass, which is frequently greater than the patient's initial functional capacity. In addition, the loading characteristics attributed to upper-body mass through the range of trunk extension have not been determined (72).

Electromyography

Electromyography (EMG) has been used extensively to quantify skeletal muscle activity associated with resistance exercise. Moritani and deVries evaluated surface integrated EMG activity (IEMG) of the elbow flexor muscles during isometric exercise and found a linear relationship between IEMG and isometric torque production with a highly significant correlation ($r = 0.99$, $p \le 0.05$) (82). While the strength and endurance characteristics of back pain sufferers is fairly well understood, the activation patterns of the lumbar muscle groups are less clear. Comparisons of surface EMG activity of the lumbar paraspinals during exercise and at rest in low back pain patients and healthy controls have yielded conflicting results. Studies have found increased activity of the lumbar paraspinal muscles (114), decreased activity (16,

127), and no difference in activity (3, 76) between patients with low back pain and healthy controls. Other EMG activity studies have found bilateral asymmetries (3) and a disappearance of the flexion-relaxation phenomena (108, 120, 121) in patients with chronic low back pain. Furthermore, patients with chronic low back pain have displayed significantly less increase in signal intensity on T2-weighted MR (magnetic resonance) images of the lumbar extensors following Roman chair exercise than have healthy subjects (27). Thus, the development of more precise measures to assess back muscle activity would be useful for clinical populations as well.

Historically, lumbar muscle function has been commonly evaluated by surface or needle electromyography (EMG). Technical limitations associated with surface EMG, such as lack of reliability (124), inability to provide an indication of specific muscle patterns (118), variability in signals from electrode type and placement (128), variability associated with subcutaneous tissue (110), and confounding of the myoelectric signal by cross talk between muscles (119), along with the invasiveness of needle EMG, limit the ability to make definitive conclusions about muscle function from electromyography. Despite these limitations, EMG has remained the procedure of choice to evaluate low back muscle activity during exercise and lifting tasks, and many researchers consider surface EMG to be representative of the "neural drive" to a given area. The following paragraphs highlight the research that has described the EMG activity of the lumbar musculature during exercise.

Tan et al. evaluated the effects of trunk position on surface EMG activation of the lumbar musculature during isometric contractions while standing and found that the erector spinae muscles are significantly more active in the flexed postures (116). This finding is consistent with research using the lumbar extension dynamometer, which has shown that isometric torque output is linear and descending from 72° to 0° of lumbar flexion (97). While standing with the trunk fully flexed, the lumbar paraspinal muscles exhibit a reduction in EMG activity. This phenomenon is commonly referred to as flexion-relaxation (121) and has been attributed to the elastic properties of the muscles and posterior vertebral connective tissues (120). Additionally, the passive torque production commonly seen during full trunk flexion when the lumbar muscles are electrically silent has been explained by these elastic properties (32).

Udermann et al. evaluated the influence of pelvic restraint during back extension exercise on EMG activation of the hamstring, gluteal, and lumbar extensor muscles using a lumbar extension dynamometer (123). In this study, 12 men completed two dynamic lumbar extension exercises of 12 repetitions with a load equaling 80% of body weight. One exercise was performed with the pelvic stabilization mechanisms intact and one with the stabilization mechanisms removed. No difference in EMG activity was observed between the restrained and unrestrained conditions in any of the muscle groups ($p > 0.05$), which supports the findings of Mayer et al. (71) that pelvic stabilization during training is not required for the recruitment of the lumbar musculature or for increases in lumbar extension strength.

Lee found that surface EMG mean power frequency patterns of muscle fatigue on a Roman chair isometric endurance test decreased after 4 weeks of resistance training on both a lumbar dynamometer and Roman chair (16.8% vs. 15.2%, respectively) (57). The investigators used these data to suggest that exercise on the Roman chair affects the lumbar extensor muscles similarly to exercise on the dynamometer.

Kearns et al. also evaluated lumbar extension muscle activation during isolated (stabilized) and nonisolated (unstabilized) lumbar extension exercises (51). Twelve male subjects completed 2 dynamic repetitions at 50% and 90% of their 1-RM on a lumbar dynamometer with its pelvic restraint mechanisms intact, using a Roman chair, and performing straight-legged dead lifts. Surface EMG activity was recorded from the gluteal, hamstring, and erector spinae muscles during exercise. At 50% of the 1-RM, erector spinae muscle activation was significantly higher during the Roman chair exercise than during the dynamometer and dead-lift exercises. At 90% of the 1-RM, erector spinae activation was significantly higher during exercises on the Roman chair and dynamometer than during dead lifts, with no significant difference between the Roman chair and dynamometer. Gluteal and hamstring activation at 50% and 90% of the 1-RM was greater during the Roman chair exercise than during dynamometer and dead-lift exercises. The investigators concluded that the differences in lumbar extensor muscle activation between exercises on the Roman chair and dynamometer may be due to loading differences attributable to the counterweight on the dynamometer designed to offset torso mass.

The 1-RM for the Roman chair and dead-lift exercises in the Kearns et al. (51) study was determined by placing handheld metal plates against the chest and gripping a metal barbell, respectively, and performing a dynamic repetition. Fifty percent and 90% of the weight of the handheld metal plates and barbell was used for the EMG analyses. The load attributed to upper-body mass was not taken into consideration for Roman chair and dead-lift exercises. Therefore, the actual loads for these two exercises probably exceeded 50% and 90% of the true 1-RM, and EMG comparisons with exercise on the dynamometer were likely not valid. However, this study still provided useful information by noting that similar muscle groups, namely the lumbar extensors, were active during trunk extension exercise on both the Roman chair and dynamometer.

Recently, a back extension machine has been developed to allow performance of progressive resistance exercise in a relatively inexpensive and portable manner. This lumbar extension machine (BackStrong International) is a variable-angle Roman chair (VARC) that can be adjusted from 75° relative to horizontal to 0° relative to horizontal in 15° increments. As the angle from horizontal decreases on the VARC, the load applied to the low back extensor muscles increases (72). Specifically, the surface EMG activity of the lumbar paraspinal muscles during exercise increases progressively and consecutively between all six angles from 75° to 0°. Furthermore, lumbar paraspinal EMG activity is increased progressively during VARC exercise by positioning the subject's hands and arms farther away from the axis of rotation in the lower lumbar spine. Since there is a strong positive linear relationship between the magnitude of EMG activity observed and the amount of muscle mass recruited during exercise (81, 82), the VARC is capable of providing a mechanism for progressive resistance lumbar extension exercise (72).

Although the VARC appears to allow for variable loading, the device lacks the sophistication to quantify load in a classical sense. Furthermore, it is not known whether progressive resistance exercise training on the VARC can accommodate the increases in training load necessary for strength gains. Therefore, there is a need for mechanisms to accurately quantify load during back extension exercise on the VARC and other Roman chair devices. Exercise training for the prevention and rehabilitation of LBP on these devices warrants further study.

Summary

Low back pain is one of the most common and costly medical problems in our society. This may be due to the fact that the muscles of the lower back, the lumbar extensors, are significantly deconditioned in most people. Training this unique and complex group of muscles with resistance exercise has been a challenge, but recent advances in resistance training equipment for the low back muscles has been fruitful. Targeting the lumbar muscles by restricting pelvic rotation on certain lumbar dynamometers and with the Roman chair has been a successful strategy for improving the functional capacity of the lower back in clinical as well as asymptomatic populations. Due to the initial weakness of these muscles, a low-frequency (one to two times per week), moderate intensity (one set, 12 to 16 repetitions) training program is recommended.

References

1. Alaranta, H., H. Hurri, M. Heliovaara, A. Soukka, and R. Harju. 1994. Non-dynamometric trunk performance tests: Reliability and normative data. *Scandinavian Journal of Rehabilitation Medicine* 26: 211-215.

2. Alaranta, H., K. Tallroth, A. Soukka, and M. Heliovaara. 1993. Fat content in lumbar extensor muscles and low back disability: A radiographic and clinical comparison. *Journal of Spinal Disorders* 6: 137-140.

3. Alexiev, A.R. 1994. Some differences of the electromyographic erector spinae activity between normal subjects and low back pain patients during the generation of isometric trunk torque. *Electromyography and Clinical Neurophysiology* 34: 495-499.

4. Allan, D.B., and G. Waddell. 1989. An historical perspective on low back pain and disability. *Acta Orthopaedica Scandinavica* 234 (suppl.): 1-23.

5. Andersson, G.B.J., M.H. Pope, J.W. Frymoyer, and S. Snook. 1991. Epidemiology and cost. In *Occupational low back pain: Assessment, treatment, and prevention,* edited by M.H. Pope, G.B.J. Andersson, J.W. Frymoyer, and D.B. Chaffin, 95-113. St. Louis: Mosby-Year Book.

6. Battie, M., S. Bigos, L. Fisher, T. Hansson, M. Jones, and M.D. Wortley. 1989. Isometric lifting strength as a predictor of industrial back pain reports. *Spine* 14 (8): 851-856.

7. Biering-Sorensen, F. 1984. Physical measurements as risk indicators for low back trouble over a one year period. *Spine* 9: 106-119.

8. Bigos, S.J., M.C. Battie, D.M. Spengler, L.D. Fisher, W.E. Fordyce, T. Hansson, A.L. Nachemson, and J. Zeh. 1992. A longitudinal, prospective study of industrial back injury reporting. *Clinical Orthopaedics and Related Research* 279: 21-34.

9. Bigos, S.J., R. Bower, G. Braen, et al. 1994. Acute low back pain problems in adults. *Clinical practice guideline, quick reference guide no. 14.* AHCPR Pub. no. 95-0643. Rockville, MD: U.S. Department of Health and Human Services, Public Health Service, Agency for Health Care Policy and Research.

10. Bogdanffy, G. 1993. Exercise physiology and fitness. In *Rehabilitation of the spine: Science and practice,* edited by S. Hochschuler, H. Cotler, and R. Guyer, 667-676. St. Louis: Mosby.

11. Bogduk, N. 1980. A reappraisal of the anatomy of the human lumbar erector spinae. *Journal of Anatomy* 131 (3): 525-540.

12. Bogduk, N., and L. Twomey. 1990. *Clinical anatomy of the lumbar spine.* New York: Churchill Livingstone.

13. Bortz, W. 1984. The disuse syndrome. *Western Journal of Medicine* 141: 691-694.

14. Cady, L.D., D.P. Bischoff, E.R. O'Connell, P.C. Thomas, and J.H. Allan. 1979. Strength and fitness and subsequent back injuries in firefighters. *Journal of Occupational Medicine* 21: 269-272.

15. Carey, T.S., A. Evans, N. Hadler, W. Kalsbeek, C. McLaughlin, and J. Fryer. 1995. Care seeking among individuals with chronic low back pain. *Spine* 20: 312-317.

16. Cassisi, J., M. Robinson, P. O'Conner, and M. MacMillan. 1993. Trunk strength and lumbar paraspinal muscle activity during isometric exercise in chronic low back pain patients and controls. *Spine* 18 (2): 245-251.

17. Chaffin, D., G. Herrin, and W. Keyserling. 1978. Preemployment strength testing. *Occupational Medicine* 20 (6): 403-408.

18. Chaffin, D., and K. Park. 1973. A longitudinal study of low back pain as associated with occupational lifting factors. *American Industrial Hygiene Association Journal,* December, 513-524.

19. Cresswell, A.G., and A. Thorstensson. 1989. The role of the abdominal musculature in the elevation of the intra-abdominal pressure during specified tasks. *Ergonomics* 32: 1237-1246.

20. Cresswell, A.G., A. Grundstrom, and A. Thorstensson. 1992. Observations on intra-abdominal pressure and patterns of abdominal intra-muscular activity in man. *Acta Physiologica Scandinavica* 144: 409-418.

21. Cresswell, A.G., L. Oddsson, and A. Thorstensson. 1994. The influence of sudden perturbations on trunk muscle activity and intra-abdominal pressure while standing. *Experimental Brain Research* 98: 336-341.

22. Cunningham, L., and J. Kelsey. 1984. Epidemiology of musculoskeletal impairments and associated disability. *American Journal of Public Health* 74: 574-579.

23. Davies, J., T. Gibson, and L. Tester. 1979. The value of exercises in the treatment of low back pain. *Rheumatology Rehabilitation* 18: 243-247.

24. Deyo, R., D. Cherkin, D. Conrad, and E. Volinn. 1991. Cost, controversy, crisis: Low back pain and the health of the public. *Annual Review of Public Health* 12: 141-156.

25. Dreisinger, T. 1994. The use and misuse of performance testing. *Orthopedics* 17: 473-477.

26. Fleck, S., and W. Kraemer. 1997. *Designing resistance training programs.* Champaign, IL: Human Kinetics.

27. Flicker, P., J. Fleckenstein, K. Ferry, J. Payne, C. Ward, T. Mayer, R. Parkey, and R. Peshock. 1993. Lumbar muscle usage in chronic low back pain. *Spine* 18 (5): 582-586.

28. Foster, D., M. Avilar, M. Pollock, J. Graves, G. Dudley, D. Woodard, and D. Carpenter. 1993. Adaptations in strength and cross-sectional area of the lumbar extensor muscles following resistance training (abstract). *Medicine and Science in Sports and Exercise* 25 (5): S47.

29. Frymoyer, J.W., and W.L. Cats-Baril. 1991. An overview of the incidences and costs of low back pain. *Orthopedic Clinics of North America* 22: 263-271.

30. Fujita, S., W.F. Brechue, C.F. Kearns, and M.L. Pollock. 1997. Effect of non-isolated lumbar extension resistance training on isolated lumbar extension strength. *Medicine and Science in Sports and Exercise* 29 (5): S166.

31. Gibbons, L., P. Latikka, T. Videman, H. Manninen, and M. Battie. 1997. The association of trunk muscle cross-sectional area and magnetic resonance imaging parameters with isokinetic and psychosocial lifting strength and static back muscle endurance in men. *Journal of Spinal Disorders* 10 (5): 398-403.

32. Graves, J.E., M.L. Pollock, D.M. Carpenter, S. Leggett, A. Jones, M. MacMillan, and M. Fulton. 1990. Quantitative assessment of full range-of-motion isometric lumbar extension strength. *Spine* 15 (4): 289-294.

33. Graves, J.E., M.L. Pollock, D. Foster, S.H. Leggett, D.M. Carpenter, R.M. Vuoso, and A. Jones. 1990. Effect of training frequency and specificity on isometric lumbar extension strength. *Spine* 15 (6): 504-509.

34. Graves, J.E., D.C. Webb, M.L. Pollock, S.H. Leggett, D.M. Carpenter, D.N. Foster, and J. Cirulli. 1994. Pelvic stabilization during resistance training: Its effect on the development of lumbar extension strength. *Archives of Physical Medicine and Rehabilitation* 75 (2): 210-215.

35. Graves, J.E., D.C. Webb, M.L. Pollock, J. Matkozich, and S.H. Leggett. 1990. Effect of training with pelvic stabilization on lumbar extension strength. *International Journal of Sports Medicine* 11: 403-404.

36. Grimby, G., and O. Hook. 1971. Physical training of different patient groups. *Scandinavian Journal of Rehabilitation Medicine* 3: 15-25.

37. Hasue, M., M. Fujiwara, and S. Kikuchi. 1980. A new method of quantitative measurement of abdominal and back muscle strength. *Spine* 5: 143-148.

38. Hemborg, B., U. Moritz, and H. Lowing. 1985. Intra-abdominal pressure and trunk muscle activity during lifting IV. The causal factors of intra-abdominal pressure rise. *Rehabilitation Medicine* 17: 25-38.

39. Hides, J., C. Richardson, and G. Jull. 1996. Multifidus recovery is not automatic after resolution of acute, first episode low back pain. *Spine* 21 (23): 2763-2769.

40. Hides, J., M. Stokes, G. Jull, and D. Cooper. 1994. Evidence of multifidus wasting ipsilateral to symptoms in patients with acute/subacute low back pain. *Spine* 19 (2): 165-172.

41. Hides, J.A. 1996. Multifidus muscle recovery in acute low back pain. Ph.D. diss., University of Queensland.

378

42. Hochschuler, S. 1993. General considerations: Stability, flexibility, strength, cardiac fitness, and aerobic capacity. In *Rehabilitation of the spine: Science and practice,* edited by S. Hochschuler, H. Cotler, and R. Guyer, 11-18. St. Louis: Mosby.

43. Hodges, P.W., and C.A. Richardson. 1998. Delayed postural contraction of transversus abdominis in low back pain associated with movement of the lower limbs. *Journal of Spinal Disorders* 11: 46-56.

44. Hodges, P.W., and C.A. Richardson. 1996. Inefficient muscular stabilization of the lumbar spine associated with low back pain: A motor control evaluation of transversus abdominis. *Spine* 21: 2640-2650.

45. Hodges, P.W., and C.A. Richardson. 1997. Relationship between limb movement speed and associated contraction of the trunk muscles. *Ergonomics* 40: 1220-1230.

46. Hultman, G., M. Nordin, H. Saraste, and H. Ohlsen. 1993. Body composition, endurance, strength, cross-sectional area, and density of mm erector spinae in men with and without low back pain. *Journal of Spinal Disorders* 6 (2): 114-123.

47. Ito, T., O. Shirado, H. Suzuki, M. Takahashi, K. Kaneda, and T. Strax. 1996. Lumbar trunk muscle endurance testing: An inexpensive alternative to a machine for evaluation. *Archives of Physical Medicine and Rehabilitation* 77: 75-79.

48. Jorgensen, K. 1997. Human trunk extensor muscles: Physiology and ergonomics. *Acta Physiologica Scandinavica,* suppl. 637: 1-58.

49. Kalimo, H., J. Rantanen, T. Viljanen, and E. Sakari. 1989. Lumbar muscles: Structure and function. *Annals of Medicine* 21: 353-359.

50. Kankaanpaa, M., D. Laaksonen, and S. Taimela. 1998. Age, sex, and body mass index as determinants of back and hip extensor fatigue in the isometric Sorensen back endurance test. *Archives of Physical Medicine and Rehabilitation* 79: 1069-1075.

51. Kearns, C., W. Brechue, J. Bauer, M. Pollock, and M. Fulton. 1997. Muscle activation during isolated and non-isolated lumbar extension exercises. *Medicine and Science in Sports and Exercise* 29 (5): S165.

52. Kirkaldy-Willis, W., ed. 1988. *Managing low back pain.* 2d ed. New York: Churchill Livingstone.

53. Kottke, F.J. 1961. Evaluation and treatment of low back pain due to mechanical causes. *Archives of Physical Medicine* 42: 426-440.

54. Kumar, S., R. Dufresne, and T. Van Schoor. 1995. Human trunk strength profile in flexion and extension. *Spine* 20 (2): 160-168.

55. Langrana, N.A., C.K. Lee, H. Alexander, and C.W. Mayott. 1984. Quantitative assessment of back strength using isokinetic testing. *Spine* 9: 287-290.

56. Leavitt, F. 1992. The physical exertion factor in compensable work injuries: A hidden flaw in previous research. *Spine* 17: 307-310.

57. Lee, S. 1996. Comparative analysis of two lumbar strength training apparatuses on low back strength. Paper presented at Comprehensive Spine and Joint Care—From Exercise to Outcomes, July 18, University of California at San Diego, LaJolla, CA.

58. Leggett, S., V. Mooney, L.N. Matheson, B. Nelson, T. Dreisinger, J. Van Zytveld, and L. Vie. 1999. Restorative exercise for clinical low back pain: A prospective two-center study with 1-year follow-up. *Spine* 24 (9): 889-898.

59. Li, Y., J. Graves, L. Ploutz-Snyder, and J. Mayer. 1998. Neuromuscular adaptations to lumbar extension strength gain. *Medicine and Science in Sports and Exercise* 30 (5): S207.

60. Linton, S. 1985. The relationship between activity and chronic back pain. *Pain* 21: 289-294.

61. Luoto, S., M. Heliovaara, H. Hurri, and H. Alaranta. 1995. Static back endurance and the risk of low back pain. *Clinical Biomechanics* 10 (6): 323-324.

62. MacIntosh, J., and N. Bogduk. 1991. The attachments of the lumbar erector spinae. *Spine* 16 (7): 783-792.

63. MacIntosh, J., and N. Bogduk. 1987. The morphology of the lumbar erector spinae. *Spine* 12 (7): 658-668.

64. Macintosh, J.E., F. Valencia, N. Bogduk, and R.R. Munro. 1986. The morphology of the human lumbar multifidus. *Clinical Biomechanics* 1: 196-204.
65. Manniche, C., G. Hesselsoe, R. Bentzen, I. Christiansen, and E. Lundberg. 1988. Clinical trial of intensive muscle training for chronic low back pain. *Lancet* 24: 1473-1476.
66. Manniche, C., E. Lundberg, I. Christiansen, L. Bentzen, and G. Hesselsoe. 1991. Intensive, dynamic back exercises for chronic low back pain. *Pain* 47: 53-63.
67. Mannion, A.F., G.A. Dumas, J.M. Stevenson, and R.G. Cooper. 1998. The influence of muscle fiber size and type distribution on electromyographic measures of back muscle fatigability. *Spine* 23 (5): 576-584.
68. Mannion, A., and P. Dolan. 1994. Electromyographic median frequency changes during isometric contraction of the back extensors to fatigue. *Spine* 19 (11): 1223-1229.
69. Mannion, A., G. Dumas, R. Cooper, E. Espinosa, and M. Faris. 1997. Muscle fibre size and type distribution in thoracic and lumbar regions of erector spinae in healthy subjects without low back pain. *Journal of Anatomy* 190: 505-513.
70. Mannion, A., B. Weber, J. Dvorak, D. Grob, and M. Muntner. 1997. Fiber type characteristics of the lumbar paraspinal muscles in normal healthy subjects and patients with low back pain. *Journal of Orthopedic Research* 15: 881-887.
71. Mayer, J., J. Graves, Y. Li, B. Udermann, and L. Ploutz-Snyder. 1998. Specificity of training and isolated lumbar extension strength. *Medicine and Science in Sports and Exercise* 30 (5): S206.
72. Mayer, J., J. Graves, V. Robertson, J. Verna, E. Pierra, and L. Ploutz-Snyder. 1999. Electromyographic activity of the lumbar extensor muscles: The effect of angle and hand position during Roman chair exercise. *Archives of Physical Medicine and Rehabilitation* 80 (7): 751-755.
73. Mayer, L., and B. Greenberg. 1942. Measurement of the strength of trunk muscles. *Journal of Bone and Joint Surgery* 4: 842-856.
74. Mayer, T., S. Smith, J. Keeley, and V. Mooney. 1985. Quantification of lumbar function. Part 2: Sagittal plane trunk strength in chronic low-back pain patients. *Spine* 10 (8): 765-772.
75. McNeill, T., D. Warwick, G. Andersson, and A. Schultz. 1980. Trunk strengths in attempted flexion, extension, and lateral bending in healthy subjects and patients with low back disorders. *Spine* 5: 529-538.
76. Miller, D. 1985. Comparison of electromyographic activity in the lumbar paraspinal muscles of subjects with and without chronic low back pain. *Physical Therapy* 65 (9): 1347-1354.
77. Mooney, V., and G. Andersson. 1994. Controversies: Trunk strength testing in patient evaluation and treatment. *Spine* 19 (21): 2483-2485.
78. Mooney, V., J. Gulick, M. Perlman, D. Levy, R. Pozos, S. Leggett, and D. Resnick. 1997. Relationships between myoelectric activity, strength, and MRI of the lumbar extensor muscles in back pain patients and normal subjects. *Journal of Spinal Disorders* 10 (4): 348-356.
79. Mooney, V., D. Kenny, S. Leggett, and B. Holmes. 1996. Relationship of lumbar strength in shipyard workers to workplace injury claims. *Spine* 21 (17): 2001-2005.
80. Mooney, V., M. Kron, P. Rummerfield, and B. Holmes. 1995. The effect of workplace based strengthening on low back injury rates: A case study in the strip mining industry. *Journal of Occupational Rehabilitation* 5: 157-167.
81. Moritani, T., and H. deVries. 1979. Neural factors versus hypertrophy in the time course of muscle strength gain. *American Journal of Physical Medicine* 58 (3): 115-130.
82. Moritani, T., and H. deVries. 1978. Reexamination of the relationship between the surface integrated electromyogram (IEMG) and force of isometric contraction. *American Journal of Physical Medicine* 57 (6): 263-277.
83. Morris, J., B. Lucas, and B. Bresler. 1961. Role of the trunk in stability of the spine. *Journal of Bone and Joint Surgery* 43A: 327-333.

84. Nachemson, A. 1981. Disc pressure measurements. *Spine* 6: 93-97.

85. Nachemson, A. 1992. Newest knowledge of low back pain. A critical look. *Clinical Orthopaedics and Related Research* 279: 8-20.

86. Nachemson, A., and M. Lindh. 1969. Measurement of abdominal and back muscle strength with and without low back pain. *Canadian Journal of Rehabilitation Medicine* 1: 60-65.

87. Nelson, B., D. Carpenter, T. Dreisinger, M. Mitchell, C. Kelly, and J. Wegner. 1999. Can spine surgery be prevented by aggressive strengthening exercises? A prospective study of cervical and lumbar patients. *Archives of Physical Medicine and Rehabilitation* 80: 20-25.

88. Nelson, B., E. O'Reilly, M. Miller, M. Hogan, J. Wegner, and C. Kelly. 1995. The clinical effects of intensive, specific exercise on chronic low back pain: A controlled study of 895 consecutive patients with 1-year follow up. *Orthopedics* 18 (10): 971-981.

89. Newton, M., and G. Waddell. 1993. Trunk strength testing with iso-machines: A decade of scientific evidence. *Spine* 18 (7): 801-811.

90. Ng, J., C. Richardson, V. Kippers, and M. Parnianpour. 1998. Relationship between muscle fiber composition and functional capacity of back muscles in healthy subjects and patients with low back pain. *Journal of Orthopedic and Sports Physical Therapy* 27 (7): 389-402.

91. Panjabi, M., K. Abumi, J. Duranceau, and T. Oxland. 1989. Spinal stability and intersegmental muscle forces: A biomechanical model. *Spine* 14: 194-200.

92. Parkkola, R., U. Kukala, and U. Rytokoski. 1992. Response of the trunk muscles to training assessed by magnetic resonance imaging and muscle strength. *European Journal of Applied Physiology* 65: 383-387.

93. Parkkola, R., U. Rytokoski, and M. Kormano. 1993. Magnetic resonance imaging of the disc and trunk muscles in patients with chronic low back pain and healthy control subjects. *Spine* 18 (7): 830-836.

94. Parnianpour, M., M. Nordin, N. Kahanovitz, and V. Frankel. 1988. The triaxial coupling of torque generation of trunk muscles during isometric exertions and the effect of fatiguing isoinertial movement on the motor output and movement patterns. *Spine* 139: 982-992.

95. Petersen, C.M., L.R. Amundsen, and M.J. Schendel. 1987. Comparison of the effectiveness of two pelvic stabilization systems on pelvic movement during isometric trunk extension and flexion muscle contractions. *Physical Therapy* 67 (March): 534-541.

96. Pollock, M.L., J. Graves, D. Carpenter, D. Foster, S. Seggett, and M. Fulton. 1993. Muscle. In *Rehabilitation of the spine: Science and practice*, edited by S. Hochschuler, H. Cotler, and R. Guyer, 263-284. St. Louis: Mosby.

97. Pollock, M.L., S.H. Leggett, J.E. Graves, A. Jones, M. Fulton, and J. Cirulli. 1989. Effect of resistance training on lumbar extension strength. *American Journal of Sports Medicine* 17 (5): 624-629.

98. Reid, J., and P. Costigan. 1987. Trunk muscle balance and muscular force. *Spine* 12 (8): 783-786.

99. Risch, S., N. Norvell, M. Pollock, E. Risch, H. Langer, M. Fulton, J. Graves, and S. Leggett. 1993. Lumbar strengthening in chronic low back pain patients: Physiological and psychosocial benefits. *Spine* 18: 232-238.

100. Rissanen, A., H. Alaranta, P. Sainio, and H. Harkonen. 1994. Isokinetic and non-dynamometric tests in low back pain patients related to pain and disability index. *Spine* 19 (17): 1963-1967.

101. Rissanen, A., H. Kalimo, and H. Alaranta. 1995. Effect of intensive training on the isokinetic strength and structure of lumbar muscles in patients with chronic low back pain. *Spine* 30 (3): 333-340.

102. Robinson, M.E., J.E. Cassisi, P.D. O'Connor, and N. McMillan. 1992. Lumbar EMG during isotonic exercise: Chronic low back pain patients versus controls. *Journal of Spinal Disorders* 5: 8-15.

103. Ross, E.C., M. Parnianpour, and D. Martin. 1993. The effect of resistance level on muscle coordination patterns and movement profiled during trunk extension. *Spine* 18: 1829-1838.

104. Russell, G.D., T.R. Highland, and T.E. Dreisinger. 1990. Changes in isometric strength and range of motion of the isolated lumbar spine following eight weeks of clinical rehabilitation. Paper presented at the North American Spine Society, Toronto.

105. Schoene, M., ed. 1991. Back machines: A waste of money? *The Back Letter* 5 (7): 8.

106. Seeds, R.H., J.A. Levene, and H.M. Goldberg. 1988. Abnormal patient data for the isostation B100. *Journal of Orthopaedic and Sports Physical Therapy* 10: 121-133.

107. Shirado, O., T. Ito, K. Kaneda, and T. Strax. 1995. Concentric and eccentric strength of trunk muscles: Influence of test postures on strength and characteristics of patients with chronic low-back pain. *Archives of Physical Medicine and Rehabilitation* 76: 604-611.

108. Shirado, O., T. Ito, K. Kaneda, and T. Strax. 1995. Flexion-relaxation phenomenon in the back muscles. A comparative study between healthy subjects and patients with chronic low back pain. *American Journal of Physical Medicine and Rehabilitation* 74 (2): 139-144.

109. Shirado, O., K. Kaneda, and T. Ito. 1992. Trunk muscle strength during concentric and eccentric contraction: A comparison between healthy subjects in patients with chronic low back pain. *Journal of Spinal Disorders* 5: 175-182.

110. Sihvonen, T., J. Paranten, and O. Hanninen. 1988. Averaged (rms) surface EMG in testing back function. *Electromyography and Clinical Neurophysiology* 28: 335-339.

111. Smidt, G., T. Herring, L. Amundsen, M. Rogers, A. Russell, and T. Lehmann. 1983. Assessment of abdominal and back extensor function—A quantitative approach and results for chronic low-back patients. *Spine* 8: 211-219.

112. Smidt, G.L., L.R. Amundsen, and W.F. Dostal. 1980. Muscle strength at the trunk. *Journal of Orthopaedic and Sports Physical Therapy* 1: 165-170.

113. Smith, S.S., T.G. Mayer, R.J. Gatchel, and T.J. Becker. 1985. Quantification of lumbar function. Part 1: Isometric and multispeed trunk strength measures in sagittal and axial planes in normal subjects. *Spine* 10: 757-764.

114. Soderberg, G., and J. Barr. 1983. Muscular function in chronic low back dysfunction. *Spine* 8: 79-85.

115. Suzuki, N., and S. Endo. 1983. A quantitative study of trunk muscle strength and fatiguability in the low back pain syndrome. *Spine* 8: 69-74.

116. Tan, J., M. Parnianpour, M. Nordin, H. Hofer, and B. Willems. 1993. Isometric maximal and submaximal trunk extension at different flexed positions in standing. *Spine* 18 (16): 2480-2490.

117. Tesh, K.M., J.S. Dunn, and J.H. Evans. 1987. The abdominal muscles and vertebral stability. *Spine* 12 (5): 501-508.

118. Thelan, D., J. Ashston-Miller, and A. Schultz. 1996. Lumbar muscle activities in rapid three-dimensional pulling tasks. *Spine* 21 (5): 605-613.

119. Thelan, D., A. Schultz, and J. Ashton-Miller. 1995. Contraction of the lumbar muscles during the development of time-varying triaxial moments. *Journal of Orthopedic Research* 13: 390-398.

120. Toussaint, H., A. de Winter, Y. de Haas, M. de Looze, J. Van Dieen, and I. Kigma. 1995. Flexion relaxation during lifting: Implications for torque production by muscle activity and tissue strain at the lumbo-sacral joint. *Journal of Biomechanics* 28 (2): 199-210.

121. Triano, J., and A. Schultz. 1987. Correlation of objective measures of trunk motion and muscle function with low back disability ratings. *Spine* 12: 561-565.

122. Tucci, J.T., D.M. Carpenter, M.L. Pollock, J.E. Graves, and S.H. Leggett. 1992. Effect of reduced frequency of training and detraining on lumbar extension strength. *Spine* 17 (12): 1497-1501.

123. Udermann, B., J. Graves, R. Donelson, J. Iriso, and J. Boucher. 1999. Effect of pelvic restraint on hamstring, gluteal, and lumbar muscle EMG activation. *Archives of Physical Medicine and Rehabilitation* 80 (4): 1176-1179.

124. Veiersted, K. 1991. The reproducibility of test contractions for calibration of electromyographic measurements. *European Journal of Applied Physiology* 62: 91-98.
125. Videman, H., T. Nurimen, S. Tola, I. Kuorinka, H. Vanharanta, and J.D. Troup. 1984. Low back pain in nurses and some loading factors of work. *Spine* 9: 400-404.
126. Videman, T., and M.C. Battie. 1996. A critical review of the epidemiology of idiopathic low back pain. In *Low back pain: A scientific and clinical overview,* edited by J.N. Weinstein and S.L. Gordon, 317-332. Rosemont, IL: American Academy of Orthopaedic Surgeons.
127. Wolf, S., and J. Basmajian. 1977. Assessment of paraspinal electromyographic activity in normal subjects and in chronic low back pain patients using a muscle biofeedback device, edited by E. Asmussen and K. Jorgensen. International Congress of Biomechanics. Baltimore: University Park Press.
128. Zedka, M., S. Kumar, and Y. Narayan. 1997. Comparison of surface EMG signals between electrode types, interelectrode distances, electrode orientations in isometric exercise of the erector spinae. *Electromyography and Clinical Neurophysiology* 37: 439-447.

20

CHAPTER

Resistance Training for the Prevention of Osteoporosis

Jennifer E. Layne, MS, CSCS
Miriam E. Nelson, PhD, FACSM
Tufts University

Introduction

This chapter focuses on the effects of resistance training on bone health. A brief review of the specifics of osteoporosis includes clinical symptoms, diagnosis, demographics, risk factors, prevention, and treatment. Bone physiology and the theoretical model by which resistance training influences bone remodeling are then discussed. Review and analysis of the most recent randomized controlled trials in the scientific literature serve as the basis for resistance training recommendations for the prevention and treatment of osteoporosis.

Specifics of the Disease and Clinical Symptoms

Osteoporosis is a systemic skeletal disease characterized by low bone mass and microarchitectural deterioration of bone tissue, with consequent increase in bone fragility and susceptibility to fracture (6). Although osteoporosis is now considered to be a highly preventable disease, it was once considered a normal consequence of the aging process. More than 28 million Americans over the age of 65 are affected by this bone disease: 10 million with osteoporosis and an additional 18 million with low bone mass termed *osteopenia* (6). Clinical symptoms include fracture, kyphosis, impaired balance, pain, and adverse psychological consequences including fear of falling and depression.

One and one half million osteoporotic fractures occur annually in the United States in people aged 50 years and older (13). The associated cost of hospitalization and nursing home care attributed to these fractures was $13.8 billion in 1995 (13). The three most common sites of fracture are the spinal vertebrae, the hip, and the wrist, although any bone can be affected by osteoporosis. Fractures may occur due to trauma, such as from a fall, or when the skeleton can no longer withstand usual loads as a result of decreased bone mass.

Fractures of the thoracic and lumbar spine account for almost half, approximately 700,000, of all osteoporotic fractures annually (13). Biconcave, wedge, and crush fractures manifest as a collapse of the middle, front or back, or entire spinal vertebrae, respectively. These types of vertebral fractures present as kyphosis and loss of height over time but do not typically require hospitalization. Osteoporotic kyphosis is associated with musculoskeletal pain, decreased back extensor strength, and decreased lung capacity (6, 46).

More than 90% of the 300,000 hip fractures that occur annually are attributed to osteoporosis (34). The Office of Technology Assessment estimates that only one-third of hip fracture patients fully recover to their prefracture level of function and ambulatory status (13, 32). Fifty thousand people die each year from complications associated with hip fracture (13, 32).

Wrist fracture occurs most frequently at the distal radius (13). This type of wrist fracture is termed Colles' fracture after the physician who first described its occurrence. Approximately one-half of the 250,000 individuals experiencing wrist fracture recover completely. Others may experience lingering symptoms, including pain, weakness, and decreased range of motion.

Diagnosis

Unfortunately, fracture is often the first indicator of osteoporosis. Osteoporosis is diagnosed as bone mineral density (BMD) that is 2.5 standard deviations below normal for healthy young adults or approximately 25% bone loss (6, 13). Several instruments are used to measure BMD and bone mineral content (BMC), diagnose osteoporosis, predict risk of a fracture, project rate of bone loss, and monitor effects of treatment. Common diagnostic techniques and the bone sites measured are included in table 20.1. Dual-energy X-ray absorptiometry (DXA) is the most widely available and precise technique. DXA uses a very low dose of radiation, approximately one-tenth of a traditional X-ray, and is much more sensitive to measuring the amount of bone.

Demographics and Risk Factors

Eighty percent of those affected by osteoporosis are women. The percentage of men who present with osteoporosis is expected to increase due to increased life expectancy. Certain risk factors for osteoporosis are nonmodifiable and are evident in individuals of all ethnic backgrounds. Some risk factors are potentially modifiable with proper treatment. For example, disordered eating and amenorrhea are treatable conditions; however, a history of disordered eating or amenorrhea during adolescence cannot be eliminated as a present risk factor. Major risk factors are summarized in table 20.2. Lifestyle factors and choice of medical treatment are highly modifiable risk factors.

Prevention and Treatment

Prevention can take place at each stage of the life cycle. Achieving peak bone mass during childhood, adolescence, and early adulthood, maintaining bone mass through middle age, and minimizing loss during old age are the cornerstones of prevention. Optimizing BMD and BMC in childhood ultimately leads to a reduction in the risk of osteoporosis (35). Weight-bearing and strengthening exercises that load the skeleton via

TABLE 20.1   Common Bone Density Tests

Abbreviated test name (full test name)	Bone sites measured
DXA (dual-energy X-ray absorptiometry)	Hip, spine, total body, wrist
DPA (dual-photon absorptiometry)	Hip, spine, total body
QCT (quantitative computed tomography)	Spine, wrist, hip
PDXA (peripheral dual-energy X-ray absorptiometry)	Finger, heel, wrist
RA (radiographic absorptiometry)	Hand
SXA (single-energy X-ray absorptiometry)	Heel, wrist
SPA (single-photon absorptiometry)	Wrist
Ultrasound	Heel, patella, tibia

TABLE 20.2   Osteoporosis Risk Factors

Nonmodifiable	*Potentially modifiable*	*Modifiable*
Age: over 65 years	Body habitus: weight gain	Alcohol: excessive intake
Body habitus: small boned, thin	Disordered eating	Diet: low calcium, vitamin D
Disordered eating	Hormone status	Lactose intolerance
Ethnicity: Asian, Caucasian	Medical conditions	Sedentary lifestyle
Family history: osteoporosis	Medication management	Smoking
Gender: female		
Medical conditions: intestinal diseases, diabetes type 1, thyroid conditions, rheumatoid arthritis		
Medications: glucocorticoids, anticonvulsants, thyroid replacement, others		
Hormone status: amenorrhea, early or surgical menopause, postmenopausal, low testosterone		

muscular contraction are powerful contributors to maximizing peak bone mass. However, evidence from randomized controlled trials examining bone accretion from exercise in addition to normal skeletal growth in children has yet to be published (35). Cross-sectional reports and nonrandomized trials suggest that rigorous exercise in childhood is optimal for maximizing the skeletal BMD and BMC (35).

Hereditary factors determine 70-80% of the variability of peak bone mass; the remaining variability is determined by dietary intake, hormone exposure, and environmental and lifestyle factors (42, 48, 49). The majority of bone mass is accumulated by 17-18 years of age; however, bone mass continues to increase between the ages of 20 and 30 years, during which time peak bone mass is achieved. During adulthood and middle age, both men and women begin to lose bone at the rate of approximately 0.5% per year. The rate of bone loss accelerates to 1-2% per year or higher in women at menopause due to decreased estrogen exposure (43). Bone continues to be lost at this higher rate for approximately five years postmenopause and then gradually slows to a rate of loss of 0.5-1% per year (43). This is the same rate of loss seen in normally aging men (43). Interestingly, both the loss of BMD and muscle mass with age are greater in the axial skeleton than in the appendicular skeleton (10).

Treatment modalities include dietary modification and nutritional supplementation to ensure optimal intake and absorption of calcium and vitamin D. Advances in pharmacological interventions include calcitonin, alendronate, and selective estrogen receptor modulators (SERMs), in addition to traditional hormone replacement therapy (HRT) (6, 8, 9, 13, 16, 23). Eliminating smoking, reducing excessive intake of alcohol, exercising regularly, and reducing the risk of falling are also important components of treatment. The overwhelming majority of hip and wrist fractures, 90%, and 50% of spine fractures occur as a result of a fall (13, 22, 34).

Treatment should also address the psychological components of osteoporosis, which include depression, anxiety, anger, fear, and loss of self-confidence (7, 13). Interestingly, resistance training can be an integral part of treatment of both the physical and psychological components of osteoporosis (7, 37). A combination of treatments—nutrition, pharmacology, exercise, lifestyle and environmental modifications, and falls reduction—is optimal for most individuals.

Bone Formation and Remodeling

Healthy bone is maintained through a continuous remodeling process during which old bone cells are removed by osteoclasts and replaced by newly formed bone cells, osteoblasts. Bone is classified as cortical and trabecular tissue. Cortical bone makes up approximately 80% of the skeleton, while trabecular bone accounts for the remaining 20%. Cortical bone is thin and dense and is found primarily in the appendicular skeleton. In contrast, trabecular bone is spongy in appearance and highly vascularized, containing red marrow and fat tissue. The greatest amount of trabecular bone is located in spinal vertebrae, the pelvis, and the ends of the long bones of the arms and legs. These are also the sites most prone to osteoporotic fracture. In one year approximately 10% of cortical bone and 40% of trabecular bone is remodeled.

Bone Response to Resistance Training

Minimal essential strain is defined as the threshold stimulus that initiates new bone formation (5). Minimal essential strain is theorized to be the force per unit area approximately equal to one-tenth the level of strain necessary to fracture the bone (18). A force that is equal or greater than the minimal essential strain and occurs repeatedly will signal osteoblasts to migrate to the region of the bone that is receiving the stimulus. Osteoblasts begin the bone formation process by deposition of collagen fibers in the bone matrix. This first step of bone accretion occurs within 8-12 weeks of mechanical loading at the minimal essential strain level. Mineralization of the collagen fibers must then occur over an additional equal time period to ultimately increase BMD and strengthen bone (14, 30). As a result, the minimum estimated time frame to increase BMD with appropriate loading conditions is four to six months.

New bone formation occurs primarily at the periosteum, or outer surface of bone (5, 53). The bone diameter and strength are thus increased without compromising the space needed for the marrow cavity and vascularization at the center of the bone (18). This pattern of increase allows force to be distributed over a greater surface area and is a protective mechanism against fracture. This process also mirrors the adaptation of muscle to training via the increase of myofilaments to the periphery of the existing myofibril (5, 29).

Bone metabolism is regulated to ensure that the forces received by each area of bone on a habitual basis do not exceed the minimal essential strain. The maximum strength of bone is maintained above the voluntary force-producing capacity of the attached musculature (5). The force of a muscle contraction is transmitted through this fascia to the bone. The fascial layers within the muscle converge at the end of the muscle to form a tendon. As bone increases in diameter, the tendon or ligament insertion becomes buried in the bone to further strengthen the junction (5).

Resistance training can increase bone by providing periodic increases greater than the habitual loads applied to bone. Thus, minimal essential strain from resistance training will vary by individual based on history of bone-loading activity and current type and level of activity. The adaptation to mechanical loading occurs at a more rapid rate in the axial skeleton than the appendicular skeleton due to the higher percentage of trabecular bone in the former (5, 10).

Bone accretion as a result of resistance training may also be attributed to the adaptive response of lower cytokine levels associated with regular exercise and the subsequent reduction in osteoclast activity (1, 26, 27, 45). Endogenous prostaglandin production by bone due to mechanical strain may mediate reduced bone resorption through cytokine activity and stimulate bone production (1, 27). Serum calcitrol levels and vitamin D levels are higher in exercise-trained individuals than in untrained individuals and may positively affect calcium balance and directly benefit bone (36). Development of a more favorable hormonal status or cytokine profile as well as the induction of bioelectric potentials may also contribute to improvements in bone density with resistance training (36, 40, 45).

Effects of Resistance Training

Cross-sectional evidence indicates that resistance training is associated with high BMD at multiple bone sites in young and old adults (5, 15, 20, 49). In addition, numerous randomized controlled trials have also demonstrated that progressive, high-intensity resistance training has significant potential in the prevention and treatment of osteoporosis (17, 24, 25, 28, 37, 39, 50, 51). The effects of resistance training on BMD appear to depend on the exercise prescription components—mode, frequency, intensity, load and duration—and the characteristics of the exercise participants—age, gender, exercise history, and nutritional status. The time frame of bone and connective tissue to adapt to resistance training is longer than muscle adaptation and may be subject to rapid effects of detraining (5). This presents an important underlying assumption in lifelong exercise participation and prescription. A threshold effect is evident for maximum BMD on an individual basis (38, 41). A site-specific effect can be observed from cross-sectional and longitudinal data as evidenced by higher BMD and muscle mass in the dominant arms of tennis players when compared to their nondominant side, or in the trained limb following unilateral resistance training (20, 24).

Resistance Training Protocols With Positive Bone Results

Resistance training interventions that have produced the greatest effect on BMD were one year in duration, conducted 2-3 times per week at 75-85% of the one-repetition maximum (1-RM). Three sets of 8 repetitions for a range of 5-12 total body exercises were performed (17, 24, 25, 28, 37, 39, 51). Women ranging in age from 20 to 74 years were the primary population studied. A minimum daily intake of calcium through diet or supplementation was required in these study participants.

These randomized controlled trials provide compelling evidence that resistance load (intensity) is more important than the number of loading cycles (repetitions) (17, 24, 25, 28, 37, 39, 51). Studies illustrating these points are described in this section. A complete list of studies reviewed and reported outcome measures is provided in table 20.3.

The results of Kerr et al. support the theory that resistance load drives bone adaptation by comparing progressive unilateral resistance training in postmenopausal women (24). Subjects were randomized to either resistance training for strength (high intensity, low repetitions) or resistance training for endurance (RTE) (low intensity, high repetitions). Within each participant one side of the body was trained and the other side served as a control. Maximal muscle strength increased significantly, 69-75%, over the year as a result of both resistance training

TABLE 20.3   Randomized Controlled Trials of Resistance Training and Bone

(Ref) Subjects	Protocol	Exercise selection	Results*
(12) Women 40-50 yr RT = 12 CON = 14 500 mg Ca daily supp	Frequency: 3×/wk 1-5 sets 4-15 reps Intensity: 4-15 RM Duration: 6 mo	1. Biceps curl 2. Calf raise 3. Front raise 4. Lat pull-down 5. Lateral raise 6. Leg press 7. Overhead press 8. Triceps extension 9. Triceps push-down 10. Upright row	1-RM strength: +101% RT, not reported CON DXA: L spine, femur, radius No significant change RT, CON
(25) Women 60-74 yr RT = 13 GRF = 14 CON = 12 1500 mg Ca daily intake	Frequency: 3-5×/wk 3-4 sets 8-11 reps Intensity: 8-12 RM Duration: 11 mo	1. Bench press 2. Biceps curl 3. Leg extension 4. Leg flexion 5. Leg press 6. Shoulder press 7. Squats 8. Triceps press	1-RM strength: +62% RT, not reported GRF, CON Isokinetic strength: +15% RT, +9% GRF, +7% CON DXA: L spine +1.5% RT, +1.8% GRF, no change CON Femoral neck −0.2% RT, +3.5% GRF, no change CON Total body +1.6% RT, +2.0% GRF Radius no change RT, GRF, CON
(24) Women 51-62 yr RT = 25 RTE = 21	Frequency: 3×/wk 3 sets 8 reps Intensity: 8-RM Duration: 1 yr	1. Biceps curl 2. Hip abduction 3. Hip adduction 4. Hip extension 5. Hip flexion 6. Leg press 7. Wrist curl 8. Reverse wrist curl 9. Wrist pronation, supination 10. Triceps push-down	1-RM strength: +75% RT, +69% RTE DXA:** Trochanter +1.7% RT, −0.6% RTE Intertrochanter +1.5% RT, −0.1% RTE Ward's triangle +2.3% RT, 0.8% RTE Distal radius +2.4% RT, −1.4% RTE Midradius +0.1% RT, −1.0% RTE
(17) Women 20-35 yr RT = 32 CON = 3 1500 mg Ca daily intake	Frequency: 3×/wk Sets, reps not reported Intensity: moderate Duration: 2 yr	1. Arm curls 2. Bent-knee dead lifts 3. Bent rows 4. Cleans 5. Military press 6. Push-ups 7. Shoulder press 8. Sit-ups	Isokinetic strength: Knee flexion +22% RT, +14% CON Knee extension +17% RT, +6% CON Trunk extension +27% RT, +15% CON DXA: I spine +1.3% RT, +0.1% CON Femoral neck +0.5% RT, −1.8% CON

(Ref) Subjects	Protocol	Exercise selection	Results*
			Trochanter +2.6% RT, +0.3% CON QCT: T spine −0.5% RT, −3.0% CON SPA: Calcaneus +5.6% RT, −0.8% CON
(28) Women 28-39 yr RT = 22 CON = 34 500 mg Ca daily supp	Frequency: 3×/wk 3 sets 8-12 reps Intensity: 75% 1-RM Duration: 18 mo	1. Biceps curl 2. Bench press 3. Lat pull-down 4. Leg curl 5. Leg extension 6. Leg press 7. Low rows 8. Military press 9. Supine fly 10. Wrist curls 11. Not reported 12. Not reported	1-RM strength: +58% RT, not reported CON Isokinetic strength: +34% RT, +11% CON DXA: L spine +1.4% RT, −0.5% CON Trochanter +2.0% RT, not reported CON
(33) Women/men 60-80 yr RT = 76 CON = 66	Frequency: 2×/wk 3 sets 10-12 reps Intensity: 50-80% 1-RM Duration: 42 wk	1. Abdominal curls 2. Ankle plantar flexion 3. Ankle dorsiflexion 4. Single-arm curls 5. Bench press 6. Unilateral leg press 7. Military press	1-RM strength: +20-65% RT, not reported CON DPA: Total body, L spine—no significant change RT, CON
(38) Women 60-84 yr RT = 9 CON = 8 800 mg Ca minimum daily intake	Frequency: 3×/wk 3 sets 8-12 reps Intensity: 80% 1-RM Duration: 1 yr	1. Back extension 2. Bench press 3. Lat pull-down 4. Leg extension 5. Leg flexion 6. Seated row 7. Shoulder press 8. Trunk flexion	1-RM strength: +15-71% RT, no change CON DXA: L spine, femoral neck, trochanter, total body—no significant change RT, CON
(41) Women 65-79 yr RTH = 8 RTL = 7 CON = 11 500 mg Ca, 200 IU vitamin D daily supp Most on HRT	Frequency: 3×/wk 3 sets 7-14 reps Intensity: 80% 1-RM Duration: 1 yr	1. Back extension 2. Bench press 3. Biceps curl 4. Lat pull-down 5. Leg abduction 6. Leg adduction 7. Leg extension 8. Leg flexion 9. Leg press 10. Military press	1-RM strength: +33% RTH, +39% RTL, +5% CON DXA: L spine, femoral neck, trochanter Ward's triangle—no significant change RTH, RTL, CON

(continued)

TABLE 20.3 *(continued)*

(Ref) Subjects	Protocol	Exercise selection	Results*
(37) Women 59-70 yr RT = 19 CON = 20	Frequency: 2×/wk 3 sets 8 reps Intensity: 84% 1-RM Duration: 1 yr	1. Abdominal flexion 2. Back extension 3. Chest press 4. Lat pull-down 5. Leg curl 6. Leg extension	1-RM strength: +54% RT, +5% CON DXA: L spine +1.0% RT, −1.8% CON Femoral neck +0.9% RT, −2.5% CON Total body—no change RT, CON
(51) Women 20 yr RT = 12 JOG = 10 CON = 8 500 mg Ca daily supp	Frequency: 3×/wk 3 sets 8-12 reps Intensity: 60-85% 1-RM Duration: 8 mo	1. Back extension 2. Bench press 3. Biceps curl 4. Hip abduction 5. Hip adduction 6. Hip extension 7. Hip flexion 8. Knee extension 9. Knee flexion 10. Lat pull-down 11. Military press 12. Sit-ups 13. Triceps press 14. Upright row	1-RM strength: +10-54% RT, no change JOG, CON DXA: L spine BMD +1.2% RT, +1.3% JOG, no change CON Proximal femur—no significant change RT, JOG, CON
(39) Women 43-46 yr RT = 9 CON = 11 ERT = 0.625 mg daily 1400 mg Ca daily intake	Frequency: 3×/wk 1 set 8 reps Intensity: 8-RM Duration: 1 yr	1. Calf raises 2. Negative chins 3. Leg extension 4. Low back 5. Torso arm	Strength: not reported RT, CON SPA: Midradius +4.1% RT, −0.3% CON DPA: Spine +8.3% RT, 1.5% CON Total body +2.1% RT, 0.6% CON
(50) Women 55-57 yr RT = 22 CON = 27 Some ERT	Frequency: 3-4×/wk 3 sets 10 reps Intensity: 70% 1-RM Duration: 1 yr	1. Double-leg raise 2. Prone trunk extension 3. Sit-up	Isokinetic strength: +28% RT, no change CON DPA: L spine no change RT, −2.3% CON Femoral neck, proximal femur— no significant change RT, CON

BMD: bone mineral density; Ca: calcium; CON: control group; DPA: dual-photon absorptiometry; DXA: dual-energy X-ray absorptiometry; ERT: estrogen replacement therapy; GRF: ground reaction force-trained group; HRT: hormone replacement therapy; I: integral (spine); IU: international units; JOG: jogging; L: lumbar (spine); QCT: quantitative computed tomography; RT: resistance-trained group; RTE: endurance resistance-trained group; RTH: resistance-trained (high intensity) group; RTL: resistance-trained (low intensity) group; SPA: single-photon absorptiometry; supp: dietary supplement; T: trabecular (spine)

*All results are statistically significant unless otherwise indicated.

**Results are significant when compared to nonexercising limb.

protocols (24). Interestingly, the magnitude of change in strength was not significantly different between the strength and endurance protocols. However, the effect on bone was remarkably different. Only the high-intensity, low-repetition resistance training group had significant increases in femoral BMD ranging from 1.5% to 2.3%, at the intertrochanter, trochanter, and Ward's triangle sites when compared to the RTE group (24). Ultradistal radius BMD also increased significantly, by 2.4% (24). The RTE group who performed 3 sets of 20 repetitions did not have a significant change in BMD at any hip site. These site-specific increases in BMD were significantly correlated to increased strength of the attached muscle groups and corresponded to the site of muscle tendon attachment (24). Increases in trochanter BMD were significantly correlated with increases in hip flexion strength and may be related to the iliopsoas insertion at the lesser trochanter. Increases in trochanter and intertrochanter BMD were significantly correlated to change in hip extension strength, potentially related to insertion of the gluteus maximus muscle on the greater trochanter. Increases in Ward's triangle BMD correlated significantly with strength gains in hip abduction and adduction.

Friedlander et al. were able to demonstrate significant increases in BMD in young women up to 35 years of age performing a moderate-intensity resistance training protocol 3 times per week over a 2-year time period when compared to a stretching control group (17). Distinct exercise programs were performed 1 time each per week: (1) circuit training emphasizing dynamic loading of the skeleton through push-ups, sit-ups, free-weight exercises, and high-impact aerobic activities; (2) a total body free-weight lifting program including structural exercises (e.g., cleans and dead lifts); and (3) a vigorous high-intensity aerobic program using step benches (17). Significant improvement in isokinetic strength for knee flexion, knee extension, and trunk extension was seen during the first year of the intervention. Strength did not continue to increase during the second year, suggesting a plateau or maintenance effect of the loading stimulus. However, significant increases in BMD of the integral spine (1.3%), femoral neck (0.5%), trochanter (2.6%), and calcaneus (5.6%) occurred after the second year but were not seen in the first year (17). In contrast, BMD at these sites decreased or was maintained in the control women.

Lohman and colleagues reported significant increases in 1-RM (58%) and isokinetic strength (34%) in previously sedentary adult women, 28-39 years of age, performing 12 resistance training exercises at 70-80% 1-RM when compared with controls (28). BMD of the lumbar spine (1.4%) and trochanter (2.0%) increased significantly after 18 months as a result of the resistance training intervention (28). The investigators propose that a site-specific redistribution of BMC may account for regional increases in BMD in this study in light of the fact that total body BMD did not increase.

Nelson et al. also reported clinically significant increases of 54% in muscle strength and approximately 1% increase in lumbar spine and femoral BMD over the course of one year in postmenopausal women. The control group had decrements in BMD of 1.8-2.5% at these sites. The resistance training protocol consisted of 3 sets of 8 repetitions at an average intensity of 84% 1-RM for 6 exercises performed 2 times per week. No plateaus in strength were seen over the course of the year, which provides further support of the progressive nature of the load stimulus on bone. Increased muscle mass, spontaneous physical activity participation, and improvement in balance were also reported (37).

Notelovitz et al. randomized surgically postmenopausal women receiving estrogen replacement therapy (ERT) to either resistance training 3 times per week of 1 set of 8 repetitions at 8-RM intensity for 5 exercises for one year or a sedentary control group (39). Significant increases of 8.3% in the spine, 4.1% at the midradius, and 2.1% total body BMD were achieved when compared to the control group receiving ERT alone (39). The increase in BMD reported by Notelovitz is approximately two times greater than that reported in other studies. The initial estrogen-depleted status of the participants and the subsequent ERT in both the resistance training and control is a probable contributor to this large positive effect. This study indicates that the combination of ERT and resistance training is more effective than either intervention alone.

Resistance Training Protocols Without Positive Bone Results

Other resistance training studies have shown significant increases in strength without concomitant increases in BMD (12, 33, 38, 41, 50). These randomized controlled trials were generally less than one year in duration and performed at moderate intensity and volume, despite study designs described as moderate to high intensity. Exercise selection and volume in these resistance training studies that did not increase BMD were similar to those in resistance training studies that reported positive effects. Study populations that did not show improvement in BMD with resistance training included postmenopausal women with high BMD compared to normative data and adults between 60-80 years of age (33, 38, 41).

Dornemann et al. reported significant increases in strength over 6 months of training in women 40-50 years old (12). No significant changes in bone occurred, although a trend toward increased BMD of the lumbar spine in the resistance training women when compared to the control group was seen (12). Nonsignificant trends toward increased femoral neck BMD and decreased radial BMD were reported for both groups. The authors suggest that the duration of the protocol was too short and potentially the limiting factor for bone outcomes. In addition, the resistance training protocol may not have provided sufficient load because it included a light, moderate, and heavy day each week instead of maintaining a consistently high-intensity stimulus.

Similarly, McCartney et al. did not detect a change in total body BMD or lumbar spine BMD in older women and men aged 60-80 years after 42 weeks of progressive weightlifting (33). Significant increases in maximal muscle strength were measured, and strength continued to increase and did not plateau in the resistance training group at any time during the intervention. Other physiological measures, maximum cycle ergometer power output, treadmill walking time, and knee extensor muscle cross-sectional area also improved in the resistance training group when compared with the control group (33). The authors suggest that the training frequency of 2 times per week, intensity ranging from 50 to 80% 1-RM, and duration were insufficient to cause measurable bone remodeling in these older men and women (33).

High initial BMD of the research participants appears to be the limiting factor in two year-long, high-intensity resistance training protocols in postmenopausal women (38, 41). Preintervention hip BMD was 105% of normative values for age-matched women in one study (38), while initially spine BMD ranged from 107% to 126% of normative in the second study (41). In addition, the intensity of the exercise was not sufficient to increase strength during the final six months of the intervention reported by Nichols et al. (38). Preintervention use of HRT may have contributed to optimal bone status and resulted in a ceiling effect for further increases in BMD (41).

Smidt and colleagues found that a home-based resistance training program tended to maintain lumbar spine BMD when compared with a 2.3% loss in the control group (50). The intervention consisted of three exercises emphasizing the abdomen and back muscles, with one supervised training session per month. The investigators hypothesized that resistance training must be performed for 2-3 remodeling cycles, between 8 and 18 months, to result in increased BMD.

Disadvantages, Contraindications, and Special Concerns

No randomized controlled trial has shown a deleterious effect of resistance training on bone. To the contrary, the overwhelming majority of these studies have reported no musculoskeletal injuries as a result of the intervention (24, 33). Minor muscular strains occurred in both the control and exercise groups and resolved quickly or were unrelated to the protocol in several other studies (17, 37, 38, 41, 50). It has been clearly demonstrated that resistance training is safe, beneficial, and enjoyable, as evidenced by high compliance for a wide range of participants with osteoporotic risk factors (12, 17, 24, 25, 28, 33, 37-39, 41, 50, 51).

While it has been proposed that those individuals with severe osteoporosis should not perform lumbar flexion exercises due to increased risk of vertebral fractures, this recommendation is based on a retrospective, nonrandomized study (47). Exercise performance of spinal extension and flexion was not supervised, nor was exercise compliance reported. Initial spine BMD was also not reported and may have been a significant independent predictor of fracture risk.

Comparison to Cardiovascular Training

Cardiovascular training must be weight-bearing, high-intensity, dynamic, and high-impact loading to have a positive effect on bone (2, 3, 5, 25, 51, 52). High-impact loading is considered to be at least three times the body weight. Human lumbar forces are approximately equal to body weight (one time body weight) during brisk walking and approximately 1.75 times body weight during running. Weightlifting in the standing position is estimated to create forces between five and six times body weight (19, 31, 52).

Low-intensity exercise such as walking has many benefits for cardiovascular and psychological health; however, it does not consistently enhance spine or hip BMD in either young or old women (4, 44, 52). Epidemiological evidence suggests that the rate of bone loss is lower in postmenopausal women who walk habitually when compared with sedentary counterparts (4, 26, 44). The intensity, impact, and direction of loading from walking must continue to increase as the skeleton adapts to the impact of walking, possibly by adding running, jumping, stepping, or resistance training to the cardiovascular training program to allow for continued adaptation of bone.

A unique cardiovascular training intervention reported by Heinonen et al. used body weight as resistance with progressive, multidirectional jumping over low hurdles and stepping up onto benches (21). Women aged 35-45 years were randomized either to cardiovascular training 3 times per week for 18 months or to a control group. Each exercise included 100-200 jumps or steps per session (21). The height of the jumps and steps gradually increased from 10 to 25 cm and resulted in increases in the magnitude of ground reaction forces (GRF) and the magnitude of loading. Peak force from jumping and stepping ranged from 2.1 to 5.6% body weight (21). Significant increases in BMD were measured at the lumbar spine, femoral neck, distal femur, patella, proximal tibia, and calcaneus in the women who exercised compared to the controls (21). No significant change was observed in the trochanter or the distal radius in either group. In addition, significant improvement in cardiovascular fitness, leg power, and dynamic balance was observed. These previously sedentary adult women performed this intense, high-impact protocol with high compliance and minimal adverse musculoskeletal side effects (21). Other investigators have also reported increased BMD in young women with jumping and running protocols (2, 51).

Specific Recommendations for Resistance Training

The primary consideration for resistance training for osteoporosis is proper medical screening and evaluation, including health history and current health status. A bone density test is essential to obtain information about the specific regions of bone and fracture risk, and to monitor change in bone over time. Assessment of exercise history, current exercise participation, joint stability, flexibility, and strength is also appropriate.

Resistance training to maximize bone health should be performed for a minimum of one year at moderate- to high-intensity 75-85% 1-RM or at 8-12 RM intensity. Three sets of 8-12 repetitions performed 3 times per week for 6-12 total body exercises provide the optimal stimulus to bone (17, 24, 25, 28, 37, 39, 51). Two exceptions of note are one study in which resistance training was performed 2 times per week and another study in which just 1 set of 8 repetitions was performed in conjunction with ERT therapy (37, 39).

Exercise Selection

Osteogenesis is mediated by the force of muscle contraction at the site of the tendon attachment to the bone (5, 24). The most beneficial exercises for bone use muscles that originate or insert at the bony landmarks of interest because they provide the most direct site-specific mechanical load on bone (table 20.4).

Hip and Femur

The six deep external rotator muscles (gemellus inferior and superior, obturator internus and externus, quadratus femoris, piriformis) originate on the hip and insert on the medial aspect of the greater trochanter at the edge of the femoral neck. The agonist adductor muscles (adductor brevis and longus, pectineus) insert on the critical area of the proximal femur. Exercises that use these muscles and joint actions include hip abduction and adduction and may have contributed to the significant increase of 2.3% in femoral neck BMD (Ward's triangle) in postmenopausal women (24).

TABLE 20.4   Exercise Selection Summary by Bone Site

Bone site	Exercise selection	Reference
Femoral neck, Ward's triangle	Hip abduction, adduction Jumping, stepping Leg extension, leg flexion	(17, 24, 25, 37)
Proximal femur: intertrochanter, trochanter	Leg extension, flexion Hip adduction, flexion Jumping, stepping Leg press, squat	(17, 24, 28, 37)
Spine	Back extension, dead lifts Rows, bent and low Cleans Hip extension Lat pull-down Trunk flexion pull-over (torso arm)	(17, 24, 25, 28, 37, 39, 51)
Wrist	Arm curl, arm curl with rotation Negative chin-up Pull-over (torso arm) Wrist curl, reverse wrist curl Wrist pronation, supination	(24, 39)

Three of the four quadriceps muscles that extend the leg originate at the critical sites of the proximal femur: intertrochanteric line, greater trochanter, lesser trochanter (supracondylar line), and linae aspera. The gluteus muscles that extend the hip insert on the proximal femur and greater trochanter. Leg extension and flexion and hip extension and flexion exercises, including leg press and squat, stimulate bone at the proximal femur. These exercises contributed to significant increases of 1.5-2.6% trochanter BMD in several studies (17, 24, 25, 28, 37, 51).

Spine

Back and hip extension exercise, lat pull-down, and rows that engage the deep muscle of the spine and the superficial muscles of the back have been shown to be effective in maintaining or increasing lumbar spine BMD up to 8.3% (24, 25, 28, 37, 39, 50, 51). Bent-knee dead lifts and cleans are advanced structural exercises incorporating back and hip extension and have been effective in young adult women (17).

Back extension exercise has also been shown to improve thoracic kyphosis; unfortunately, it may also exacerbate lordosis and sacral inclination (46). Ideally, back extension should be combined with exercises to decrease lumbar lordosis such as trunk flexion.

Wrist

The brachioradialis and pronator quadratus are the two muscles that insert on the distal radius. The actions of these muscles pronate the forearm and flex the forearm at the elbow, and pronate and supinate the forearm to the midposition. Exercises that use these muscles and joint actions are the arm curl, arm curl with forearm rotation, wrist pronation, and supination (24, 39). A resistance strength training protocol using these specific exercises as well as wrist curl and reverse wrist curl resulted in significant increase in wrist BMD of +2.4%, when compared to a decrease of −1.4% with resistance endurance training (24). The torso arm exercise (pull-over), which exerts forces with the forearm supinated to the midpoint, may have contributed to the significant 4.1% midradius BMD increase in conjunction with ERT when compared to a 0.3% decrease with ERT only (39).

Conclusion

Resistance training is a potent prevention and treatment strategy for osteoporosis and may be most successful when combined with adequate intake of calcium and vitamin D, lifestyle modification, and medication (6, 11, 13, 17, 25, 28, 39, 51). Resistance training must be performed at the proper intensity, volume of loading (number of exercises, sets, repetitions), and be of sufficient duration to increase BMD. High-intensity resistance training interventions greater than two years in duration have not been reported. It may not be feasible or optimal to maintain training at a high intensity over a long period of time even in highly conditioned elite athletes. Varying exercise selection, changing the direction of the force applied, including structural exercises, and exercises that allow greater absolute loads may be of additional benefit to bone (5). Further resistance training research is needed to investigate the effect of manipulating training variables after an initial one- to two-year period of primarily high intensity to maximize and maintain BMD and bone health.

References

1. Aggarwal, B., and R. Puri. 1995. *Human cytokines: Their role in disease and therapy.* Cambridge, MA: Blackwell.
2. Bassey, E., and S. Ramsdale. 1994. Increase in femoral bone density in young women following high-impact exercise. *Osteoporosis International* 4 (2): 72-75.
3. Bassey, E., and S. Ramsdale. 1995. Weight-bearing exercise and ground reaction forces: A 12-month randomized controlled trial of effects on bone mineral density in healthy postmenopausal women. *Bone* 16: 469-476.
4. Cavanaugh, D., and C. Cann. 1988. Brisk walking does not stop bone loss in postmenopausal women. *Bone* 9: 201-204.

5. Conroy, B.P., and R.W. Earle. 1994. Bone, muscle, and connective tissue adaptations to physical activity. In *Essentials of strength training and conditioning*, edited by T.R. Baechle, 51-66. Champaign, IL: Human Kinetics.

6. Consensus Development Conference. 1993. Diagnosis, prophylaxis and treatment of osteoporosis. *American Journal of Medicine* 94: 646-650.

7. Cook, D., G.H. Guyatt, J.D. Adachi, J. Clifton, L.E. Griffith, R.S. Epstein, et al. 1993. Quality of life issues in women with vertebral fractures due to osteoporosis. *Arthritis and Rheumatism* 36 (6): 750-756.

8. Cummings, S.R., D.M. Black, D.E. Thompson, W.B. Applegate, E. Barrett-Connor, T.A. Musliner, et al. 1998. Effect of alendronate on risk of fracture in women with low bone density but without vertebral fractures: Results from the Fracture Intervention Trial. *Journal of the American Medical Association* 280 (24): 2077-2082.

9. Cummings, S.R., S. Eckert, K.A. Krueger, D. Grady, T.J. Powles, J.A. Cauley, et al. 1999. The effect of raloxifene on risk of breast cancer in postmenopausal women: Results from the MORE randomized trial. *Journal of the American Medical Association* 281 (23): 2189-2197.

10. Davies, C., D. Thomas, and M. White. 1986. Mechanical properties of young and elderly human muscle. *Acta Medica Scandinavica,* suppl. 711: 219-226.

11. Dawson-Hughes, B., S.S. Harris, E.A. Krall, and G.E. Dallal. 1997. Effect of calcium and vitamin D supplementation on bone density in men and women 65 years of age or older. *New England Journal of Medicine* 337: 670-676.

12. Dornemann, T., R.G. McMurray, J.B. Renner, and J.J. Anderson. 1997. Effects of high-intensity resistance exercise on bone mineral density and muscle strength of 40-50-year-old women. *Journal of Sports Medicine and Physical Fitness* 37: 246-251.

13. Eddy, D.M., C.C. Johnston Jr, S.R. Cummings, B. Dawson-Hughes, R. Lindsay, L.J. Melton III, and C.W. Slemenda. 1998. Osteoporosis: Review of the evidence for prevention, diagnosis and treatment and cost-effectiveness analysis. *Osteoporosis International* 8 (S4): 1-88.

14. Eriksen, E., H.J. Gundersen, F. Melsen, and L. Mosekilde. 1984. Reconstruction of the formative site in iliac trabecular bone in 20 normal individuals employing a kinetic model for matrix and mineral apposition. *Metabolic Bone Disease and Related Research* 5: 243-252.

15. Ernst, E. 1998. Exercise for female osteoporosis: A systematic review of randomised clinical trials. *Sports Medicine* 25 (6): 359-368.

16. Ettinger, B., D.M. Black, B.H. Mitlak, R.K. Knickerbocker, T. Nickelsen, H.K. Genant, et al. 1999. Reduction of vertebral fracture risk in postmenopausal women with osteoporosis treated with raloxifene: Results from a 3-year randomized trial. *Journal of the American Medical Association* 282 (7): 637-645.

17. Friedlander, A., H.K. Genant, S. Sadowsky, N.N. Byl, and C.C. Gluer. 1995. A two-year program of aerobics and weight training enhances bone mineral density of young women. *Journal of Bone and Mineral Research* 10 (4): 574-585.

18. Frost, H.M. 1990. Skeletal structural adaptations to mechanical sage (SATMU): 1. Redefining Wolff's law: The bone modeling problem. *Anatomical Record* 226: 403-413.

19. Granhed, H., R. Jonson, and T. Hansson. 1987. The loads on the lumbar spine during extreme weight lifting. *Spine* 12: 146-149.

20. Gutin, B., and M. Kasper. 1992. Can vigorous exercise play a role in osteoporosis prevention? A review. *Osteoporosis International* 2: 55-69.

21. Heinonen, A., P. Kannus, H. Sievanen, P. Oja, M. Pasanen, M. Rinne, et al. 1996. Randomised controlled trial of effect of high-impact exercise on selected risk factors for osteoporotic fractures. *Lancet* 348: 1343-1347.

22. Kannus, P., J. Parkkari, H. Sievanen. A. Heinonen, I. Vuori, and M. Jarvinen. 1996. Epidemiology of hip fractures. *Bone* 18 (1S): 57S-63S.

23. Keating, N., P.D. Cleary, A.S. Rossi, A.M. Zaslavsky, and J.Z. Ayanian. 1999. Use of hormone replacement by postmenopausal women in the United States. *Annals of International Medicine* 130: 545-553.
24. Kerr, D., A. Morton, I. Dick, and R. Prince. 1996. Exercise effects on bone mass in postmenopausal women are site-specific and load-dependent. *Journal of Bone and Mineral Research* 11 (2): 218-225.
25. Kohrt, W., A. Ehsani, and S. Birge. 1997. Effects of exercise involving predominantly either joint-reaction or ground-reaction forces on bone mineral density in older women. *Journal of Bone and Mineral Research* 12 (8):1253-1261.
26. Krall, E., B. Dawson-Hughes, K. Hirst, J.C. Gallagher, S.S. Sherman, and G. Dalsky. 1997. Bone mineral density and biochemical markers of bone turnover in healthy elderly men and women. *Journal of Gerontology* 52A: M61-M67.
27. Kunkel, S., and D. Remick. 1992. *Cytokines in health and disease.* New York: Marcel Dekker.
28. Lohman, T., S. Going, R. Pamenter, M. Hall, T. Boyden, L. Houtkooper, et al. 1995. Effects of resistance training on regional and total bone mineral density in premenopausal women: A randomized prospective study. *Journal of Bone and Mineral Research* 10 (7): 1015-1024.
29. MacDougall, J. 1986. Morphological changes in human skeletal muscle following strength training and immobilization. In *Human muscle power,* edited by N. Jones, N. McCarthy, and A. McComas, 269-285. Champaign, IL: Human Kinetics.
30. Marcus, R., ed. 1994. *Osteoporosis,* vol. 1. Boston: Blackwell.
31. Marcus, R., B. Drinkwater, and G. Dalsky. 1992. Osteoporosis and exercise in women. *Medicine and Science in Sports and Exercise* 24: 5301-5307.
32. Martottoli, R., L. Berkman, and L. Cooney. 1992. Decline in physical function following hip fracture. *Journal of the American Geriatric Society* 40: 861-866.
33. McCartney, N., A.L. Hicks, J. Martin, and C.E. Webber. 1995. Long-term resistance training in the elderly: Effects on dynamic strength, exercise capacity, muscle and bone. *Journals of Gerontology* 50A (2): B97-B104.
34. Melton, L. 1996. Epidemiology of hip fractures: Implications of the exponential increase with age. *Bone* 18 (3S): 121S-125S.
35. Morris, F.L., G.A. Naughton, J.L. Gibbs, J.S. Carlson, and J.D. Wark. 1997. Prospective ten-month exercise intervention in premenarcheal girls: Positive effects on bone and lean mass. *Journal of Bone and Mineral Research* 12 (9): 1453-1462.
36. Nelson, M.E., C.N. Meredith, B. Dawson-Hughes, and W.J. Evans. 1988. Hormone and bone mineral status in endurance trained and sedentary postmenopausal women. *Journal of Clinical Endocrinology and Metabolism* 66: 927-933.
37. Nelson, M., M.A. Fiatarone, C.M. Morganti, I. Trice, R.A. Greenberg, and W.I. Evans. 1994. Effects of high-intensity strength training on multiple risk factors for osteoporotic fractures: A randomized controlled trial. *Journal of the American Medical Association* 272: 1909-1914.
38. Nichols, J.F., K.P. Nelson, K.K. Peterson, and D.J. Sartoris. 1995. Bone mineral density responses to high-intensity strength training in active older women. *Journal of Aging and Physical Activity* 3 (36): 26-38.
39. Notelovitz, M., D. Martin, R. Tesar, F.Y. Khan, C. Probart, C. Fields, et al. 1991. Estrogen therapy and variable resistance weight training increases bone mineral in surgically menopausal women. *Journal of Bone Mineral and Research* 6: 583-590.
40. Pollack, S. 1994. Bioelectrical properties of bone. *Orthopedic Clinics of North America* 15 (1): 3-13.
41. Pruitt, L.A., D.R. Taaffe, and R. Marcus. 1995. Effects of a one-year high-intensity versus low-intensity resistance training program on bone mineral density in older women. *Journal of Bone Mineral Research* 10 (11): 1788-1795.
42. Recker, R., K.M. Davies, R.M. Dowd, and R.P. Heaney. 1999. The effect of low-dose continuous estrogen and progesterone therapy with calcium and vitamin D on bone in

elderly women: A randomized, controlled trial. *Annals of International Medicine* 130: 897-904.

43. Riggs, B., and L. Melton. 1986. Involutional osteoporosis. *New England Journal of Medicine* 314: 1676-1686.

44. Riggs, B., and L. Melton. 1995. The worldwide problem of osteoporosis: Insights afforded by epidemiology. *Bone* 17 (5, suppl.): 505S-511S.

45. Roubenoff, R., T.B. Harris, L.W. Abad, P.W. Wilson, G.E. Dallal, and C.A. Dinarello. 1998. Monocyte cytokine production in an elderly population: Effect of age and inflammation. *Journals of Gerontology* 53A (1): M20-M26.

46. Sinaki, M., E. Itoi, J.W. Rogers, E.J. Bergstrahl, and H.W. Wahner. 1996. Correlation of back extensor strength with thoracic kyphosis and lumbar lordosis in estrogen-deficient women. *American Journal of Physical Medicine and Rehabilitation.* 75: 370-374.

47. Sinaki, M., and B.A. Mikkelsen. 1984. Postmenopausal spinal osteoporosis: Flexion versus extension exercises. *Archives of Physical Medicine and Rehabilitation* 65: 593-596.

48. Slemenda, C., and D. Heilman. 1998. Reduced quadriceps strength relative to body weight. *Arthritis and Rheumatism* 41 (11): 1951-1959.

49. Slovik, D. 1999. Osteoporosis. In *Exercise in rehabilitation medicine*, edited by W. Frontera, 313-348. Champaign, IL: Human Kinetics.

50. Smidt, G.L., S.Y. Lin, K.D. O'Dwyer, and P.R. Blanpied. 1992. The effect of high-intensity trunk exercise on bone mineral density of postmenopausal women. *Spine* 17 (3): 280-285.

51. Snow-Harter, C., and M. Bouxsein. 1992. Effects of resistance and endurance exercise on bone mineral status of young women: A randomized exercise intervention trial. *Journal of Bone and Mineral Research* 7 (7): 761-769.

52. Swezey, R. 1996. Exercise for osteoporosis—Is walking enough? *Spine* 21 (23): 2809-2813.

53. Uhthoff, H., and Z. Jaworski. 1985. Periosteal stress-induced reactions resembling stress fractures: A radiologic and histologic study in dogs. *Clinical Orthopaedics and Related Research* 199: 284-291.

Index

Tables and figures are indicated with an italic *t* and *f*.

Contributors

Matthew D. Beekley, MS, Department of Kinesiology, Indiana University, Bloomington.

Michael J. Berry, PhD, Department of Health and Exercise Science, Wake Forest University, Winston-Salem, North Carolina.

Randy W. Braith, PhD, Center for Exercise Science, College of Health and Human Performance, College of Medicine, University of Florida, Gainesville.

William F. Brechue, PhD, Department of Kinesiology, Indiana University, Bloomington.

James B. Brown, MS, Department of Kinesiology, Indiana University, Bloomington.

Ash Contractor, MBBS, MEd, Center for Heart Disease Prevention, Saint Joseph's/Candler Health System, Savannah, Georgia.

Ted Dreisinger, PhD, Progressive Spine Care and Rehabilitation, Columbia, Missouri.

Walter H. Ettinger, MD, Executive Vice President for Physician Services, Virtua Health, Inc., Marlton, New Jersey.

William J. Evans, PhD, Nutrition, Metabolism, and Exercise Laboratory, Donald W. Reynolds Department of Geriatrics, University of Arkansas for Medical Sciences, and Geriatric Research, Education, and Clinical Center, VA Medical Center, Little Rock, Arkansas.

Matthew S. Feigenbaum, PhD, Department of Health and Exercise Science, Furman University, Greenville, South Carolina.

Maria A. Fiatarone Singh, MD, School of Exercise and Sport Science, University of Sydney, Australia, and Nutrition, Exercise Physiology, and Sarcopenia Laboratory, Jean Mayer USDA Human Nutrition Research Center on Aging at Tufts University, Boston, Massachusetts.

James G. Garrick, MD, Director, Center for Sports Medicine, Saint Francis Memorial Hospital, San Francisco, California.

Neil F. Gordon, MD, PhD, MPH, Center for Heart Disease Prevention, Saint Joseph's/Candler Health System, Savannah, Georgia.

Jennifer E. Layne, MS, CSCS, Nutrition, Exercise Physiology, and Sarcopenia Laboratory, Jean Mayer USDA Human Nutrition Research Center on Aging at Tufts University, Boston, Massachusetts.

Richard F. Leighton, MD, Center for Heart Disease Prevention, Saint Joseph's/Candler Health System, Savannah, Georgia.

Arthur S. Leon, MD, Laboratory of Physiological Hygiene and Exercise Science, Division of Kinesiology, and Heart Disease Prevention Clinic, Department of Medicine, University of Minnesota, Minneapolis.

Peter M. Magyari, MS, Center for Exercise Science, College of Health and Human Performance, College of Medicine, University of Florida—Gainesville.

John Mayer, DC, PhD, Department of Exercise Science, Syracuse University, Syracuse, New York.

Neil McCartney, PhD, Department of Kinesiology, McMaster University, Hamilton, Ontario.

Vert Mooney, MD, U.S. Spine and Sport, San Diego, California.

Miriam E. Nelson, PhD, Nutrition, Exercise Physiology, and Sarcopenia Laboratory, Jean Mayer USDA Human Nutrition Research Center on Aging at Tufts University, Boston, Massachusetts.

Lori Ploutz-Snyder, PhD, Department of Exercise Science, Syracuse University, Syracuse, New York.

Ralph K. Requa, MSPH, Research Director, Center for Sports Medicine, Saint Francis Memorial Hospital, San Francisco, California.

James H. Rimmer, PhD, Center on Health Promotion Research, Department of Disability and Human Development, University of Illinois at Chicago.

Otto A. Sánchez, MD, Laboratory of Physiological Hygiene and Exercise Science, Division of Kinesiology, University of Minnesota, Minneapolis.

Ray W. Squires, PhD, Mayo Clinic, Rochester, Minnesota.

Kerry J. Stewart, EdD, Johns Hopkins University School of Medicine, Baltimore, Maryland.

Lorelee L. Stock, MD, Center for Sports Medicine, Saint Francis Memorial Hospital, San Francisco, California.

About the Editors

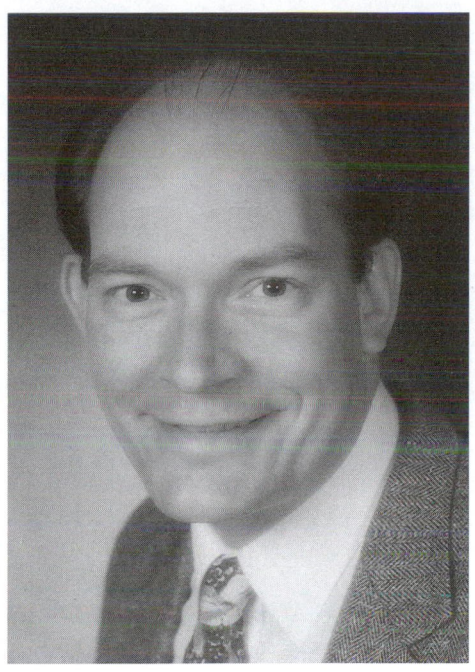

James E. Graves, PhD, is professor of exercise science and associate dean for graduate studies and research at Syracuse University where his accomplishments include the establishment of the Musculoskeletal Research Laboratory. He also developed the Center for Exercise Science at the University of Florida in Gainesville. Coauthor of *The Lumbar Spine*, Dr. Graves' research interests and experience include the prescription of resistance training for the prevention and rehabilitation of orthopedic problems. He earned his PhD from the University of Massachusetts at Amherst.

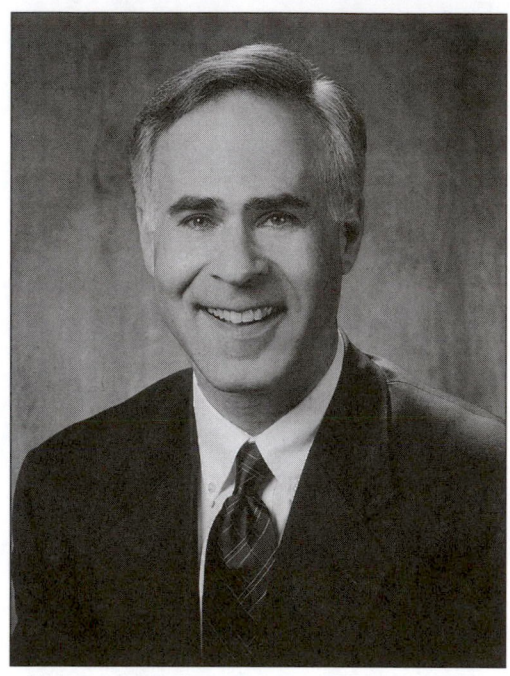

Barry A. Franklin, PhD, has been director of the Cardiac Rehabilitation and Exercise Laboratories at William Beaumont Hospital in Royal Oak, Michigan, since 1985. He is also professor of family medicine at the University of Michigan at Ann Arbor, and he served as president of the American College of Sports Medicine from 1999 to 2000. A prolific writer, he has authored or coauthored more than 300 scholastic papers. He earned his PhD in physiology from Pennsylvania State University and a master's degree from the University of Michigan.

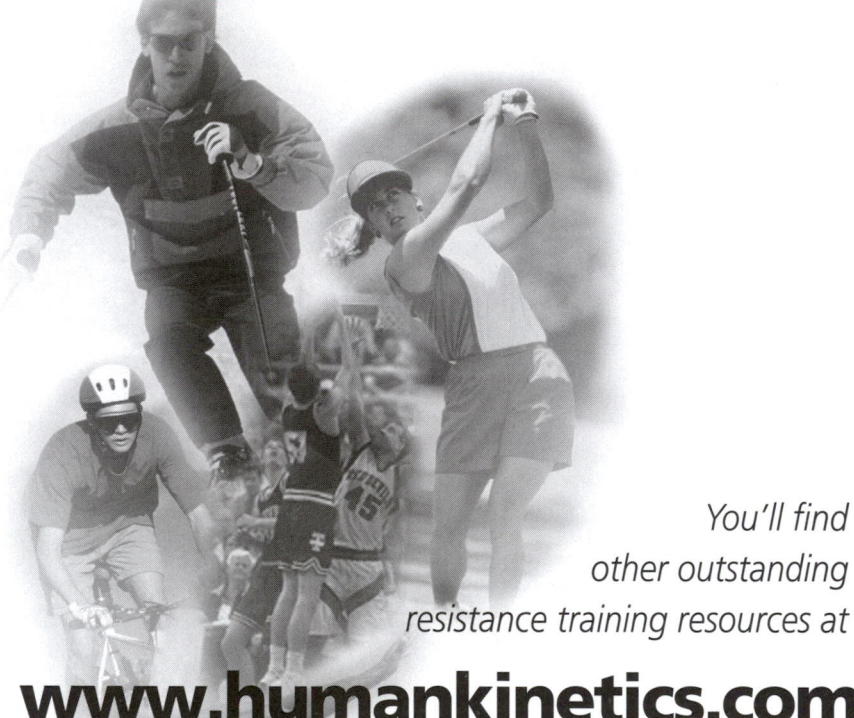
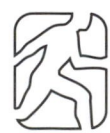